DREAMS, HEALING, AND MEDICINE IN GREECE

Dreams, Healing, and Medicine in Greece

From Antiquity to the Present

Edited by
STEVEN M. OBERHELMAN
Texas A&M University, USA

ASHGATE

Published by
Ashgate Publishing Limited
Wey Court East
Union Road
Farnham
Surrey, GU9 7PT
England

Ashgate Publishing Company
110 Cherry Street
Suite 3-1
Burlington, VT 05401-3818
USA

www.ashgate.com

British Library Cataloguing in Publication Data
Dreams, healing, and medicine in Greece : from antiquity to
the present.
1. Dreams – Therapeutic use – Greece – History.
2. Medicine, Magic, mystic, and spagiric –Greece –
History. 3. Dreams – Religious aspects – Christianity.
4. Medicine, Greek and Roman.
I. Oberhelman, Steven M.
615.8'52'09495-dc23

Library of Congress Cataloging-in-Publication Data
Dreams, healing, and medicine in Greece : from antiquity to the present / edited by
Steven M. Oberhelman.
pages cm
Includes bibliographical references and index.
ISBN 978-1-4094-2423-9 (hardcover) – ISBN 978-1-4094-2424-6 (ebook)
1. Medicine, Ancient. 2. Medicine – Greece. 3. Medical innovations – History.
I. Oberhelman, Steven M., editor of compilation.
R135.D74 2013
610.938–dc23

2012034182

ISBN 9781409424239 (hbk)
ISBN 9781409424246 (ebk –PDF)
ISBN 9781409474395 (ebk –ePUB)

MIX
Paper from
responsible sources
FSC® C018575

Printed and bound in Great Britain
by MPG PRINTGROUP

Contents

List of Illustrations

Notes on Contributors

Jovan Bilbija is a former Ph.D. student in the Department of Greek Language and Literature at Vrije Universiteit, Amsterdam. His main research interests include divination in the ancient Mediterranean world and oneirology in Graeco-Roman antiquity. In April 2012, he defended his dissertation entitled "The Dream in Antiquity: Aspects and Analyses."

Louise Cilliers was for many years Head of the Department of Latin and then of the Department of Classical Languages at the University of the Free State in Bloemfontein, South Africa, and is at present an honorary research fellow of that university. She regularly reads papers at international conferences and was for many years the editor of the national journal *Acta Classica*. Her main research interest is the texts of the fourth- and fifth-century AD North African medical writers, on which she has published various articles, as well as a critical edition with translation and commentary of Vindicainus' *Gynaecia*. At present she is working on a critical edition of another North African medical physician, Theodorus Priscianus, and has recently contributed lemmas to various international encyclopedias. A second research project is that on ancient medicine with a colleague, François Retief, which has to date produced some 70 articles in accredited and international journals, and for which they were awarded the Stals Prize for Interdisciplinary Teamwork by the South African Academy of Arts and Science.

Stavroula Constantinou is Assistant Professor of Byzantine Literature at the Department of Byzantine and Modern Greek Studies, University of Cyprus. Her research interests include literary theory and Byzantine literature, especially hagiography and fictional narrative. She has published a book on female holiness and the body (*Female Corporeal Performances: Reading the Body in Byzantine Passions and Lives of Holy Women* [Uppsala, 2005]), and a number of articles on genre, performance, gender, ritual, punishment, and friendship in Byzantine literature. She is currently working on a monograph on the genre of miracle collection and is co-editing a volume on court ceremonies and rituals of power in the medieval Mediterranean.

Ildikó Csepregi is a postdoctoral researcher at the Medieval Studies Department, Central European University in Budapest. She is a member of the European Science Foundation/OTKA research team studying medieval saints' cult and miraculous healing. She has published on Greek and Christian incubation; her book on temple sleep in Byzantium is due to be published in 2013 by Cambridge University Press. Her research interests include dreams in Greek and early Christian literature, illness interpretations, nonmedical healing, and the formation of miracle narratives, as well as the emergence and history of healer saints' cults in Byzantium and Central Europe.

Janet Downie is Assistant Professor of Classics at Princeton University. Her research interests are in Greek literature, including Greek prose of the Roman Imperial era, the history of rhetoric and oratory, the figure of the author, issues of professional self-presentation, and also ancient medical writers, including Galen. She has written a forthcoming book on Aelius Aristides' *Hieroi Logoi* (*Sacred Tales*) and is now beginning a new project on the intersections of mythic, cultural, and intellectual geography in the physical landscape of Imperial-era Asia Minor, starting from Philostratus' third-century dialogue *On Heroes*.

Jill Dubisch, Regents Professor of Anthropology at the Department of Anthropology at Northern Illinois University, is currently researching contemporary spiritual pilgrimage and "New Age" energy healing. Her research interests have included Greece, pilgrimage, gender, ritual, and healing. These have resulted in several books, including two edited volumes *Gender and Power in Rural Greece* (Princeton, 1986) and (with M. Winkelman) *Pilgrimage and Healing* (Tucson, 2005), and ethnographic studies, in particular *In a Different Place: Pilgrimage, Gender and Politics at a Greek Island Shrine* (Princeton, 1995).

Maithe A.A. Hulskamp is Lecturer and Researcher in Ancient History at the University of Amsterdam. She has published a number of articles in the field of ancient medicine. Her research interests include ancient medical and philosophical matters pertaining to mind, soul, and body. She is currently working on sleep and coma in Galen's oeuvre, and on Galen's views on *pneuma* as a mediator between body and soul.

Timothy S. Miller is Professor of History at Salisbury University, Maryland. His research has been in the history of Byzantine philanthropy, beginning with *Birth of the Hospital in the Byzantine Empire* (Baltimore, 1985). Almost 20 years later, he finished *Orphans of Byzantium: Child Welfare in the Christian Empire*

(Washington, D.C., 2003) and is currently working on a book about medieval leprosy together with John Nesbitt, an expert on Byzantine sigillography and numismatics.

Steven M. Oberhelman is Professor of Classics and Cornerstone Faculty Fellow of Liberal Arts at Texas A&M University. His fields of research are Greek and Roman cultural studies, ancient and Byzantine medicine, and medieval dream texts. He has in print six books and over 75 articles, conference papers, and reviews, including *Rhetoric and Homiletics in Fourth-Century Christian Literature: Prose Rhythm, Oratorical Style, and Preaching in the Works of Ambrose, Jerome, and Augustine* (Atlanta, 1991); *The Oneirocriticon of Achmet: A Medieval Greek and Arabic Treatise on the Interpretation of Dreams* (Lubbock, TX, 1991); and *Dreambooks in Byzantium: Six Oneirocritica in Translation, with Commentary and Introduction* (Aldershot, 2008). He is currently working on a monograph (as part of the Medieval Medicine in the Mediterranean series) which deals with a medical *iatrosophion* (practical healing book) from Western Crete dated to the later Ottoman Greek period.

Lee T. Pearcy is Research Associate in the Department of Greek, Latin, and Classical Studies at Bryn Mawr College and recently retired from a career in teaching and administration at the Episcopal Academy in Newtown Square, Pennsylvania. His research focuses on ancient medical texts and theories, Latin poetry, and classical reception. He is the author of articles on "Dreams and Dream Interpretation" and "Apparition" in the forthcoming *Virgil Encyclopedia*, edited by Richard Thomas and Jan Ziolkowski (Malden, MA), and is currently working on a book about the uses of the Graeco-Roman past in the poetry and prose of Ralph Waldo Emerson, Walt Whitman, and Frederick Douglass. His most recent book is *The Grammar of Our Civility: Classical Education in America* (Waco, TX, 2005).

François Pieter Retief was Director General of the Department of Health and Population Development, and then Rector and Vice-Chancellor of the University of the Free State. After his retirement, his interest in diseases in antiquity developed into a joint research project with Professor Louise Cilliers (which has produced more than 70 articles) for which they were awarded the Stals Prize for Interdisciplinary Teamwork by the South African Academy of Arts and Science.

Charles Stewart teaches in the Department of Anthropology at University College London. He has conducted long-term field research on the island of

Naxos. He is the author of *Demons and the Devil: Moral Imagination in Modern Greek Culture* (Princeton, 1991) and *Dreaming and Historical Consciousness in Island Greece* (Cambridge, MA, 2102).

Christine Walde is Chair of the Department of Classics and Latin Studies at the Johannes Gutenberg University, Mainz. Her research interests include exile literature (antiquity to the current day), scientific aspects of ancient culture, ancient dreams and dream interpretation, the history of science, and literary theory and interpretation methods (e.g., psychoanalysis and literature). Among her many publications are *Herculeus Labor: Studien zum pseudosenecanischen Hercules Oetaeus* (Frankfurt, 1992), *Die Traumdarstellungen in der griechisch-römischen Dichtung* (Munich and Leipzig, 2001), and *Antike Traumdeutung und moderne Traumforschung* (Düsseldorf, 2001). She has served as editor of *Der Neue Pauly: Enzyklopadie* and has edited volumes on Lucan, reception, and dreams, including (with E. Scioli) *Sub imagine somni: Dreams and Other Nocturnal Phenomena in Greco-Roman Antiquity* (Pisa, 2009).

Barbara Zipser is Researcher at Royal Holloway University of London, funded by a Wellcome Trust University Award. A classicist by training, she obtained her Ph.D. from Heidelberg University. She works on the transmission of Greek medical texts. Her book on John the Physician was published by Brill. Currently, she is working on an edition of Theophanes Nonnos. She also runs a collaborative online edition project of Simon of Genoa's *clavis sanationis*, a Greek-Latin-Arabic medical dictionary.

Acknowledgements

This project was conceived during an extended trip to Greece in the late spring of 2008. Before attending a conference in Athens on dreams and visions in the Byzantine world, I decided to drive a rental car around much of the Peloponnesus and visit as many classical Greek sites as possible. I used ancient Corinth, where I had excavated as a regular member of the American School of Classical Studies in 1978–1979, as my base of operations. Corinth has always held a special place for me, as I spent many afternoons of my graduate student days climbing the precipitous slopes of Acrocorinth, picnic lunch in hand and camera bouncing off my hip and against the Venetian fortification walls. Atop the remains of the Temple of Aphrodite, I would look south toward Mycenae and Sparta, east back to Athens, north in the direction of Delphi, and west to Patrae and then Olympia. For a classicist, there is no better view.

The morning before returning to Athens, I decided to drive to Epidaurus to examine the artifacts in the archaeological museum and revisit the dream-healing sanctuary. It was while I was reading the accounts of miraculous dream cures on a stele inside the museum that I formed the idea of a volume on dreams and medicine in Greece. I knew that studies on dreams as they relate to Greek medicine had been published, but they were synchronic, not diachronic, in scope. I was interested in investigating how dreams formed part of formal and informal medicine in Greece over the past two millennia—from the classical period of Greece to the Hellenistic and Byzantine eras and then to the Tourkokratia (Turkish occupation of Greece) and the modern period. As no such book had yet been written, I was excited to get started on assembling a distinguished group of scholars on historical dreams. First, though, I needed encouragement; this was provided by colleagues whose work has served to inspire my own research: Christine Angelidi, George Calofonos, Catia Galatariotou, Maria Mavroudi, Margaret Mullett, Charles Stewart, and Barbara Tedlock. Second, I required the advice of someone skilled in the publication of books that are interdisciplinary and multidisciplinary, and widely disparate in methodology. I found that person in Jo Josyln, who provided constructive advice and assistance at the critical initial steps and therefore made this volume possible.

I am also thankful to the people at Ashgate Publishing. Jon Lloyd was a superb and conscientious copy-editor whose careful eye made the manuscript much better than what it was and who caught the many errors that I missed. Pamela Bertram was unfailing in her help and technical expertise during the final stages of preparation. Finally, John Smedley has been the ideal editor; his support and shaping of the book have been fundamental in bringing it to press.

Chapter 1

Introduction: Medical Pluralism, Healing, and Dreams in Greek Culture

Steven M. Oberhelman

The history of medicine, in both diachronic and synchronic terms, has traditionally been marked by binary oppositions. The most common opposition was "rational" medicine versus "irrational" medicine. "Rational" was associated with the scientific and the logical, with Western allopathy, while "irrational" denoted empirical and non-scientific medical practices marked by magic and primitivism. In recent years, however, scholars have argued that a medical system is culturally constructed, that is, it reflects the values and structures of the society in which it exists. Etiology of disease, treatment of disease, methods of self- and communal assessment of ill health, preventative care, types and effectiveness of medical practitioners—all are but a few facets of healing that vary across cultures and even coexist, differentially or to similar degrees, within the same culture. Medical anthropologists, employing an ethnographic approach to the social history of medicine, have shown that in a society, there exists not a single medical system, but multiple systems. Individuals resort to one or another of these systems for a variety of reasons, such as economic means, accessibility of medical practitioners, the form of illness, the healer's past success or his reputation for dealing with specific ailments, and previous experiences of the patient and her family and friends.

Scholars have now proposed a number of intriguing methodological models for studying medical pluralism in a society. Matthew Ramsey, in his analysis of eighteenth- and nineteen-century French medicine, sees a variety of healers operating beyond elite medical professionals.[1] Ramsey distinguishes between professional medicine and popular medicine, and argues that popular medicine is manifested by folk and empirical medicine and even magical practices. He does not see practitioners of popular medicine working in isolation from the medical

[1] M. Ramsey, *Professional and Popular Medicine in France, 1770–1830: The Social World of Medical Practice* (Cambridge, 1988) and "Magical Healing, Witchcraft and Elite Discourse in Eighteenth- and Nineteenth-Century France," in M. Gijswijt-Hostra (ed.), *Illness and Healing Alternatives in Western Europe* (London, 1997), pp. 14–37.

profession, but healers of all sorts overlapping and interacting in their medical knowledge and practices. Healers are cast in social as well as economic terms: the folk healer, forming a popular culture, is part of a traditional economy; the professional physician belongs to the city and reflects "corporatism"; and the empiric healer operates on the fringes of other healing practices and participates in a market economy.[2]

Arthur Kleinman has created a sector model for understanding how multiple healing systems coexist in a society through three overlapping sectors of health care.[3] Each sector uniquely explains disease and treats health-related problems; determines the healer(s) and the patient and the ways in which they interact; and fixes on the course of treatment. The sectors are not isolated loci of healing, for people may move freely from one sector to the next and even to a third and then back again, especially when a cure is not effective or when a combination of approaches may seem optimal. The key here is the overlap and intersections of the three sectors, for a health care system in its totality is the interworkings and relationships of the sectors. As Kleinman states, health care may be "described as a *local cultural system composed of three overlapping parts: the popular, the professional and folk sectors.*"[4] These sectors and their activities may be cast in the following Venn diagram:

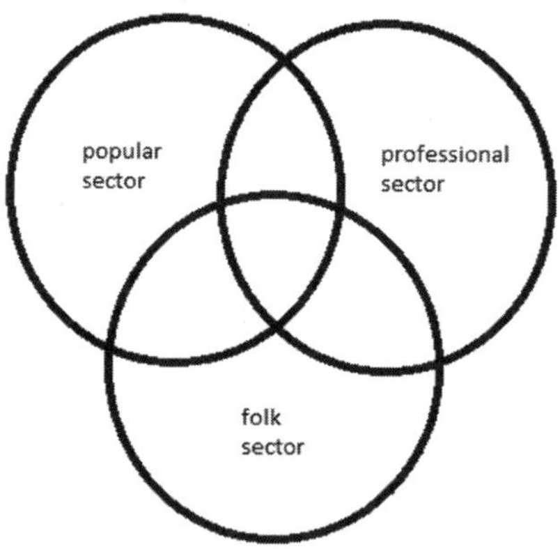

Figure 1.1 Venn Diagram of Kleinman's Medical Pluralism

[2] I owe much of the wording here to D. Gentilcore, *Healers and Healing in Early Modern Italy* (Manchester, 1998), pp. 2–3.

[3] *Patients and Healers in the Context of Culture: An Exploration of the Borderland between Anthropology, Medicine, and Psychiatry* (Berkeley, 1980).

[4] Ibid., pp. 49–50; emphasis in original. In societies lacking professionalization, however, the folk and the popular may constitute the entire health care system.

The professional sector consists of organized, legally sanctioned healing professions. As Kleinman points out: "so dominant has the modern medical profession become in the health care systems of most societies (developing and developed) that studies of health care often equate modern medicine with the entire system of health care."[5] This sector includes physicians of every ilk, but also those who support them (nurses, technicians, etc.) or who complement their activities (e.g., paramedical professionals like midwives). The term "professional" is not limited to training in Western scientific medicine or the possession of credentials (say, a university diploma); it describes anyone acknowledged, or perceived, in a culture as belonging to a professional group. Of course, in many cultures, professional healers are those people recognized by law and enjoying the power of the medical establishment behind them, but in other cultures no formal licensure exists. We may think of classical Greece as an example; no doctor had a diploma or was accredited, and his reputation ultimately rested on his successes and failures.[6]

In the folk sector, healers are non-professional, non-bureaucratic specialists; they have received little or no training in professional medicine.[7] Their knowledge of healing often comes from serving as an apprentice to another folk healer; they are viewed as important healers because they have an inborn or special healing power and/or have been the recipient of her or his master's knowledge. Folk healers are, according to Kleinman, frequently classified into sacred and secular, but these are blurred in practice and usually overlap. Folk healers usually approach healing in a holistic way, dealing with a person's interactions with the natural and the supernatural realms and with a person's physical, emotional, and even spiritual problems. They practice herbalism and concoct recipes consisting of plant and animal and mineral substances (hence some are herbalists and root-cutters); they also use traditional surgical and manipulative treatments, recommend special systems of exercise, and advocate "symbolic non-sacred healing" (hence some may be termed shamans). Because of folk healers' methods and their intermediary position between the popular and professional sectors, professional healers view them with distrust and suspicion (although the feeling is often reciprocal), even as charlatans and quacks who pose a danger to those whom they treat.

The popular sector is non-professional and non-specialist.[8] It is at this level where medical problems and ill health are first recognized and defined. The

---

5 Ibid., p. 56.

6 See the comments of G.E.R. Lloyd, *Magic, Reason and Experience: Studies in the Origin and Development of Greek Science* (Cambridge, 1979), pp. 38–9.

7 Kleinman, *Patients and Healers*, pp. 59–60.

8 Ibid., pp. 50–53.

popular sector includes all the healing options that people freely make use of without recourse to folk healers or medical professionals. Most illnesses, as Kleinman points out, are self-diagnosed, and methods for treating them are based on this self-assessment or on the advice of a relative, friend, or neighbor. Healing and treatment may also be carried out in a religious setting or by consulting a layperson possessing special experience or knowledge. As Kleinman argues, the main arena of health care in the popular sector is the family, and it is here where most illnesses (70, even 90, percent)[9] are evaluated and treated, usually by women like mothers and grandmothers. The popular sector is usually overlooked in medical literature, but for many cultures this is the predominant form of care and the first therapeutic intervention. This sector also emphasizes prophylaxis or preventative medicine. People learn healthy lifestyles through informants at this level: what foods to eat or to avoid; appropriate levels of drinking, sleeping, working; the role of spirituality; and interpersonal relationships. Even so-called magical means like charms and amulets may constitute acceptable prophylaxis if they can ward off disease or maintain good health.

Sick people, at the individual or family level, make choices about whom in the three sectors they should consult for help if their own self-treatment fails. In some cultures (and, as we will see, this was and is still true for parts of Greece), a person may consult healers from several sectors at the same time; for example, one may seek the help of a doctor while also seeing a priest, especially if the source of the illness is seen by the patient in supernatural terms. Or a patient may act sequentially: after self- or familial help has failed, one may consult a folk healer like a root-cutter and then, if that course of treatment fails, a licensed physician. Ill people will not only choose the sector for treatment, but will even, at times, determine which course of treatment to follow among the options provided by that sector. Many factors go into this decision-making process. A healer in one sector may diagnose or offer therapeutics that seem nonsensical to the patient or run contrary to her expectations, and so the next option may be best. Other deciding factors include the unavailability of a sector (for example, only folk healers may live in the village); a lack of economic means (an inability to pay or travel distances); the (real or imagined) success and reputation of the healer; or the patient's self-assessment of the problem or the assessment of the problem by others. When an ill person resorts to a folk or a professional healer, the choice is determined by the popular sector. The person self-assesses the problem or uses the assessment of others in his circle (immediate family, extended family, friends, neighborhood, church, etc.), and

9 Ibid., p. 50 with bibliography.

proceeds to treatment. If that course of action is insufficient, then the patient moves to the folk or professional sector (or even to both simultaneously). After treatment, the patient returns to the popular sector for evaluation and decides if further steps are needed and whether the care has worked and was of quality; that experience, in turn, determines future action when illness recurs. Therefore, the popular sector is the nexus of the boundaries between the other sectors; one enters into, exits from, and interacts with the other two sectors from the popular sector.

The attraction of Kleinman's theory is that it demonstrates the existence of medical pluralism, and how competing and coexistent medical traditions operate, in a culture. There is a weakness to the model is that categorization is not always so neat; for example, herbalists in a culture may have a professional status, while a midwife may employ Western drugs as quickly as a magical amulet. Moreover, one sector may achieve such a dominant status that the other sectors are marginalized or even proscribed.[10] Indeed, in many developed countries, the professional sector is so entrenched that folk healing is viewed as superstitious, irrational nonsense, and the popular sector, with its emphasis on self-assessment and self-treatment, is strongly discouraged (unless done in the context of the professional, such as the dispensing of over-the-counter, sanctioned pharmaceuticals).

For our purposes in this volume, Kleinman's model is insufficient in another respect: the religious is a subset of the popular category. Religion, whether the belief-systems of ancient and Hellenistic Greece or the Eastern Orthodox Christianity of Byzantium and post-Byzantium, has always formed an integral part of Greek culture and everyday life. Thus, in a model of medical pluralism, the

[10] See, e.g., the situation in England, as described in L.S. King, *The Medical World of the Eighteenth Century* (Chicago, 1958), pp. 1–25. See also T.D. Walker's *Doctors, Folk Medicine and the Inquisition: The Repression of Magical Healing in Portugal during the Enlightenment* (Leiden and Boston, 2005). Walker examined Inquisition trials during the period 1563–1818 that concerned healing done through (allegedly) sorcery and witchcraft. He notes the wide range of conventional and nonconventional medicine available to ill people of the time. While physicians and surgeons, as well as priests and saints, could heal, so did "wise" women, who were folk healers. Many of these women, of the poorest social classes and viewed as outsiders, offered cures for their consultants; many of these remedies were a combination of prayers, incantations, dietary regimen, and vegetable and plant concoctions. Peasants used these healers because they possessed a centuries-long tradition of folk remedies, but also because professional healers were few and most lived far away. Folk healers, most of them poor women, were persecuted by Inquisition Tribunals; the purpose was to discredit these healers and their healing methods, and to establish "rationalized scientific" medicine. Thus, the church joined with university-trained physicians and surgeons, e.g., those on the Faculty of Medicine at the University of Coimbra.

religious must be accorded a prominent place. Here David Gentilcore's medical pluralism model for early modern Italy (*Healers and Healing*) works beautifully. Gentilcore saw in Matthew Ramsey's model of medical practitioners an absence of religious healing and proposed a Venn diagram that comprises three sectors—medical, ecclesiastical, and popular—to explain medical pluralism for a country (Italy) not dissimilar to Greece:

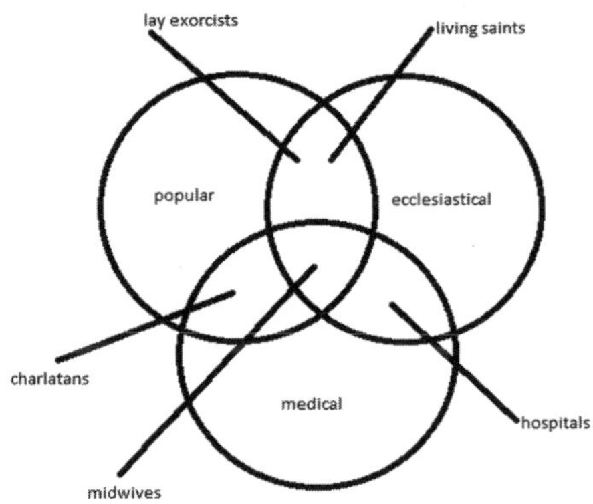

Figure 1.2 Venn Diagram of Gentilcore's Medical Pluralism

Like Kleinman, through his model, Gentilcore leads us to see how various forms of medical healing overlap and intersect, and how practitioners of different backgrounds and orientation function in a culture of medical pluralism. For Gentilcore, the medical sphere includes apothecaries, physicians and surgeons, midwives, and itinerant doctors; the ecclesiastical sphere comprises priests, ordained exorcists, living saints, and healing shrines and religious objects (relics, icons, etc.); and the popular sphere "cunning folk." Gentilcore's model also allows us to see how activities of a healer in one category may overlap with those in another. Thus, hospitals fit into the intersection of the medical and the ecclesiastical: many monasteries functioned both as a hospital, with physicians and surgeons on staff, and as a place of spirituality, with clergy in residence. The cunning folk of Gentilcore's study, often village women knowledgeable in health and healing, used religion: prayers, the sign of the cross, and items like holy oil and holy water, in conjunction with herbal concoctions. Their knowledge of remedies came from a shared network, the observation of the properties of local flora, and empiricism.[11]

[11] Gentilcore, *Healers and Healing*, pp. 22–3. A similar situation appears in the anthropological research of modern Greece and other Mediterranean countries; see below.

A priest may be involved in healing through prayers and rituals, but he could also run an apothecary shop that offered for sale spells that are decidedly magical in nature.[12] Another priest could rely on religious exorcism to conjure disease from a body, but then turn around and resort to bleedings, fumigation, regimen, poultices, and purgatives.[13] Midwives placed magical amulets on the abdomen of a woman in delivery, but they could just as quickly place on her an icon.[14] There were, then, in early modern Italy no absolute distinctions between the professional practitioner, the religious healer, and the wise (cunning) woman. This is not to say, however, that antagonism did not exist or certain limitations were not placed on activities of certain healers. For example, clerics, if they used magical forms of healing, were prosecuted, and they were forbidden from performing surgery or having a medical practice. Also, since some diseases can be caused by demonic forces or sorcery, physicians did not treat them and referred the patient to trained and licensed clergy for exorcism; however, since lay exorcists also performed this ritual, they were attacked by the church hierarchy. Charlatans, that is, healers who practiced as professionals but who lacked the requisite training (formal and even folk), dispensed drugs; however, they were censured on the grounds that they did not know the true properties and effects of plants, the ingredients of medical recipes, and which drugs were appropriate to certain illnesses.[15]

Gentilcore's model of overlapping, though at times competing, areas of health care and healing—popular, professional, and ecclesiastical—with points of intersection like hospitals, charlatans, exorcists or dispensers of spells, and midwives fits Greek medicine in praxis from antiquity into the twentieth century. As G.E.R. Lloyd has demonstrated in many publications, Greek medicine in the ancient world was a pluralism that included, of course, the well-known temple medicine (the cult of Asclepius) and physicians like the Hippocratics, Herophilus, and Galen.[16] But other approaches to healing were available to the sick. One could self-treat, making use of the many herbs and plants in one's gardens and growing wild in the fields and mountains nearby. Itinerant sellers of charms and incantations moved from village to village; many

12 Ibid., pp. 14–15, 56–7.

13 Ibid., pp. 162, 182.

14 Ibid., p. 191.

15 Ibid., p. 16. Gentilcore's model and discussions apply equally well to Walker's *Doctors, Folk Medicine and the Inquisition*; see note 10 above.

16 Lloyd, *Magic, Reason and Experience*, pp. 295–6, 421–2 and *In the Grip of Disease: Studies in the Greek Imagination* (Oxford, 2003), pp. 40–83. See also L. McNamara, "'Conjurers, Purifiers, Vagabonds, and Quacks'?: The Clinical Roles of the Folk and Hippocratic Healers of Classical Greece," *Iris: Journal of the Classical Association of Victoria*, 16–17 (2003–2004): pp. 2–25, who offers excellent primary sources on this topic.

sold amulets and phylacteries for medical uses. Magicians offered hope to the sick through their spells; surviving Greek magical papyri offer for many physical ailments curative treatments that combine *materia medica* with magical names and characters and exorcism prayers.[17] Midwives and other female healers practiced health care; most women in antiquity, in fact, probably received their maternity care from midwives.[18] Root-cutters (ῥιζοτόμοι) and drug-sellers (φαρμακοπῶλαι) could be consulted, and it is not unlikely that most rural people saw them first for treatment.[19] Root-cutters collected plants and herbs that were medically beneficial and then sold them at county fairs. The drug-sellers hawked their compounds to country and city people alike, while emphasizing the efficacy of the herbs and plants they had in hand.[20] Botanists like Theophrastus and Dioscorides recorded in many volumes the properties and actions of plants, minerals, and animals, and how they worked in medical recipes.[21] Some of their

---

[17] The bibliography is immense. I direct the reader to the following outstanding essay for its extensive notes and contemporary scholarship contained therein: R. Kotansky, "Incantations and Prayers for Salvation on Inscribed Greek Amulets," in C.A. Faraone and D. Obbink (eds), *Magika Hiera: Ancient Greek Magic and Religion* (New York and Oxford, 1991), pp. 107–37; cf. R. Kotansky, "An Early Christian Gold *Lamella* for Headache," in P. Mirecki and M. Meyer (eds), *Magic and Ritual in the Ancient World, Part 4* (Leiden, 2002), pp. 37–46. The Greek magical papyri are now easily accessible in English translation in H.D. Betz, *The Greek Magical Papyri in Translation, Including the Demotic Spells*, 2nd edn with an updated bibliography (Chicago and London, 1992); this edition contains many medical recipes and medical spells (check the handy table of contents of spells). See also McNamara, "'Conjurers, Purifiers, Vagabonds, and Quacks'?," p. 2.

[18] V. French, "Midwives and Maternity Care in the Greco-Roman World," *Helios*, 13 (1986): pp. 69–84.

[19] G.E.R. Lloyd, *Science, Folklore and Ideology* (Cambridge, 1983), pp. 119–35.

[20] H. King, *Hippocrates' Woman: Reading the Female Body in Ancient Greece* (New York, 2001), p. 122 with bibliography; Lloyd, *Science, Folklore and Ideology*, pp. 120–25; McNamara, "'Conjurers, Purifiers, Vagabonds, and Quacks'?," pp. 3, 7, 14–15, 19–20. For a modern Greek parallel, see D. Vokou, "Ethnobotanical Survey of Zagori (Epirus, Greece): A Renowned Centre of Folk Medicine in the Past," *Journal of Ethnopharmacology*, 39 (1993): pp. 87–196; and E. Hanlidou, "The Herbal Market of Thessaloniki (N Greece) and Its Relation to the Ethnobotanical Tradition," *Journal of Ethnopharmacology*, 91 (2004): pp. 281–99, where the authors examined medicinal plants found in the herbal market of Thessalonica, which consists of traditional shops, modern shops, and open-air market stalls. A vast majority of the herbs (93) can be found in Dioscorides' work and are applied to the same aliments and diseases, suggesting that intersection between the herbal trade and folk medical usage has remained uninterrupted since antiquity.

[21] L.M.V. Totelin, "A Recipe for a Headache: Translating and Interpreting Ancient Greek and Roman Remedies," in A. Imhausen and T. Pommerening (eds), *Writings of Early Scholars in the Ancient Near East, Egypt, Rome, and Greece* (Berlin and New York), pp. 219–40, at pp. 224–5; J. Scarborough, "Theophrastus on Herbals and Herbal Remedies," *Journal*

knowledge came from their experiments and from samples they collected while traveling, but another critical source was the root-cutter and the drug-seller, although Theophrastus writes that he also interrogated farmers about flora and crops.[22] Finally, gymnastic trainers and dieticians dispensed medical advice, especially with regards to regimen, diet, and exercise.[23]

These various medical practitioners often overlapped in theory and praxis. In the healing cult of the god Asclepius, sick patients would come and sleep at night in a sleeping chamber.[24] The god visited the sick person and healed by direct intervention (laying on of hands, applying medicines, even performing surgery) or indirectly by sending a dream in which he recommended a treatment. The instructions in the latter case were often straight out of Hippocratic medicine: bloodletting, baths, diet, exercise, drugs, poultices, emetics, and the like. Hippocratic writers, on their part, possessed a religious outlook; they invoked the gods and called on their patronage, and recommended prayers as a useful companion to medical treatment. Professional doctors like Rufus of Ephesus and Galen accepted amulets, although they saw naturalistic reasons for their efficacy.[25] The pharmacology of ancient physicians and the great botanists includes magic and religion as well as good folk medicine, and in this respect we see nothing dissimilar in the Greek magical papyri, where we have many spells and incantations, amulets, and phylacteries directed toward healing. Some spells contain excellent medicinal ingredients, and even if the accompanying spoken incantation (which often included a jumble of Christian, Jewish, and pagan religious elements) and some extraneous or non-efficacious materials in the drug

of the History of Biology, 11 (1978): pp. 353–85; cf. the older but useful contribution of M. Wellmann, "Das älteste Kräuterbuch der Girechen," in *Festgabe für Franz Susemihl* (Leipzig, 1898), pp. 22–31. For Dioscorides, I refer the reader to J. Riddle, *Dioscorides on Pharmacy and Medicine* (Austin, 2011).

[22] See S. Amigues, *Théophraste: Recherches sur les plantes: Tome V, Livre IX* (Paris, 2006), for a discussion of Theophrastus' sources; cf. McNamara, "'Conjurers, Purifiers, Vagabonds, and Quacks'?," p. 3.

[23] V. Nutton, *Ancient Medicine* (London, 2004), p. 96; P.J. van der Eijk, "Divination, Prognosis and Prophylaxis: The Hippocratic Work 'On Dreams' (*De Victu* 4) and Its Near Eastern Background," in H.F.J. Hostmanshoff and M. Stol (eds), *Magic and Rationality in Ancient Near Eastern and Graeco-Roman Medicine* (Leiden, 2004), pp. 187–218, at pp. 202–3; McNamara, "'Conjurers, Purifiers, Vagabonds, and Quacks'?," p. 5.

[24] See most recently H. Versnel, *Coping with the Gods: Wayward Readings in Greek Theology* (Leiden, 2011), pp. 400–421 with bibliography; and the chapters in this volume by Cilliers and Retief, Downie, and Pearcy. See also J. Bilbija, "The Dream in Antiquity: Aspects and Analyses" (Ph.D. dissertation, Vrije Universiteit, 2012), pp. 250–56.

[25] J.G. Gager, *Curse Tablets and Binding Spells from the Ancient World* (New York, 1999), p. 221; and Lloyd, *Magic, Reason and Experience*, p. 42.

compound (e.g., nasal mucus, mule's earwax, menstrual blood) added nothing in a medical sense, some ingredients appear in the best ancient pharmacology.[26]

This same pattern of medical pluralism appears in the Byzantine period of Greece (c. 330–1453 AD), although here the healing cult of Asclepius has been replaced by the incubation practiced at saints' shrines and in Christian churches. Professional doctors were later trained in medical schools or at hospitals, which were attached to monasteries, but in early Byzantium they learned their trade through apprenticeship. Some of the more illustrious physicians in Greek medical history lived during the Byzantine era: Oribasius (329–403), Alexander of Tralles (525–605), Aëtius of Amida (502–575), Paul of Aegina (seventh century), Simeon Seth (twelfth century), and Michael Psellus (1018–c. 1078). Many of the doctors wrote encyclopedias to transmit the great body of medical knowledge from antiquity. Paul of Aegina's *Epitome* (in seven books) is a perfect example of the encyclopedic fervor of Byzantine savants. Like other Byzantine medical writers, Paul aimed to preserve and pass down the best of Greek medical knowledge, in particular Dioscorides' *Pharmacology* and Galen's theories, and added material drawn from the works of Hippocrates, Oribasius, and Aëtius. Paul quotes his classical, Hellenistic, and early Byzantine sources nearly verbatim in his meticulous catalog. For example, Book 7 is a precise cataloging of *materia medica* drawn from Dioscorides' *Pharmacology*; Paul describes about 600 botanicals, 80 non-botanicals, and 170 animal products, and carefully notes their properties and effectiveness in medical recipes.[27]

During this same period, miraculous cures were occurring throughout the eastern Mediterranean. Former pagan temples and healing centers were transformed into Christian places of healing performed by saints or by Jesus and the Theotokos.[28] The church of Cosmas and Damian in Constantinople

---

26 J. Scarborough, "The Pharmacology of Sacred Plants, Herbs, and Roots," in Faraone and Obbink (eds), *Magika Hiera*, pp. 138–74, at pp. 154–61. As we have seen in other instances of cultural medical pluralism, tensions did exist between the various areas. Lloyd (*Magic, Reason and Experience*, pp. 45–6), for example, notes the antagonism of the Hippocratics towards charlatans, quacks, and sellers of spells, and the subtle jabs at the medical profession in the *iamata* (inscriptions of cures) at the sanctuary of Asclepius at Epidaurus; see too Versnel, *Coping with the Gods*, pp. 404–21.

27 J. Scarborough, "Early Byzantine Pharmacology," *Dumbarton Oaks Papers*, 38 (1984): pp. 213–32, at pp. 228–32.

28 D. Krueger, "Christian Piety and Practice in the Sixth Century," in M. Maas (ed.), *The Cambridge Companion to the Age of Justinian* (Cambridge, 2005), pp. 291–315; see also most recently the essays in J. Chirban (ed.), *Holistic Healing in Byzantium* (Brookline, 2010); and especially A.-M. Talbot, "Pilgrimage to Healing Shrines: The Evidence of Miracle Accounts," *Dumbarton Oaks Papers*, 56 (2002): pp. 153–73, with a lengthy and impressive

was the site of numerous miracles and cures accomplished for the faithful who slept in its porticoes and atrium.[29] Justinian the Great himself was cured through a dream vision at this church. Cosmas and Damian's fame spread throughout Greece and Crete, with even the Asclepian sanctuary on the south slope of the Athenian acropolis converted in the fifth or sixth century into a healing shrine for the pair.[30] The saints conducted business just as Asclepius had done, in that they appeared in a dream to a suppliant; they either cured the suppliant with unguents or surgery, or gave instructions for a cure that he was to follow the next day. Another famous healing pair of saints, Cyrus and John, healed worshippers through personal touch or by prescribing remedies in dreams. The cult was originally based in Egypt, but after that country fell to the Arabs in the seventh century, it moved to Rome and Constantinople.[31] The Greek writer Sophronius records 70 miracle cures performed by the two saints.[32] Other famous sites of incubation were the shrine of Artemius, whose specialty seems to have been male genital ailments, at the church of John Prodromus in Oxeia;[33] the shrine of Saint Simeon the Younger, near Antioch;[34] and the shrine of Thecla at Seleucia.[35]

---

list of healing shrines throughout the Byzantine world; at pp. 155–67, she surveys the newest excavations of dream-healing sanctuaries in the Byzantine world. See also the bibliography in the chapters by Constantinou, Csepregi, and Miller in this volume.

[29] The saints' specialty were eye diseases: J. Lascaratos, "Miraculous Ophthalmological Therapies in Byzantium," *Documenta Ophthalmologica*, 81 (2004): pp. 145–52; and S. Efthymiadis et al., "Greek Hagiography in Late Antiquity (Fourth–Seventh Centuries)," in S. Efthymiadis (ed.), *The Ashgate Research Companion to Byzantine Hagiography, vol. 1: Periods and Places* (Aldershot, 2011), pp. 35–94, at p. 66.

[30] L. Deubner, *De incubatione capita quattuor* (Leipzig, 1900), pp. 68–79 and *Kosmas und Damian: Texte und Einleitung* (Leipzig, 1907).

[31] D. Frankfurter, *Religion in Roman Egypt: Assimilation and Resistance* (Princeton, 2000), pp. 165–6.

[32] For healing done by the two saints, see D. Montserrat, "Pilgrimage to the Shrine of SS Cyrus and John at Menouthis in Late Antiquity," in D. Frankfurter (ed.), *Pilgrimage and Holy Space in Late Antique Egypt* (Leiden/Boston/Cologne, 1998), pp. 257–80; cf. J. Duffy, "Some Observations on Sophronius' Miracles of Cyrus and John," *Journal of Theological Studies*, 35 (1984): pp. 71–90.

[33] *The Miracles of St Artemios* records 45 cures that took place in an incubation center in seventh-century Constantinople. This saint seems to have specialized in curing scrotal hernia and disorders of the male genitals. See V.S. Crisafulli and J.W. Nesbitt, *The Miracles of St. Artemios* (Leiden/New York/Cologne, 1996).

[34] G. Vikan, "Art, Medicine, and Magic in Early Byzantium," *Dumbarton Oaks Papers*, 38 (1984), pp. 65–86, at p. 73; see also his *Sacred Images and Sacred Power in Byzantium* (Aldershot, 2003), p. 63.

[35] S.F. Johnson, *The Life and Miracles of Thekla: A Literary Study*, Hellenic Studies, 13 (Cambridge, MA and London, 2006).

These places demonstrate that healing through dreams was a very important component of Byzantine religion and society.

Healing could be achieved through means other than religious and professional medicine. Amulets were used in healing,[36] and magical textbooks included sections on magical medicine and *materia magica* for cures. A prominent example is the *Cyranides*, a book on natural and talismanic magic dating from the first or second century AD but copied and recopied for use in Byzantium.[37] The author discusses the magical and occult properties of animals, birds, plants, and stones, and how to make amulets from plants, animals, and stones.[38] Also, diseases were often attributed to demonic forces or to astrological influences; for example, most of the 36 decans of small constellations were associated with specific diseases, a concept borrowed from Egyptians but repeated in Byzantine magical treatises.[39] Folk medicine worked itself into the writings of the Byzantine doctors.[40] Alexander of Tralles, for example, listened to folk healers and lay healers for new drugs and recipes, and in an instance of the intersection of various modes of healing, he approved the use of amulets and charms in treating illness.[41] Women formed the first line of medical defense in the treatment of disease. Mothers and wives concocted cures for ailments and illness, and we know that in Byzantium there were women medics such as nurses and midwives.[42]

---

36 Vikan, "Art, Medicine and Magic in Early Byzantium"; and J. Spier, "Medieval Byzantine Magical Amulets and Their Tradition," *Journal of the Warburg and Courtauld Institutes*, 56 (1993): pp. 25–62.

37 I refer the reader to the edition by D. Kaimakis, *Die Kyraniden* (Frankfurt am Main, 1980); and translations and discussion in M. Waegeman, *Amulet and Alphabet: Magical Amulets in the First Book of Cyranides* (Amsterdam, 1987).

38 See M. Mavroudi, "Occult Science and Society in Byzantium: Considerations for Future Research," in P. Magdalino and M. Mavroudi (eds), *The Occult Sciences in Byzantium* (Geneva, 2007), pp. 39–95.

39 R.P.H. Greenheld, "A Contribution to the Study of Palaeologan Magic," in H. Maguire (ed.), *Byzantine Magic* (Washington, D.C., 1995), pp. 117–53, at p. 137.

40 Scarborough, "Early Byzantine Pharmacology"; J. Stannard, "Aspects of Byzantine Materia Medica," *Dumbarton Oaks Paper*, 38 (1984): pp. 205–11; D. Bennett, "Medical Practice and Manuscripts in Byzantium," *Society for the Social History of Medicine*, 13 (2000): pp. 279–91.

41 J. Scarborough, "The Life and Times of Alexander of Tralles," *Expedition*, 39 (1997): pp. 51–60, at p. 55.

42 V. Nutton, "Healers in the Medical Market Place: Towards a Social History of Graeco-Roman Medicine," in Andrew Wear (ed.), *Medicine in Society* (Cambridge, 1992), pp. 15–58, at p. 54; and G. Clark, *Women in Late Antiquity* (Oxford, 1994), pp. 63–93.

Byzantine hospitals were another place where medical pluralism is clearly in evidence.[43] The hospital (ξενών), an invention of the Byzantines, arose from the Eastern Orthodox Christian tradition of houses of philanthropy for the poor and homeless. The hospital was attached to a monastery and accommodated patients who were treated by an extensive medical staff. A famous hospital was the Christ Pantokratôr, which was located in Constantinople and built in the early twelfth century by Emperor John II Comnenus (1118–1143). The hospital could house 50 patients (38 males, 12 females) and had a staff of 47 physicians and surgeons, assistants, and nurses. But physical ailments were not the only focus of the complex, as there was a chapel as well as priests to look after the spiritual needs of patients. Moreover, as Alain Touwaide has argued, doctors at these hospitals were extensively involved in the transmission of medical knowledge. Each hospital had collections of medical recipes and formulas copied from ancient authors (Hippocrates, Dioscorides, and Galen). Physicians, individually or as a group, recopied these formularies but also edited them on the basis of their own clinical experience and observations. They saw the course of diseases and the effect of certain drugs on those diseases, and revised or updated (in the case of new epidemiology) their texts. New *materia medica*, thanks to trade and exploration, became available to the doctors, who then incorporated these substances into existing praxis. Thanks to the hospitals at the monasteries, the medical body of knowledge was constantly revised.[44]

All these forms of healing (folk, magical, pharmacological, professional, and religious) appear in the medical handbooks used by priests, practical doctors, and other medical healers of Byzantium, and down into the twentieth-century. This type of handbook is called *iatrosophion*.[45] An *iatrosophion* is a collection of

---

[43] The classic study, in my opinion, is T.S. Miller, *The Birth of the Hospital in the Byzantine Empire* (Baltimore, 1997); see also the cautionary remarks in P. Horden, "How Medicalised Were Byzantine Hospitals?," *Medicina e Storia*, 10 (2006): pp. 45–74. An intermediary position is sought by D. Krueger, "Healing and the Scope of Religion in Byzantium: A Response to Miller and Crislip," in Chirban (ed.), *Healing in Byzantium*, pp. 119–30. See also A. Touwaide, "Byzantine Hospital Manuals (*Iatrosophia*) as a Source for the Study of Therapeutics," in B. Bowers (ed.), *The Medieval Hospital and Medical Practice* (Aldershot, 2007), pp. 147–73.

[44] Touwaide, "Byzantine Hospital Manuals"; see also C. Papadopoulos, "Post-Byzantine Medical Manuscripts: New Insights into the Greek Medical Tradition, Its Intellectual and Practical Interconnections, and Our Understanding of Greek Culture," *Journal of Modern Greek Studies*, 27 (2009): pp. 107–30.

[45] Basic studies on the *iatrosophion* for the English reader are Touwaide, "Byzantine Hospital Manuals"; Papadopoulos, "Post-Byzantine Medical Manuscripts"; and P.A. Clark, "Landscape, Memories, and Medicine: Traditional Healing in Amari, Crete," *Journal of Modern Greek Studies*, 20 (2002): pp. 339–65 and *A Cretan Healer's Handbook in the*

medical recipes taken from classical and Byzantine medical treatises (for example, the writings of Hippocrates and Galen or the writings of Paul of Aegina and Alexander of Tralles) and from pharmacological works like Dioscorides' massive work on plants. *Iatrosophia* were constantly updated by new medical knowledge and new medical substances. Thus, the texts gradually incorporated discussions of the "French disease" (i.e., syphilis) and new *materia medica* like coffee, quinine, and tobacco, which took their place alongside rosemary and oregano and other garden herbs that had formed medical recipes for millennia.

There were two basic types of *iatrosophia*. One, linked particularly to monasteries and penned by monks, contained only medical recipes and therapeutics. Most recipes in the texts consisted of herbal concoctions, with others containing mineral or animal substances. The majority of recipes derived from ancient and Byzantine formal medicine, but we also have the pharmacopoeia of folk healing. The second, and more prevalent, type, and the one I wish to discuss here briefly, also contains remedies drawn from folk medicine and classical Greek medicine; but besides the medical recipes and treatments, the text contains sections on a variety of topics like agricultural and veterinarian matters, astrology, exorcisms and spells, magic, and religion.[46]

The *iatrosophion* was a popular form of medical writing. Evangelia Varella has noted that from the Ottoman period of Greece, over 700 medical manuscripts and books have survived. Of that number, approximately nearly half are *iatrosophia*.[47] Agamemnon Tselikas offers a lower number of approximately 150.[48] *Iatrosophia*

Byzantine Tradition: Text, Translation and Commentary (Aldershot, 2011), especially pp. 1–22. Clark's 2011 bibliography has extensive references to the substantial body of modern Greek scholarship which must be consulted by those specializing in this area of the history of Greek medicine.

46 An example of the first type is the *iatrosophion* that A. Lardos is currently publishing; his preliminary results are to be found in "The Botanical *Materia Medica* of the *Iatrosophion*—A Collection of Prescriptions from a Monastery in Cyprus," *Journal of Ethnopharmacology*, 104 (2006): pp. 387–406. The latter is best seen in N.E. Papadogiannakês' *Κρητικὸ Ιατροσόφιον του 19ου αιώνα* (Rhethymno, 2001); see also Clark's iatrosophic text (*A Cretan Healer's Handbook*).

47 E. Varella, "La thérapeutique byzantine dans le monde grec d'époque ottoman," *Medicina nei secoli*, 11 (1999): pp. 577–84.

48 A. Tselikas, "Τα Ελληνικά γιατροσόφια: Μία Περιφρονημένη Κατηγορία Χειρογράφων," in T. Diamantopoulos (ed.), *Ιατρικά Βυζαντινά Χειρόγραφα* (Athens, 1995), pp. 57–69; cf. Papadopoulos, "Post-Byzantine Medical Manuscripts," p. 109. It is difficult to determine the exact number for several reasons. First, many simply have not been inventoried; far too many are in private collections or remain uncataloged in libraries. I have counted 22 *iatrosophia* among the codices at Mount Athos alone. Second, copyists borrowed extensively from other manuscripts they had access to, and so sometimes only an exhaustive

may be found all over Greece—in monasteries, libraries, and private collections.[49]

With these iatrosophic texts, medical healers can access a plethora of cures for ailments, which are listed *a capite ad calcem* ("from the top of the head to the toe"). The recipes for a specific disease are listed one after another, giving the impression that the healer should decide which recipe would be most effective or most appropriate in the situation, or that if one course of treatment failed, then others were available for restoring health. For example, for migraine headaches, a Cretan *iatrosophion*, dated to around 1800 but based on longstanding local traditions, offers these methods of treatment:

> Take "the guts of the earth," that is, worms. Simmer them in a fire along with 15 crushed peppercorns. Mix these with vinegar and apply to the head. Grind the dung of wild pigeon and mix with vinegar; smear on. Boil seeds of monk's pepper in anointing oil. Beat and then apply to the forehead and temples. Soften quicklime with honey and apply. Take the fruit of the rue and place in the ears and on the head; press it firmly [onto the skin] and then cover [with cloth]. Pestle bitter almonds and kneaded mastic gum; mix with vinegar and smear on the forehead. Pestle the tender buds of ivy. Mix the juice with rose oil and vinegar and apply. Put dry oleander leaves into burning coals and have the patient breathe the fumes through his nose. Ground a fresh root of the caper plant and smear on. Pestle rue and mix with vinegar. Place on the area where the head aches. Boil oakum in vinegar; extract the pitch and sprinkle it with salt. Cover the head with this. Turn a hedgehog's skin into ash; mix with oil and apply. Take the leaves and root of an asphodel and turn into ash. Mix with oil and apply. (Papadogiannakês, *Κρητικὸ Ιατροσόφιον*, pp. 57–9)[50]

Many of these recipes have been culled from the medical texts of ancient Greek and Byzantine doctors like Alexander of Tralles and Galen, and the botanist Dioscorides. Further recipes for migraines use folk medical practices:

> Take the rust from an iron object and pestle it well. Place it in three cups of vinegar and boil this well, however long it takes for the mixture to thicken. Then spread [the concoction] on a cloth so as to make a plaster. Place this plaster on the person's eyelids. You should do this for 3 days ... Take a bird's egg, making sure it is fresh, and then remove the white from it. Beat the white in a cup with

comparative analysis can determine whether two *iatrosophia* are actually separate texts or one is a reproduction of the other.

49 Clark, "Landscape, Memories, and Medicine"; Papadopoulos, "Post-Byzantine Medical Manuscripts" with literature; cf. Touwaide, "Byzantine Hospital Manuals," pp. 155–7.

50 All translations are my own, unless otherwise noted.

> a little rosewater and saffron. Get a linen cloth and make a plaster. Then place it on the spot [of the pain] ... Take the hurting person to a stone trough filled with water that mules and horses drink; let him drink from this after [the animals have drunk]. If you do this, his head will be rid of pain, and his teeth will too. (Papadogiannakês, *Κρητικὸ Ιατροσόφιον*, pp. 51–2)

Hippocratic theory is usually cited in *iatrosophia* when the etiology of disease is discussed. So, in the section on headaches, the iatrosophic writer of the Cretan text above follows Hippocratic theory that cephalalgia is the result of humors arising from the body and settling in the head; these humors must be purged to restore proper humoral balance. Methods for purgations are as follows:

> Crush leaves of the pine tree and place the juice in the person's nose. Grind black cumin finely; stir in woman's breast milk and place this [mixture] in the patient's nose. Pestle cyclamen and place the juice in the nostrils. Crush black cumin finely and then mix it with anointing oil; let it sit and then smear it in the nose. (Papadogiannakês, *Κρητικὸ Ιατροσόφιον*, pp. 61–2)

An accumulation of phlegm can also cause headaches and must be purged too:

> Take a jar of vinegar and boil it along with hyssop, pennyroyal, oregano, and marjoram. Let these juices ferment. [Place and] keep in the mouth to draw out many fluids. Mix crushed ginger and stavesacre; one should then chew this. Crush very finely stavesacre and pepper and then add mastic gum. Chew this in order to expel many fluids. Take stavesacre, vinegar, pennyroyal, thyme, and oregano. Seethe these and then keep in the mouth so as to produce much sputum and spittle. (Papadogiannakês, *Κρητικὸ Ιατροσόφιον*, pp. 60–61)

In many *iatrosophia*, disease may be exorcised through spells of the sort that we see in magical texts. For each type of ailment, the iatrosophic writers offer recipes, spells, prayers, and instructions for phylacteries and amulets. Every method has been tried and tested, so they claim, and will amaze healer and patient alike in its efficacy. One text offers this exorcism for releasing a sufferer from every demon-caused illness:

> I adjure you, all unclean spirits, male and female demons, to depart from this slave of God and from his house, his head, his forehead, brain, stomach, tongue, temples, eyelids, bones, intestines, shoulders, midriff, arms, hands, feet, belly, from his head to his toenails, his knees, ankles, fingernails, kidneys, back, from the right side and the left side of his body, from all his blood and his entire body ...

> Every evil, flee and make your escape from this servant of God who has the cross as his protector. [Pray:] "God is my hope, Christ is my refuge, the Holy Spirit is my shelter. Praise to you, Holy Trinity. Jesus Christ conquers. In the name of the Father and Son and Holy Spirit, now and always and forever and ever. Amen." (*Codex Bibliothèque de la Société Historique*, fol. 210)

Binding spells may use Christian theology and Christian holy objects; so, for migraines and other diseases:

> [A spell]: "Just as Solomon the Wonderful crushed the evil spirits of deception, so too I in the name of our Lord Jesus Christ bind you. [A long list of diseases is then given.] Our Lord Jesus Christ enjoins you, O evil spirits, to go away into the wild mountains where no sounds of birds are heard, to enter where neither sun nor moon shines, and to withdraw from NN, who is God's slave. On Golgotha the Lord was crucified, on the [wood of the] cypress and pine and cedar trees,[51] so that by His abrogating every action of the devil we may be well off, so that we may remain firm in the fear of God. Amen." Make the sign of the cross over [the ill person] with the holy spear three times, and say [the following] each time: "Christ was crucified at the place of the Skull, Christ was buried, Christ was raised from the dead. I adjure you, [pain in the] skull and migraine, by the Lord who was crucified and was buried and raised from the dead, by the Son and the Word of the Living God. O evil one, stop causing pain in the skull. The place of the Skull has become Paradise. You only had to bring forward, O Christ, the wood of your cross and immediately the tree of life sprouted with the smell of overwhelming delight. Glory to you, Christ, our God." (Papadogiannakês, *Κρητικὸ Ιατροσόφιον*, pp. 59–60)

Another iatrosophic text offers this remedy that contains folk medicine, a magical incantation, and an act of sympathetic magic:

> For someone who has a stone and cannot urinate. If a person wants to achieve health, write on his pubic area the following letters in red ink: "The Lord said, 'He who believes in me will have rivers of living water flowing from his belly.'" But if [it is not possible to do this] in his pubic area because of a sense of modesty, write [those words] on a piece of paper with red ink and attach the paper to his pubic area. Take the root of the mallow and boil it. He should drink the broth with a small amount of salt on an empty stomach and he should then urinate;

[51] These three types of wood comprised the cross of Jesus, according to Greek Orthodox tradition.

> then take away his shoes and have him walk barefoot to a wild fig tree. There take off the bark, however much of it is dark in color. Then take four or six nails and nail them into the place where you had stripped the bark; while you are nailing them have another person ask you, "Why are you nailing?" [Respond to him:] "I am nailing here the gallbladder of NN." Next hang over smoke the bark that you had removed. And just as the bark dries out, so too will the gallbladder. (*Codex Bibliotheque de la Société Historique*, fol. 210)

In this recipe, we have first a biblical verse (John 7:38) to be written on the sufferer's pubic area. This verse carries with it the power of the divine word to effect healing: just as living waters flow from the stomach of a Christian believer, so the patient's urinary tract will be cleared of any stone or blockage. But the physician should also apply a recipe containing mallow. Mallow is used in folk pharmacology for curing problems of the urinary, as well as respiratory, organs and the alimentary canal. Herbal books specifically recommend the plant's root boiled in water and then drunk so as to relieve pain of the urinary organs. As if more help is needed, though, the healer undertakes a sympathetic magical ritual. He removes the bark of a wild fig tree and drives nails (perhaps symbolic of Christ's crucifixion); as we know of ancient cursing tablets, this action binds the disease.[52] Next the healer speaks a charm involving *similia similibus*, that is, just as I do to this object, so may the same happen to the bodily organ. The result is that the bark, which has been bound by the nails, will dry up and so the stones in the gallbladder or bile ducts, similarly bound by the ritual, will dry up. One may wonder whether the biblical verse and the magical ritual were meant for the patient's benefit or whether the healer actually believed that they were necessary to supplement the natural healing properties of the mallow plant. Regardless, religious words, a magical incantation, a binding ritual, and folk medicine are all employed in this act of healing.

Another example of syncretism of various belief systems and approaches to healing appears in the instructions that iatrosophic writers give a healer on how to collect plant roots for use in medical cures. Greek magical texts had since ancient times advised people on the spells they were to utter while cutting roots and gathering plants for their recipes and charms. The following is from the *Greek Magical Papyri*:

> **Spell for Picking a Plant**: Use it before sunrise. **The Spell to be spoken**: "I am picking you, such and such a plant, with my five-fingered hand, I, NN, and I am

52 See J.M. Marston, "Language of Ritual Cursing in the Binding of Prometheus," *Greek, Roman and Byzantine Studies*, 47 (2007): pp. 121–33 with bibliography; see also Gager, *Curse Tablets and Binding Spells*; H. Versnel, "Beyond Cursing: The Appeal to Justice in Judicial Prayers," in Faraone and Obbink (eds), *Magika Hiera*, pp. 60–106.

> bringing you home so that you may work for me for a certain purpose. I adjure you by the undefiled name of the God: if you pay no heed to me, the earth which produced you will no longer be watered as far as you are concerned—ever in life again, if I fail in this operation, MOUTHABAR NACH BARNACHÔCHA BRAEÔMENDA LAUBRAASSE PHASPHA BENDEÔ; fulfill for me the perfect charm!" (*Papyri Graecae Magicae* IV.286–95; translation from Betz, *Greek Magical Paypri*, pp. 43–4)

It may come as a bit of surprise that our iatrosophic texts, written in a Christian environment, include similar instructions, including invocations of the various planets:

> **The plants in accordance with the planets:** The plant of Hermes is the cinquefoil. Extract this plant in the first hour of Wednesday with an oath to Hermes. If you boil this plant, it is efficacious in many ways ... The plant of Aphrodite is the male orchid. Extract it during the first hour of Friday; first swear an oath to Aphrodite three times. Pull the plant out along with its root, fruit, and flowers. Fray the plant into a deer skin. Wear this skin on your right shoulder; if you do, everyone will love you. Pestle the male orchid's leaves into a powder; if you apply it to your face, you will be amazed. (Papadogiannakês, *Κρητικὸ Ιατροσόφιον*, pp. 175–6)

We are not told here what the healer is supposed to say when swearing the "oaths," whether the words consist of non-Christian or Christian prayers or *voces magicae*.[53] However, elsewhere the same author makes it clear that the prayer to be spoken while cutting the roots of the ribwort plantain plant for curing hemorrhoids should be Christian:

> Take a newly made knife—one that has never been used to cut anything before—and on the fifth day of the moon's waning and draw binding circles with it around three roots of ribwort plantain. [While doing this,] say: "In the name of the Father, the Son, and the Holy Spirit." Then cut out the roots with the knife and recite this prayer: "O God of heaven and earth and everything in them, holy trinity rulers of life, have mercy on us. Holy Lady Theotokos, Saint Lucian, Paul, the healing saints Cosmas and Damian, intercede with Holy God so that He may cause the internal and external hemorrhoids, as well as any other ailment, to shrivel up and vanish for NN, the son of NN [masculine] and son of NN [feminine]. And just

[53] *Voces magicae* are typically untranslatable words and/or demonic names that are Egyptian, Jewish, Christian, and Near Eastern in origin but often meaningless; see H. Versnel, "The Poetics of the Magic Charm: An Essay in the Power of Words," in Mirecki and Meyer (eds), *Magic and Ritual*, pp. 105–58.

> as this knife made shavings on this plant, so may God shave away the internal and external hemorrhoids and perforations of the intestines and all diseases afflicting NN, the slave of God; by the intercession of the Blessed Theotokos and all the saints, we glorify and give thanks to the Father, Son, and Holy Spirit, now and always, forever and ever. Amen." (Papadogiannakês, *Κρητικὸ Ιατροσόφιον*, p. 128)

Here we have acts of sympathetic magic (*similia similibus*): just as the roots are shaved by the knife, so God is asked to shave away the swollen hemorrhoids; and just as the plantain roots wither over a fire and its smoke, so too God will cause the hemorrhoids to wither. Notice, though, that even within this magical context, religion pervades and is critical for the effectiveness of the treatment. This is a clear example of how faith in Christianity can exist alongside with magic (cutting herbs on moonlit nights while chanting exorcisms) and with good pharmacology, since plantain is often used to treat intestinal problems according to pharmacopeias.

Iatrosophia have been disparaged by many medical historians on the grounds that the texts are filled with superstition and magic.[54] Granted, some texts contain passages on medical astrology, releasing married couples from binding spells, exorcisms, magical curses against thieves, and divination, but these texts only reflect the worldview of both the people whom the healers treated and the healers themselves. Healing always was the prime concern. Thus, if the prevention of disease or the restoration of it could be achieved through a religious prayer, an exorcism spell, a magical ritual, a medical recipe based on traditional healing, or a concoction taken from Galen or Dioscorides, then healer and patient tried it. All curative methods were deemed valid; the healer or the sufferer would move from one to another as needed, or would even use several modes of treatment simultaneously.

Anthropological research of rural Greece, conducted in the mid- and late twentieth century, demonstrates that the medical pluralism so evident in antiquity and Byzantium had changed little.[55] Nonurban people typically resort

---

[54] See Clark, "Landscape, Memories, and Medicine," p. 341; Touwaide, "Byzantine Hospital Manuals," pp. 146–8; Papadapoulos, "Post-Byzantine Medical Manuscripts," pp. 107–8.

[55] I cite here R. Blum and E. Blum, *Health and Healing in Rural Greece: A Study of Three Communities* (Stanford, 1965) and *The Dangerous Hour: The Lore of Crisis and Mystery in Rural Greece* (London, 1970); Y. Beyene, *From Menarche to Menopause: Reproductive Lives of Peasant Women in Two Cultures* (Albany, 2001); L.M. Danforth, *Firewalking and Religious Healing the Anastenaria of Greece and the American Firewalking Movement* (Princeton, 1989).

to multiple health care providers.[56] Older married women often handle healing for the household, but other women (μάγισσαι) are consulted for their ability to use magical-ritual spells or incantations along with folk remedies and herbal recipes; such women are viewed in positive terms. At the opposite end of the spectrum are sorcerers and witches who inflict physical harm. Occupying the intermediary position are priests who also heal, but use sacred objects, prayers, snippets of liturgy, and exorcisms. Closer to the wise woman is the practical doctor (πρακτικὸς ἰατρός), trained in centuries-old pharmacology, often the possessor of an *iatrosophion*, a knowledgeable expert in local flora. An example is Nikolaos Konstantinos Theodorakis (1891–1979), who autographed the notebook he had written on medical therapeutics on 10 August 1930.[57] Theodorakis was a well-known herbalist and expert in local flora. He collected plants and tried out different combinations, dispensing them in his home and at his tobacconist shop to patients. All these various healers are seen by ill villagers; one-third to one-half of all families in the Blums' survey had gone to a magician, wise woman, practical doctor, or priest in the previous 12 months. Professional doctors are viewed with suspicion and mistrust because of an outsider status,[58] and folk healers are usually the first to be consulted. But professional health care providers are still deemed to be viable alternatives, especially if other means of healing fail, and doctors are used in conjunction with folk therapies advocated by wise women.[59]

---

[56] Blum and Blum, *Dangerous Hour*, pp. 269–70.

[57] P.A. Clark (*A Cretan Healer's Handbook*) has published his notebook (with translation and commentary); see her remarks on Theodorakis' life and work at pp. 31–45.

[58] Blum and Blum, *Dangerous Hour*, pp. 211–13. C. Stewart (*Demons and the Devil: Moral Imagination in Modern Greek Culture* [Princeton, 1991], p. 93) discusses the intersection of professional medicine and religion in his anthropological study of the island of Naxos. Also very useful is his Chapter 9 (pp. 222–43, notes on pp. 286–92) which deals with spells; see also the notes on p. 287 for spells directed against ailments like migraines.

[59] Blum and Blum, *Dangerous Hour*, pp. 158–9, 243, 255. Other Mediterranean countries offer similar multiple approaches to healing. In a village near Sofia, Bulgaria, Irwin Sanders (*Balkan Village* [Lexington, 1949]) found much of the healing done through priests and religious acts (prayers, burning candles) and religious materials (holy water), and through *babi* (grandmothers or wise old women), who use incantations and spells to help with cures. Midwives also function as folk healers. Patience Kemp (*Healing Ritual: The Technique and Tradition of the Southern Slavs* [London, 1935]) studied Slavic villages. Since many diseases are thought to be caused by spirits, magic, or the evil eye, there is an emphasis on propitiation, exorcism, and religious rituals. Doctors are consulted, as are priests, but magical methods and folk drugs are also used (convenience often dictates which approach is used). Phyllis Williams (*South Italian Pathways in Europe and America* [New Haven, 1938]) likewise discovered many healing specialists: witches, barbers, midwives, and herbalists; all these use folk remedies composed of foods and drinks and animal substances. Professional doctors and

One constant for all the areas of healing in Greece from ancient times through the twentieth century has been dreams. Dreams have played a role in how physicians have treated the diseases suffered by their patients, how religious authorities have dealt with the illnesses of worshippers and suppliants, and how folk healers (of every ilk) have assessed and cured ailments of family members, consultants, and villagers. The importance of dreams in medical healing is an extension of how dreams have functioned in Greek culture through the ages.[60] Divinatory dreams, which impart knowledge of future events to individuals and states, are the most well-known aspect of dreaming in the Greek world. Divine beings send prophetic visions or prognosticative dreams, which may be straightforward, devoid of symbolism, or enigmatic, thereby requiring interpretation.[61] But less well studied are dreams that signify a dreamer's current physical condition and emotional state.[62] The chapters in this volume aim to contribute to our knowledge of these types of dreams and

---

modern medical treatment were not neglected but were used in conjunction with the folk healing. J.A. Pitt-Rivers (*The People of the Sierra* [London, 1954]) surveyed an Andalusian village. The *sabia* (wise woman) has special powers to help people, including the knowledge of herbs and minerals for healing. Female folk healers dispense medicines and male healers set bones. As opposed to the other cultures, physicians and pharmacists, although viewed unfavorably because of their charging of fees, are consulted first; folk healers and the *sabia* are seen when "formal" medicine fails.

[60] For dreams in antiquity, the bibliography is considerable. The works I have found most useful are: G. Weber, *Kaiser, Träume und Visionen in Prinzipat und Spätantike* (Stuttgart, 2000); C. Walde, *Die Traumdarstellungen in der griechisch-römischen Dichtung* (Munich, 2001); B. Näf, *Traum und Traumdeutung im Altertum* (Darmstadt, 2004); William V. Harris, *Dreams and Experience in Classical Antiquity* (Cambridge, MA and London, 2009); Bilbija, "The Dream in Antiquity." For further reading, see Walde's chapter in this volume. For dreams in Byzantium, see: M. Mavroudi, *A Byzantine Book on Dream Interpretation: The Oneirocriticon of Achmet and Its Arabic Sources* (Leiden/Boston/Cologne, 2002); S.M. Oberhelman, *Dreambooks in Byzantium: Six Oneirocritica in Translation, with Commentary and Introduction* (Aldershot, 2008); the forthcoming volume by C. Angeliki and G. Calofonos (eds), *Dreaming of Byzantium and Beyond* (Aldershot). The study of dreams in post-Byzantine and early modern Greece has yet to be written; a brief survey may found in the section of divination in P. Koukoules, *Βυζαντινῶν βίος καὶ πολιτισμός*, 6 volumes in 7 parts (Athens, 1948–1957), vol. 1.2, pp. 155–226.

[61] An excellent study of religious (pagan and Christian) dreams in this context is P.C. Miller, *Dreams in Late Antiquity: Studies in the Imagination of a Culture* (Princeton, 1994). Individuals often used handbooks on the interpretation of dreams, called *oneirocritica*, or consulted professional diviners like Artemidorus (see Walde's chapter in this volume) for deciphering the dream. See also Oberhelman, *Dreambooks in Byzantium*, Chapters 1–3.

[62] The Greeks had little, if any, concern with how dreams may provide a glimpse into a person's past and formation of her or his psyche.

how they have functioned in healing and medicine at various times of Greek history.

Healing dreams may have different etiologies. Some dreams are non-natural in origin, in that they come from gods, saints, and angels, or the dreamer may be in a certain spiritual state that allows her to be the recipient of a healing dream.[63] Several chapters in this volume deal with the phenomenon of healing dreams in pagan and Christian religion. Louise Cilliers and François Pieter Retief discuss the Asclepian cult, which was so popular from the fifth century to the end of the Roman Empire. In their chapter, Cilliers and Retief seek to understand how suppliants could have had the dreams in ancient *testimonia* or preserved on stelae erected at Epidaurus. They investigate various theories (for example, did the patients ingest opium before going to sleep at night in the god's sleeping-chambers?) and the records of surgeries being performed at the cult centers. The authors demonstrate the cultural patterning and social construction of the medical dreams, as does Lee Pearcy in his analysis of medical dreams in the works of ancient physicians and in the Epidaurian inscriptions. The narratives in Christian dream healings also reflect social and cultural patterns and conditioning. Ildikó Csepregi, in her study of the role of hagiographers in incubation healing collections, argues that the Christian patient was conditioned by stories they had heard or read of saints' miraculous powers and the wondrous healings they performed. Some of these narratives were recorded in the sanctuary or were discussed by religious authorities and suppliants alike. These narratives then fed back into the ill person's dream narrative during the night and/or the next morning on awakening. What occurred in the church basilica or at the saint's shrine was a mirror, then, of what had transpired centuries earlier in the Asclepian pagan healing cult, where sick patients read the miracle cures on the inscriptions and heard stories of healing from cured patients and priests. In her contribution, Stavroula Constantinou investigates healing dreams in Byzantine hagiographical narratives, especially in the miracle collection, which includes a number of independent stories describing posthumous miracles performed by a saint or a pair of saints. Like the Asclepian cures, many of which were in accordance with treatments recommended by physicians, the healing means and practices performed or suggested by the saints were compatible with contemporary medical and health practices. Charles Stewart, in a chapter surveying the dreams of the inhabitants of the island of modern Naxos, mentions contemporary miracles performed by Panaghia (the Virgin Mary), religious icons, and saints, especially Nectarius and Eirini Khryssovalandou. The latter

[63] See the exhaustive survey in Bilbija, "The Dream in Antiquity," pp. 163–85 with Appendices A–B (see pp. 75–86 for Judaism, which serves as a background for Christian attitudes).

saints have monasteries near Athens, and suppliants come looking for miraculous cures. As Stewart mentions, the followers of Eirini Khryssovalandou even publish newsletters about people cured from illnesses and injuries.[64] In a chapter that focuses on the revival of the Asclepian healing cult in contemporary Greece, Jill Dubisch describes the dream-healing pilgrimages she has taken to Greece with Edward Tick, a Jungian psychotherapist. Tick conducts these journeys with groups seeking to connect to ancient sites and mythology in order to effect healing at the physical, psychological, and spiritual levels. Unlike contemporary Greek Orthodox pilgrims, however, who openly conduct rituals and even stay overnight at churches to connect with healing saints, pilgrims on Tick's journeys not only seek to imagine and connect with the past by visiting ancient sites and reading or hearing about the classical past, but also create their own sacred space. Dubisch describes how pilgrimages conclude with a dream-healing incubation, which takes place in a hotel room, converted, through ritual and sacred objects, into a healing dream space. Within this space, those pilgrims who wish to experience dream healing undergo individual dreaming, while watched over by the rest of the group. These dream experiences, and the experiences of those in attendance, are then discussed and analyzed the following day. Interestingly, although this Asclepian ritual was initially conceived of and carried out by non-Greeks, some Greeks are now designing their own dream-healing journeys. At Agios Nikolaos in the southern Peloponnesus, dream-healing pilgrimages based around the traditions of Asclepius are offered. The self-discovery and the self-growth achieved thanks to Tick's trips and at places like Agios Nikolaos fit neatly into the dream journeys of Aelius Aristides (Downie), Christian suppliants (Constantinou, Csepregi), and modern Greek islanders (Stewart).

Other healing dreams have a natural causation, and this is where medical professionals offered their theories.[65] As Pearcy shows in his chapter, Hippocratic writers viewed medical as nondivine dreams, as opposed to divine dreams that

---

64 This is the picture that other modern scholars have painted. See, e.g., M.H. Jameson et al., *A Greek Countryside: The Southern Argolid from Prehistory to the Present Day* (Stanford, 1994), p. 610; C. Ballas and S. Marketos, "The Survival of Aesculapian Tradition and Cult in Trikka of Thessaly," *Materia Medica Greca*, 9 (1981): pp. 340–46; A.A. Diamandopoulos and S. Marketos, "Votive Offerings and Other Magicoreligious Health Practices in Modern Greece," *Humane Medicine*, 9(4) (1993): pp. 296–302; D. Constantelos, "The Interface of Medicine and Religion in the Greek and Christian Greek Orthodox Tradition," in J.T. Chirban (ed.), *Health and Faith: Medical, Psychological, and Religious Dimensions* (Lanham, 1991), pp. 13–24; K. Patton, "'A Great and Strange Correction': Intentionality, Locality, and Epiphany in the Category of Dream Incubation," *History of Religions*, 43(3) (2004): pp. 194–223, at p. 196; E. Diamond, *The Science of Dreams* (London, 1962), pp. 215–16; and of course the works of the Blums referenced in note 55 above.

65 Bilbija, "The Dream in Antiquity," pp. 280–83.

prognosticate future events. The medical dream, which describes both the physical state of the body and the regimen needed to restore health, occurs when the soul, while the body is asleep, performs through its own agency all the acts of the body, such as sight, touch, perception of pain, and reflection. During the body's sleep, a displacement of perception takes place: the soul's cognitive and sensory processes shift inwardly, to the body, whereby the soul perceives the conditions of the body, including diseases. These perceptions constitute the dream's images and offer information on the dreamer's state of health.

Maithe Hulskamp, in her study of dream diagnosis in the Hippocratic corpus and in the second-century AD doctor Galen, argues convincingly that many Hippocratic writers, although they considered dreams a part of their medical practice, did not pay much attention to the *contents* of the dreams; rather, the writers focused on the *occurrence* and *types* of dreams (e.g., troubled dreams) and used this information as a diagnostic tool. The author of the Hippocratic *Regimen*, however, combined a physiological and a hermeneutic approach to the dream, seeing significance not only in the dream event but also in its contents; thus, dreams can have a dual purpose—medical diagnosis (what is happening to the body) *and* medical prognosis (what is going to happen to the body).

A medical dream, for the author of *Regimen* and subsequent Greek physicians like Rufus of Ephesus and Galen, should be analyzed according to a microcosm-macrocosm analogy. The human body is the microcosm of the universe (the macrocosm) and so the circulations in the outer, middle, and hollow parts of the body are analogous to the outer, middle, and hollow circuits (the stars, sun, and moon). Thus, according to this model of analogy, if someone dreams of a star (outer circuit) disappearing or suffering some sort of harm, this means that a moist and phlegm-like secretion has fallen to the body's outer circulation; the dreamer must then undergo a medical regimen to remove the excess moisture from the body, for example, by inducing perspiration. Dream images involving terrestrial phenomena are analogous to parts of the human body. For example, the earth is analogous to the dreamer's skin; a tree to the penis; cisterns to the bladder; and rivers to the blood's circulation and quantity. Thus, a dream of seeing the earth flooded with water indicates that the body is excessively moist, and the patient must take steps to promote drying. In my own contribution on dream interpretation and popular healing manuals of the early modern Greek period in this volume, I quote Philip van der Eijk's analysis of the steps that the author of *Regimen* took in deciphering the significance of a dream image: (1) the signs (τεκμήρια), that is, the dream images themselves; (2) the significance of the dream, that is, whether it is good or bad and whether it indicates particular bodily affections or disorders, etc.; (3) explanations of the relationship between sign and significance; (4) prophylactic (dietetic) measures; and (5) instructions as to the gods one should pray to in order to prevent disease.[66] The audience of *Regimen* 4 was composed mainly of dieticians and fitness trainers so that they could make diagnostic or prognostic determinations of a person's health and then offer an appropriate regimen.[67] The most common regimens were vapor baths, drying and cooling, alterations in a patient's food and drink, emetics, hellebore, and conducting exercises or avoiding them.

Galen, the most famous physician of antiquity after Hippocrates, was a fervent follower of the god Asclepius and used dreams in his personal and professional life.[68] Both Downie and Hulskamp discuss how dreams figure in the Galenic corpus. Hulskamp argues that although dreams were an important component of Galen's personal life, he did not give them as primary a place in his practice as past scholars have surmised. She demonstrates that Galen relegated dreams to a low place among his diagnostic procedures and employed them only occasionally for diagnosis and prognosis. Galen did agree with the author of *Regimen* 4 in seeing the need to develop a typology of dreams for helping the physician to distinguish between dreams that are medically significant and those that are not. For Galen, some dreams are divine and have nothing to do with illness; others simply repeat a dreamer's waking-state thoughts or the actions that he undertakes in everyday life; still others come from the soul's own innate ability to foretell the future. Medically significant dreams occur during disturbances in the body impact dream imagery. During sleep the soul goes into the depths of the body; having been isolated from outside stimuli and perceptions, the soul senses the body's dispositions and forms (although we are not told how) images of what it senses. The body's humors (yellow bile, black bile, blood, and phlegm, and their qualities), in turn, influence these soul-images. Thus, excess blood will cause an image of standing in a cistern of blood; a fever on the verge of crisis an image of swimming or bathing in hot water; too much sperm an image of having sexual intercourse; a large quantity of feces or foul humors an image of sitting in filth and dung; and a plethora of humors the impression of scarcely being able to move one's body or of carrying heavy burdens.[69] But Galen, as Hulskamp notes, admits that it is difficult for even trained professionals (medical or lay) to determine whether a dream is medically significant or has no value for diagnosis

---

66 Van der Eijk, "Divination, Prognosis and Prophylaxis," p. 198.

67 See ibid., pp. 195–6, 202–3.

68 S.M. Oberhelman, "Dreams in Graeco-Roman Medicine," in W. Haase and H. Temporini (eds), *Aufstieg und Niedergang der römischen Welt* (Berlin, 1993), part II, vol. 37.1, pp. 121–56, at p. 139.

69 For similar analogies in the corpus of the second-century AD Greek physician Rufus of Ephesus, see Oberhelman, "Dreams in Graeco-Roman Medicine," p. 138.

or prognosis of the body. The views of Hippocrates and Galen were followed by physicians of the Byzantine and early modern Greek eras. Byzantine scholars collected Galen's theories and published excerpts of them,[70] while *iatrosophia* and post-Byzantine *oneirocritica*, as I here show, preserve Hippocratic and Galenic theory.

Dreams may also arise naturally from plants, minerals, animals, foods, and drinks, or preternaturally from the manipulation of natural objects and substances in conjunction with spells and incantations. In his chapter, Jovan Bilbija inventories the *materia* in the botanical, medical, and pharmacological literature of the Roman Empire and Byzantium, and also magical stones and magical papyri, as all these substances cause, prevent, or neutralize certain types of dreams (sometimes as one of several symptoms in a clinical picture). Bilbija discusses problems in differentiating between *materia medica* and *materia magica*. Although the boundaries between these domains are somewhat vague, some differentiation can be made. For example, there are differences in application (for example, wearing something/sleeping on something versus drinking a liquid or rubbing an ointment), in complexity (magical rituals tend to be much more complex than medical applications of drugs), and in availability of the *materia* (e.g., the right fin of a hyena-fish versus garden lettuce). Bilbija shows how in medical literature some foods, herbs, and meats when eaten, and animal parts when applied to the body, cause disagreeable dreams. Medical texts also deal with nocturnal emissions; some substances may cause them and others may prevent them. In medical literature, herbal substances can prevent nightmares, but so can engraved stones, phylacteries, and magical spells.

A similar interconnection in dream healing between folk medicine, professional medicine, and magic also appears in the iatrosophic texts discussed by me and Barbara Zipser. Zipser's chapter focuses on manuscript MSL 14 of the Wellcome Library in London. The manuscript contains, in 23 folios, an idiosyncratic collection of remedies, prognostic signs, and magical incantations written in a mixture of vernacular and classical Greek. Ultraviolet examination reveals in the margins another text that contains magical incantations, parts of the Greek liturgy, and a few therapeutic instructions written in invisible ink. The reason behind the use of invisible ink was to give the collection greater magical properties. Zipser discusses the diseases mentioned in the manuscript, the purpose of the magical incantations, and the relationship between magic and medicine in this and other contemporary texts. Dreams and their interpretation figure prominently in the manuscript and, as Zipser points out, sections show

---

70 G. Guidorizzi, " L'opuscolo di Caleno 'De dignotione ex insomniis,'" *Bollettino per la preparazione dell'edizione nazionale dei classici greci e latini*, 21 (1973): pp. 81–105.

that oneirocritic theory had worked its way into medical training in the Middle Ages. I examine an eighteenth-century dreambook that incorporates material from *iatrosophia*; the *iatrosophion*, as defined above, is a physician's notebook of recipes and treatments or the collective compendium of classical and Byzantine medical and pharmacological texts consulted in hospital settings. While some *iatrosophia* contain only medical recipes, others (like Zipser's text) also have spells, exorcisms, magic, astrology, and practical advice (ridding houses of snakes, veterinarian care, etc.). I demonstrate how the author of the dreambook discusses the significance of dreams for physical, emotional, and spiritual wellbeing; the author recommends prophylaxis (diet and regimen), magical spells and exorcisms, and religious prayers for restoring or maintaining health. After an evaluation of some of the treatments in the dreambook, I conclude that the author consulted iatrosophic texts that preserved Hippocratic and Galenic medical theory and praxis, as well as folk medicine.

The authors of the chapters in this volume also demonstrate how various forms of healing overlapped. According to the medical anthropological models discussed at the start of this introduction, medical pluralism displays interactions and interconnections, but also tensions as certain practitioners claim their own superior healing ability. Cilliers and Retief show that at the Asclepian healing cult centers, a combination of clinical and religious medicine was practiced. They argue that lay doctors and Asclepius ordered many of the same recipes and regimens, but patients were probably more attentive to following the god's advice because of his divine status. Tensions did exist between temple medicine and secular medicine. Downie describes how the second-century AD devotee of Asclepius, Aelius Aristides, wrote of dreaming of physicians debating over a "Hippocratic" prescription (*Orations* 51.49ff). Since the doctors appear within the dream world that is Aristides' customary line of communication with Asclepius, the passage subordinates the prescriptive voice of professional medicine to the authority of the god. Pearcy discusses, on the other hand, the great lengths to which Hippocratic writers went in distancing medical prognosis from divinatory prognosis. The writers separated god-sent (Asclepian) dreams and the prophetic dreams, which are appropriate to the realm of diviners, from the medical dream that formed part of their medical praxis and is to be understood in the context of medical theory. Pearcy demonstrates how the writer of the Hippocratic *Epidemics* framed his case histories so as to distinguish them from the miracle stories on the Epidaurian stelae, even though the two sets of narratives have points of commonality. Walde shows the intersection between popular dream interpretation (Artemidorus), religious medicine, and formal medicine. Artemidorus often assumed the role of physician—a profession he recommended to his son to become knowledgeable in—and interpreted dreams that featured Asclepius offering poultices, plant remedies, and surgeries. Walde mentions how Artemidorus went so far as to claim that medicine developed out of the Asclepian incubation practice, as doctors committed to memory the god's advice on cures and treatment. This is certainly not true, but the statement shows the ancients' association of the medical profession with religious medicine. The two do share methodology of interpretation. As Hulskamp points out, both physician and dream interpreter were faced with problems of validating and verifying prognostic dreams and in developing a reliable methodology. Galen based his interpretation of medical dreams on factors external to the dream, such as the dreamer's surroundings, habits, and regimen. In popular dream interpretation too, dreams have significance unique to each dreamer. Artemidorus instructed an interpreter to analyze a dream through six *stoicheia* (elements of analysis): nature, convention, habit, occupation, name, and time; the interpreter then must determine whether the dream is *kata* (in accordance with) or *para* (in opposition to) each of those elements. The two principle *stoicheia*, however, are *phusis* (nature) and *nomos* (convention), with the latter category subdivided into unwritten social rules (*ethē*) and written laws (*nomoi*). Thus, a dream that is *kata phusin* (in accordance with nature) foretells something good, while a dream *para phusin* (contrary to nature) signifies something evil. The interpreter must be especially careful in how he collects and evaluates information concerning the dreamer and dream. Absolutely crucial is the interpreter's knowledge of a consultant's life and habits, for the images in a dream must be compared to the dreamer's biographical data: gender, number of children, marital status, social position, economic means, and so forth. Since the meaning of a dream depends on the circumstances of each dreamer, the interpreter must question the dreamer about his or her life and then decode the dream's significance based on those answers. In this methodology Artemidorus approximates that of Galen.

Timothy Miller's chapter on Byzantine hospitals offers an especially clear example of the intersection of formal medicine, popular medicine, and religion. Despite the scientific orientation of hospitals, dreams played a role in healing just as they had at the Asclepian healing centers of antiquity. Miller notes that although Byzantines hospitals were attached to monasteries and had clerical staff on duty to see to the patients' spiritual needs, hospitals were exclusively medical and supervised by physicians. The institutions not only provided access to professional medical care for their patients, but also served as pharmacies. Drawing his evidence from collections of miracles performed by the healing saints/doctors Cosmas and Damian (primarily the sixth century), Saint Artemius (seventh century), and Saint Sampson (tenth century), Miller shows how these collections include stories about hospital patients who dreamt while being treated at a hospital. Some patients awoke and found themselves miraculously cured, while others received in their dreams information that brought about a cure. As may be expected of the usual tension between religion and formal medicine, the saints in the dreams occasionally attacked human physicians as being ineffective in their healing powers when compared to God's power to cure. But we read of many instances where the saints recommended therapies that the hospital physicians then used, thus showing positive responses on the part of hospital physicians and other staff members to patients who had claimed to have received healing dreams.

The chapters in this volume are organized into three chronological periods: antiquity, Byzantium, and post-Byzantium to the current day. However, these are artificial constructs, since, as I hope to have shown in this introduction, healing dreams in formal medicine, popular medicine, and religious medicine display continuity and interconnectedness through the centuries. While differences did exist, the overlaps and interrelations dominate to a far greater extent. The chapters here are offered in the hope that they will contribute to a better understanding of how dreams have played a vital role in healing among Greeks for over two-and-a-half millennia.

PART ONE
Antiquity

Chapter 2

The Value of Dream Diagnosis in the Medical Praxis of the Hippocratics and Galen

Maithe A.A. Hulskamp

In antiquity, the significance of dreams, as a means of communication for the gods, as divine indicators of present or future events, or providing guidance after some fashion, was widely accepted: dreams and their content could be associated with almost every aspect of ancient society.[1] In medicine too, dreams played a role. On the one hand, dreams were used in a religious medical setting in the practice of incubation, the cult of the healing god Asclepius being the most famous example;[2]

---

[1] See, for example, G. Björck, "ONAP IΔEIN: De la perception de rêve chez les anciens," *Eranos*, 44 (1946): pp. 306–14, at p. 307; E.R. Dodds, *The Greeks and the Irrational* (Berkeley, 1951), p. 108; A.H.M. Kessels, "Ancient Systems of Dream Classification," *Mnemosyne*, 22 (1969): pp. 389–424, at p. 390; D. Del Corno, "Dreams and Their Interpretation in Ancient Greece," *Bulletin of the Institute of Classical Studies*, 29 (1982): pp. 55–62, at p. 55; J.J. Winkler, *The Constraints of Desire* (London and New York, 1990), p. 25; S.M. Oberhelman, "Dreams in Graeco-Roman Medicine," in W. Haase and H. Temporini (eds), *Aufstieg und Niedergang der römischen Welt* (Berlin, 1993), part II, vol. 37.1, pp. 121–56, at p. 122; P.J. van der Eijk, "Divination, Prognosis and Prophylaxis: The Hippocratic Work 'On Dreams' (*De Victu* 4) and Its Near Eastern Background," in H.F.J. Horstmanshoff and M. Stol (eds), *Magic and Rationality in Ancient Near Eastern and Graeco-Roman Medicine* (Leiden, 2004), pp. 187–218, at p. 192. Due to their divine origin, dreams were of special interest in cult life; cf. J.S. Hanson, "Dreams and Visions in the Graeco-Roman World and Early Christianity," in Haase and Temporini (eds), *Aufstieg und Niedergang der römischen Welt*, part II, vol. 23.2, pp. 1395–427, at p. 1398. In his book on dreams and experience in classical antiquity, W.V. Harris points out that dreams were not as important and widely valued as previous scholarship has led us to believe: *Dreams and Experience in Classical Antiquity* (Cambridge, MA and London, 2009), pp. 2, 123–228.

[2] In a few isolated areas, this cult is already attested in the Greek world in the sixth century BC. It really took flight toward the end of the fifth century, after the god had been introduced into Athens around 420 BC—surely not unrelated to impact of the great plague of Athens in 430–427/425 BC. Cf. *Inscriptiones Graecae* II^2, no. 4960a (= T 720 in E.J. Edelstein and L. Edelstein [eds], *Asclepius: Collection and Interpretation of the Testimonies*

on the other hand, a more "rational" approach was adopted by physicians, who believed that dreams could divulge important medical information about the condition of the body. The latter of these approaches will be the topic of the current chapter. Two relatively elaborate sources on the use of dream interpretation in medical diagnosis are usually put forward to corroborate the existence of such a practice: the Hippocratic *Regimen* 4 and the treatise *On Diagnosis from Dreams*, attributed to Galen. As we shall see, both treatises deal explicitly with medical diagnosis through the interpretation of dreams and provide examples regarding specific dream images and their meaning, thus creating the impression that dreams were an integral part of ancient medical diagnosis. The immediate context of these treatises has, however, until now been largely ignored or considered only superficially: there are other Hippocratic treatises in which dreams are featured, and there are many Galenic treatises and case studies that can be used as a touchstone for Galen's confidence in dream diagnosis. By considering these texts alongside *Regimen* and *On Diagnosis from Dreams*, we may gauge the importance of dreams in relation to other diagnostic tools and uncover the true value of dream diagnosis to the Hippocratics and Galen.

The Hippocratic Corpus

The Hippocratic Corpus contains the earliest known text that comprises a systematic account of medical dream interpretation: *Regimen* 4.[3] It has often been considered an oddity, not only in relation to the rest of the treatise—for a long time, this fourth book was thought to be only loosely connected to the rest of *Regimen*[4]—but also within the wider context of the Hippocratic Corpus.

[2 vols, Baltimore, 1945], vol. 1, pp. 374–5); cf. Edelstein and Edelstein, *Asclepius*, vol. 2, p. 55; and J. Longrigg, *Greek Medicine: From the Heroic to the Hellenistic Age* (London, 1998), pp. 11–17. For more information on the Asclepian healing cult, see Edelstein and Edelstein, *Asclepius*; L.R. LiDonnici, *The Epidaurian Miracle Inscriptions: Text, Translation and Commentary* (Atlanta, 1995); G.D. Hart, *Asclepius, The God of Medicine* (London, 2000); and of the course the chapters by Cilliers and Retief, Downie, and Pearcy elsewhere in this volume. Other healing deities with similar practices are, for instance, Amphiaraus of Oropus and Sarapis; cf. F.T. van Straten, "Gifts for the Gods," in H.S. Versnel (ed.), *Faith, Hope and Worship* (Leiden, 1981), pp. 65–151, at p. 98.

3 Cf. R.G.A. van Lieshout, *Greeks on Dreams* (Utrecht, 1980), p. 100; S.M. Oberhelman, "The Diagnostic Dream in Ancient Medical Theory and Practice," *Bulletin of the History of Medicine*, 61 (1987): pp. 47–60, at p. 49. *Regimen* (*De Victu*) 4 is also known as *On Dreams*.

4 As Book 4 does have the appearance of a separate discussion, some scholars have typified its structure as "compilatory" in the past. Cf., for instance, C. Fredrich, *Hippokratische Untersuchungen* (Berlin, 1899), pp. 221–2, 226–8; and A. Palm, "Studien zur

As regards the latter point, however, the truth is that insufficient research has been conducted into the position of *Regimen*—and especially the ideas voiced in its fourth book—within the Corpus. If little to nothing is known of other Hippocratic authors' ideas on dreams, how are we to assess whether or not the ideas postulated by the author of *Regimen* were alien to those of his fellow physicians? As Philip van der Eijk rightly asserts, "It would be a gross exaggeration to say that in his overall medical outlook, the author of *On Regimen* is completely at odds with what we find elsewhere in the Hippocratic writings."[5] In the following, views on dreams held by *Regimen*, as well as those held by other Hippocratic authors, will be considered in order to illuminate the theoretical environment within which the author of *Regimen* conceived of his system of dream interpretation, and to verify to what extent this system was indeed the novel invention its author claimed it to be.

The Hippocratic *Regimen* 4

As its title suggests, *Regimen* is concerned with the protection of people's health by means of careful regulation of their lifestyle. To this end, the author argues, one must of course have a thorough knowledge of human nature in general, and of the things regimen comprises: food and exercise. When these two are well balanced, they produce health. In addition, it is necessary to be aware of all things internal and external which may have a bearing on either the amount of food or the amount of exercise required. But, the author adds, even when all of this is known, it is not enough; if it were, illness would no longer exist (*Regimen*

Hippocratischen Schrift 'Peri Diaitês'" (Ph.D. dissertation, University of Tübingen, 1933), p. 99. Recent scholarship shows that *Regimen* 1–4 are all part of one coherent argument; cf. H. Diller, "Der innere Zusammenhang der hippocratischen Schriften De Victu," *Hermes*, 87 (1959): pp. 39–56; R. Joly, *Recherches sur le Traité pseudo-Hippocratique De Régime* (Paris, 1960), pp. 172–9 and *Hippocrate: Du Régime* (Paris, 1967), p. xxii; R. Joly and S. Byl, *Hippocrate: Du Régime* (*Hippocratis De Diaeta*), *Corpus Medicorum Graecorum*, 1.2, 4 (Berlin, 1984), pp. 20–22; Oberhelman, "Dreams in Graeco-Roman Medicine," p. 129; J. Jouanna, "L'interpretation des rêves et la théorie micro-macrocosmique dans le traité Hippocratique *Du Regime*: semiotique et mimesis," in K.-D. Fischer, D. Nickel, and P. Potter (eds), *Text and Translation* (Leiden, 1998), pp. 161–74; A.M. Holowchak, "Interpreting Dreams for Corrective Regimen: Diagnostic Dreams in Greco-Roman Medicine," *Journal of the History of Medicine and Allied Sciences*, 56 (2001): pp. 382–99, at p. 388 note 15; van der Eijk, "Divination, Prognosis and Prophylaxis," pp. 193–4.

[5] Van der Eijk, "Divination, Prognosis and Prophylaxis," pp. 189–90. Cf. also Palm, "Studien," pp. 99–124; Joly, *Recherches*, pp. 183–203; Joly and Byl, *Hippocrate: Du Régime*, pp. 36–44.

1.2 [p. 124, 17–19 Joly and Byl; vol. 6, p. 470 Littré; E. Littré (ed.), *Hippocrate, Oeuvres complètes* (10 vols, Paris 1839–1861)]). In light of this realization, the author is proud to present a solution: he boldly states that he has discovered a way to tailor patients' regimens exactly to their needs and, what is more, that he has discovered a way to predict illness:

> ἐμοὶ δὲ ταῦτα ἐξεύρηται, καὶ πρὸ τοῦ κάμνειν τὸν ἄνθρωπον ἀπὸ τῆς ὑπερβολῆς, ἐφ' ὁπότερον ἂν γένηται, προδιάγνωσις. Οὐ γὰρ εὐθέως αἱ νοῦσαι τοῖσιν ἀνθρώποισιν ἐπιγίνονται, ἀλλὰ κατὰ μικρὸν συλλεγόμεναι ἀθρόως ἐκφαίνονται. Πρὶν οὖν κρατεῖσθαι ἐν τῷ ἀνθρώπῳ τὸ ὑγιὲς ὑπὸ τοῦ νοσεροῦ, ἃ πάσχουσιν ἐξεύρηταί μοι, καὶ ὅπως χρὴ ταῦτα καθιστάναι ἐς τὴν ὑγιείην. (*Regimen* 1.2 [p. 124, 28–p. 126, 3 Joly and Byl; vol. 6, p. 472 Littré])

> What has revealed these things to me—even before a man falls ill due to excess (in whichever direction that excess might occur [sc. too much or too little])—is *prodiagnôsis*. For diseases do not surface in people all of a sudden, but they develop little by little, without being noticed, and then suddenly appear. Thus I have discovered what people suffer before health is mastered by disease, and how one should change these things into a state of health.

The only way to prevent disease, the author declares, is to cast a *prodiagnôsis*, an evaluation of the patient's condition and an identification of the excesses within his body concerning the humors[6] and their primary qualities (hot, cold, wet, and dry) *before* any disease has had a chance to manifest itself.[7] Central to the author's invention of *prodiagnôsis* is the interpretation of dreams, to which the whole fourth book of *Regimen* is devoted.[8] Through these medical dreams, the (as yet) invisible becomes visible and enables a physician to adjust his patients' regimen according to their bodies' exact needs.[9] Such a treatment is not meant

[6] The most famous combination of humors is that of black bile, yellow or red bile, blood, and phlegm, adopted from the Hippocratic *On the Nature of Man*. However, one must bear in mind that in other Hippocratic treatises, other combinations—and indeed other humors and other bodily components—are also to be found.

[7] Apparently, it is also possible to detect desire of the soul (cf. *Regimen* 4.93 [p. 228, 27 and p. 230, 2 Joly and Byl; vol. 6, p. 660 Littré]), but the author seems to do no more than take note of this; there does not seem to be any treatment.

[8] For a more elaborate discussion of the links between Books 1–3 and Book 4 and the indirect references in the first three books to dream interpretation, see van der Eijk, "Divination, Prognosis and Prophylaxis," pp. 194–5.

[9] However, this *prodiagnôsis* does not consist of an exact indication of a specific illness. Van der Eijk ("Divination, Prognosis and Prophylaxis," p. 202) remarks that "it is striking that the author is using a very descriptive, if not rather 'primitive' nosology: technical terms for

to cure disease. It is even better: it will correct a condition that might otherwise have led to disease.

In Chapter 86, the first chapter of our Hippocratic dreambook, the author explains the origin of medical dreams. In sleep, when the body is at rest, the soul is active: it is aware of everything (γινώσκει πάντα) and on its own performs all the acts it would perform together with the body during the day, such as seeing, hearing, walking, touching, feeling, and thinking.[10] These acts are, literally, the stuff of dreams.[11] How exactly this works the author does not explain, but his views on sense perception give us some small insight into the process. Beate Gundert paraphrases: "Sense-perception takes place when the sensations coming into the body through sight, hearing, and touch meet the soul on its revolutions, mix with it, shake it, and thus are sensed by it."[12] In sleep, while there is still perception by the soul, there is no *sense* perception: there are no sensations

---

diseases, e.g. phrenitis, pneumonia, ileus etc. are absent, and the terms in which the author's pathology is cast—belly, blood, flesh, 'periods'—are very similar to those he used in his anatomical and physiological theories in Books 1-3." If, however, one considers what the author claims to have invented, his great personal discovery, it will become clear that it is not surprising to find no disease names in *Regimen* 4. Incidentally, one is strongly reminded of the closing remark of *Prognostic*: Ποθεῖν δὲ χρὴ οὐδενὸς νουσήματος τοὔνομα, ὅτι μὴ τυγχάνῃ ἐνθάδε γεγραμμένον (It is not necessary to wish for the name of any disease, just because it happens not to have been written here, *Prognostic* 25 [p. 231, 6–7 Alexanderson; vol. 2, p. 190 Littré]).

[10] *Regimen* 4.86 (p. 218, 7–12 Joly and Byl; vol. 6, p. 640 Littré). There is some discussion as to the origin of this idea. For arguments in favor of an Orphico-Pythagorean theory, cf. Palm, "Studien," pp. 62–9; Joly, *Hippocrate: Du Régime*, p. 97 note 1; Joly and Byl, *Hippocrate: Du Régime*, pp. 27–30; Oberhelman, "Dreams in Graeco-Roman Medicine," p. 131; J. Godderis, *Een Arts is Vele Andere Mensen Waard* (Leuven, 2000), pp. 588–90. For the Orphic view, see Dodds, *The Greeks and the Irrational*, p. 119. For Pythagorean roots, see: Kessels, "Ancient Systems," p. 415; F. Hoessly, *Katharsis: Reinigung als Heilverfahren: Studien zum Ritual der archaischen und klassischen Zeit sowie zum Corpus Hippocraticum* (Göttingen, 2001), p. 298. For arguments against the Orphic element, see: G. Cambiano, "Une interprétation 'materialiste' des rêves: Du Régime IV," in M.D. Grmek (ed.), *Hippocratica: Actes du Colloque Hippocratique de Paris, (4–9 septembre 1978)* (Paris, 1980), pp. 87–96, at pp. 91–3; Palm, "Studien," pp. 62–9; Joly, *Hippocrate: Du Régime*, p. 97, note 1; Joly and Byl, *Hippocrate: Du Régime*, pp. 27–30, 92; Dodds, *The Greeks and the Irrational*, p. 119; Oberhelman, "Dreams in Graeco-Roman Medicine," p. 131.

[11] The author points out that there is a direct link between the things the soul does and experiences during sleep, and the things one sees in dreams: ποῖα γάρ τινα πάσχει τὸ σῶμα, τοιαῦτα ὁρᾷ ἡ ψυχὴ κρυπτομένης ὄψιος ([A]s the experiences of the body are, so are the visions of the soul when sight does not function, *Regimen* 3.71 [p. 204, 5–6 Joly and Byl; vol. 6, p. 610 Littré]).

[12] B. Gundert, "Soma and Psyche in Hippocratic Medicine," in J.P. Wright and P. Potter (eds), *Psyche and Soma* (Oxford, 2000), pp. 13–35, at p. 23.

coming into the body from without. When sleep sets in, a change takes place regarding the *object* of perception: sleep severs the connection between the soul and the outside world, so the object of perception for the soul becomes only the body and all that goes on within it.[13]

At the beginning of *Regimen* 4, the author explains that there are different dream types. Divine, prophetic dreams are the first type (4.87 [p. 218, 14–15 Joly and Byl; vol. 6, p. 640 Littré]). He distances himself from these, as there are other professionals who are able to interpret them. A clever move: by acknowledging dream interpretation as a true *technê* (profession), our author paves the way to the creation of a specialization within this *technê*, which is to be occupied only by those who also possess the skills of his own *technê*—that of medicine.[14] According to him, only medical professionals should interpret dreams in which:

> ὅσα δὲ ἡ ψυχὴ τοῦ σώματος παθήματα προσημαίνει, πλησμονῆς ἢ κενώσιος ὑπερβολὴν τῶν συμφύτων, ἢ μεταβολὴν τῶν ἀηθέων. (*Regimen* 4.87 [p. 218, 16–17 Joly and Byl; vol. 6, p. 642 Littré])
>
> the soul foretells affections of the body, surfeit, or depletion of things that are natural, or change into unaccustomed things.

Thus, while nonmedical dream interpreters may have the ability to see that something is wrong—and, if we may believe the author, even this is not always the case—they do not possess the (medical) skill to do anything useful with this information. The only help they can provide their clients will consist of a general warning or at best the advice to pray to the gods (*Regimen* 4.87 [p. 218, 16–17 Joly and Byl; vol. 6, p. 642 Littré]). However, the expert insights of a professional physician will truly aid the dreamer and send him on his way back to health. To help those who wish to approach dreams from a medical perspective, the author of *Regimen* provides a guide to the interpretation of medical dreams which comprises the entire fourth book.[15]

---

[13] Cf. Cambiano, "Une interpretation," p. 93.

[14] On the acceptation of dream interpretation as a *technê*, cf. G.E.R. Lloyd, *Magic, Reason and Experience* (Cambridge, 1979), p. 227; on the creation of a division of labor, cf. van der Eijk, "Divination, Prognosis and Prophylaxis," pp. 197–8.

[15] It has been argued that the author of *Regimen* took old, existing dream imagery from the Greek nonmedical oneirocritic tradition and fitted it with a new, rational background to match his medical purposes. Cf. Fredrich, *Hippokratische Untersuchungen*, pp. 206–17; Dodds, *The Greeks and the Irrational*, p. 119; Joly, *Recherches*, pp. 168–78; Oberhelman, "The Diagnostic Dream," p. 54; Godderis, *Een Arts*, p. 591; Holowchak,

The Hippocratic Regimen*: How to Interpret Dreams*

In Chapter 88 of Book 4, the author introduces one of the most basic principles in the interpretation of medical dreams—similarity of dream images to normality is good, and dissimilarity to it is bad:[16]

> ὅσα τῶν ἐνυπνίων τὰς ἡμερινὰς πρήξιας τοῦ ἀνθρώπου ἢ διανοίας ἐς τὴν εὐφρόνην ἀποδίδωσι κατὰ τρόπον γινομένας, ὥσπερ τῆς ἡμέρης ἐπρήχθη ἢ ἐβουλεύθη ἐν δικαίῳ πρήγματι, ταῦτα τῷ ἀνθρώπῳ ἀγαθά· ὑγείην γὰρ σημαίνει, διότι ἡ ψυχὴ παραμένει ἐν τοῖσιν ἡμερινοῖσι βουλεύμασιν, οὔτε πλησμονῇ κρατηθεῖσα οὔτε κενώσει οὔτε ἄλλῳ οὐδενὶ ἔξωθεν προσπεσόντι. Ὅταν δὲ πρὸς τὰς ἡμερινὰς πρήξιας ὑπεναντίωται τὰ ἐνύπνια καὶ ἐγγίνηται περὶ αὐτῶν ἡ μάχη ἢ νίκη, τοῦτο σημαίνει ταραχὴν ἐν τῷ σώματι· καὶ ἢν μὲν ἰσχυρὴ ᾖ, ἰσχυρὸν τὸ κακὸν, ἢν δὲ φαύλῃ, ἀσθενέστερον . . . τὸ δὲ σῶμα τοῦ ἀνθρώπου θεραπεύεσθαι ξυμβουλεύω· πλησμονῆς γάρ τινος ἐγγενομένης ἀπόκρισις ἐγένετό τις, ἥτις ἐτάραξε τὴν ψυχήν. (*Regimen* 4.88 [p. 220, 1–7, 9–10 Joly and Byl; vol. 6, p. 642 Littré])

> Those of the dreams that at night repeat someone's daytime actions or thoughts in the way they occurred, just as they were done or planned with regard to an appropriate action during the day, these are good for a man. For they signify health, because the soul persists in the ventures of the day, and is overpowered neither by surfeit nor depletion nor by any other external occurrence. But when dreams are contrary to the acts of the day, and there occurs about them a battle or a triumph, this signifies trouble in the body; if it [sc. the battle] is violent, [it signifies] violent trouble, if moderate, feebler trouble ... I advise treatment of the body. For the occurrence of some surfeit has resulted in a secretion that has disturbed the soul.

In other words, the soul normally relives the past day, unless it is disturbed by something unusual within the body—which, as we have seen, is the only possible source of any impressions available to the soul in sleep.[17] The advised treatment in

---

"Interpreting Dreams," pp. 395, 398. Potential parallels with divinatory material from other cultures have also been put forward: W. Capelle, "Ältesten Spuren der Astrologie bei den Griechen," *Hermes*, 60 (1925): pp. 381–7; Palm, "Studien," pp. 83–93; van der Eijk, "Divination, Prognosis and Prophylaxis," pp. 206–15. I believe a combination of these two approaches is very likely.

[16] Holowchak ("Interpreting Dreams," pp. 394–5) points out that Artemidorus adheres to a similar principle in his *Oneirocritica*. The principle is much older, though, dating back to pharaonic Egyptian, Assyrian, and Babylonian dream texts; see Oberhelman's chapter in this volume.

[17] There is great similarity to Aristotle's ideas on dreams here, as Cambiano ("Une interpretation," p. 94) has already noted.

this case is to purge the body and adjust the balance between exercise and food, so that the effects of surfeit, indicated by the dream, are overcome. Depending on the severity of the disturbance—the extent of which can be derived from specific aspects of the dream imagery—an emetic is suggested, accompanied by a light diet and relatively arduous exercises.[18]

The principle of similarity-good/dissimilarity-bad applies to most of the dream imagery described in the treatise, most notably to Chapters 89 and 90, both of which are to be interpreted following an analogy between a *microkosmos* (the body) and the *macrokosmos* (the world and the universe) which is based on a generational theory expounded in Chapters 9 and 10 of Book 1.[19] The author also recommends treatments that are to follow each dream type and often provides a theoretical background to such treatment based, first of all, on his *microkosmos/macrokosmos* understanding of the body. In addition to this micro/macro approach, the application of a number of other medical theories that are encountered elsewhere in the Hippocratic Corpus is in evidence in Chapter 89. Foremost is the acceptance of the existence of various bodily humors, including a belief in their potentially injurious influence on a person's health when present in the body in excess.[20] In addition, we discern the theory of fluxes,[21] the author's

[18] *Regimen* 4.88 (vol. 6, p. 644 Littré). There is a clear parallel in this chapter with *Regimen* 3.71 (p. 204, 1–6 Joly and Byl; vol. 6, p. 610 Littré): ὅταν δὲ μὴ δέχηται ἔτι τὸ σῶμα τὴν πλησμονὴν, ἀπόκρισιν ἤδη ἀφίησιν ἔσω ὑπὸ βίης τῆς περιόδου, ἥτις ὑπεναντιουμένῃ τῇ τροφῇ τῇ ἀπὸ τῶν σίτων ταράσσει τὴν ψυχήν. οὐκ ἔτι δὴ κατὰ τοῦτον τὸν χρόνον ἡδεῖς οἱ ὕπνοι, ἀλλ' ἀνάγκη ταράσσεσθαι τὸν ἄνθρωπον, καὶ δοκεῖν μάχεσθαι (But when the body can no longer contain the surfeit, it incites a secretion inward due to the force of the revolution [περιόδου], which, opposing the nourishment from food, disturbs the soul. At that moment, sleep is no longer agreeable, but the patient is inevitably disturbed, and thinks he is battling).

[19] In Chapters 9 and 10 of Book 1, the author explains the parallels between the generation of the body and the structure of the *kosmos*. For this link between Books 1 and 4, see also Cambiano, "Une interpretation," p. 96; van der Eijk, "Divination, Prognosis and Prophylaxis," p. 200; Hoessly, *Katharsis*, pp. 301–2; Oberhelman, "The Diagnostic Dream," p. 59 and "Dreams in Graeco-Roman Medicine," p. 132. For a more elaborate discussion of the analogy between *microkosmos* (the body) and *macrokosmos* (the world and the universe) in *Regimen*, see Joly, *Recherches*, pp. 37–45; and Jouanna, "L'interprétation des rêves."

[20] The author speaks of the "disruption of the outer circuit by a moist and phlegmatic secretion" and prescribes purgation by means of specific types and quantities of food, emetics, and exercise.

[21] Mentioned are "fluxes of the head." V. Nutton (*Ancient Medicine* [London and New York, 2004], p. 78) explains fluxes as follows. Fluids or humors, when visible, were seen as indicators of illness: "Like a spring, they could be depicted as flowing down from the top of the body, the brain, through its other parts, bringing down with them as they did so material that would reveal an inner state otherwise invisible to the eye." For a succinct explanation

strong belief in the adverse effects of surfeit and depletion, purity/impurity,[22] and even the potentially healthy or detrimental influence of the air surrounding us.[23] In Chapter 90 especially, we encounter the basic principle of "opposites cure opposites." The author also postulates a remarkably modern notion, namely a concern for someone's state of mind or, rather, soul (ψυχή); a disturbance of the soul can originate in sorrow. Apparently, it is possible for the soul to become ill and require healing. The preferred treatment in such cases consists in turning the mind to comical or pleasurable things for two or three days.

The dream images described in Chapters 91–3 are decidedly more symbolical in character, but here too, the normal-good/abnormal-bad principle applies. Chapter 91 deals with clothing, while Chapter 92 deals with the dead; when dreams of the dead indicate illness, it is because something harmful has entered the body, and the proper treatment involves different ways of purging. Chapter 93 comprises a range of wholly different images, some of which are a step beyond the relatively clear-cut and direct metaphors of the previous chapters, while others are of a novel character entirely. While the other chapters seem to be arranged around a central theme, Chapter 93 elicits the impression of being a collection of the interpretational indications that were left over and did not fit in anywhere else.[24] The measures prescribed in this last chapter are difficult to understand, mainly because the text lacks an explanation of what the author assumes is happening in the patient's body (a practice usually in evidence in the previous chapters). Nonetheless, it is clear that the author believes there to be a correlation between the *way* in which something is represented and the meaning of the dream for its dreamer.

---

of the theory of fluxes, see E.M. Craik, "Thucydides on the Plague: Physiology of Flux and Fixation," *Classical Quarterly*, 51(1) (2001): pp. 102–8, at pp. 104–8.

22 Images of pure things indicate health of the body; impure things are seen as foreign bodies that cause disruption and thus illness. Hoessly (*Katharsis*, pp. 298–309) argues that the tradition of *katharsis* takes up an important position in *Regimen*.

23 The author refers to "well-proportioned and pure air" and "disease that is due to inhaled breath." This of course immediately brings to mind the Hippocratic treatise *Breaths*.

24 This of course begs the question "Left over from what?" Was there a limited set of dream images the author had to discuss? Theories have been proposed as to the origin of the medical dream imagery discussed in *Regimen* 4 (see note 15 above) and these could also account for the *choice* of dream images: if it is true that the author used the limited number of images within an existing corpus that point towards physical danger or trouble, and if, in addition, it is true that there is no evidence of an empirical study (as contended in Holowchak, "Interpreting Dreams," pp. 395, 398), what reason then would there be to discuss imagery outside of that limited set? Others who have noticed the eclectic nature of Chapter 93 are van Lieshout, *Greeks on Dreams*, p. 189; and Oberhelman, "Dreams in Graeco-Roman Medicine," p. 132.

All things considered, there is no doubt that the author of *Regimen* was convinced that dream interpretation was a great, if not the best, aid in creating a healthy, tailored-to-fit regimen and thus in enabling one to lead a life free of disease (*Regimen* 4.93 [p. 230, 11 Joly and Byl; vol. 6, p. 662 Littré]). It is in a dream that the soul speaks to the dreamer, as it were, and forewarns him of any impending bodily problems or informs him of needs that have arisen.

Hippocratic Authors in Agreement

If this *prodiagnôsis* was a new medical trick, what did the other Hippocratics think of it? In the Corpus, there are two passages that display resemblances to some of the imagery described in *Regimen* 4.92 and 4.93. One is the case of anxiety (φροντίς) described in *Diseases* 2. The symptoms seem to manifest themselves both physically and psychologically:

> δοκεῖ ἐν τοῖσι σπλάγχνοισιν εἶναι οἷον ἄκανθα καὶ κεντεῖν, καὶ ἄση αὐτὸν λάζυται, καὶ τὸ φῶς φεύγει καὶ τοὺς ἀνθρώπους, καὶ τὸ σκότος φιλεῖ, καὶ φόβος λάζεται, καὶ αἱ φρένες οἰδέουσιν ἐκτὸς, καὶ ἀλγεῖ ψαυόμενος, καὶ φοβεῖται, καὶ δείματα ὁρᾷ καὶ ὀνείρατα φοβερὰ καὶ τοὺς τεθνηκότας ἐνίοτε. (*Diseases* 2.72 [p. 211, 15–20 Jouanna; vol. 7, pp. 108–10 Littré])
>
> In the viscera there seems to be a thorn pricking, and nausea attacks him, and he flees the light and people, and he loves the dark, and he is attacked by fear, and the diaphragm is distended, and he suffers when touched, and he is scared, and he sees frightening things and scary dreams and sometimes the dead.

Although most of the symptoms described do not occur in a state of sleep, the correspondences with *Regimen* 4.92 and 4.93 are striking, as will become clear below. The second passage in question is Chapter 48 from *Internal Affections*, which offers a description of a "thick disease" (παχύ), the cause of which is an accumulation of bile in the liver and in the head.[25] As a result of this, the liver swells up and starts to exert pressure on the diaphragm (ἀναπτύσσεται πρὸς τὰς φρένας). The patient also experiences severe pain in the head, especially in the area of the temples; his perception is impaired, there is fever and shivering, and carphology (*Internal Affections* 48 [p. 230, 18–p. 232, 14 Potter; vol. 7, p. 284 Littré]).[26] The point in the disease when things start to become interesting from

[25] Interestingly, in *Critical Days*, a compilatory treatise, this disease description appears practically verbatim, but typifies acute diseases: τὰ δὲ ὀξέα τῶν νοσημάτων (*Critical Days* 3 [vol. 9, pp. 300–302 Littré]).

[26] Carphology is a sort of "plucking" at things that are not there.

an interpretive point of view is when the build-up of bile continues and the liver expands even further against the diaphragm. Now the patient begins to display symptoms of a more psychological nature:

> καὶ ὅταν τὸ ἧπαρ μᾶλλον ἀναπτυγῇ πρὸς τὰς φρένας, παραφρονέει· καὶ προφαίνεσθαί οἱ δοκέει πρὸ τῶν ὀφθαλμῶν ἑρπετὰ καὶ ἄλλα παντοδαπὰ καὶ θηρία καὶ ὁπλῖται μαχόμενοι, καὶ αὐτὸς ἐν αὐτοῖσι δοκέει μάχεσθαι· τοιαῦτα λέγει ὡς ὁρῶν καὶ ἐπέρχεται, καὶ ἀπειλεῖ, ἢν μή τις αὐτὸν ἐᾷ ἔξω ἐξιέναι· ... καὶ ὅταν καθεύδῃ, ἀναΐσσει ἐκ τοῦ ὕπνου ὅταν ἐνύπνια ἴδῃ φοβερά. τῷδε δὲ γιγνώσκομεν, ὅτι ἀπὸ ἐνυπνίων ἀΐσσει καὶ φοβεῖται· ὅταν ἔννοος γένηται, ἀφηγεῖται τὰ ἐνύπνια τοιαῦτα ὁρᾶν ὁποῖα καὶ τῷ σώματι ἐποίει καὶ τῇ γλώσσῃ ἔλεγε. (*Internal Affections* 48 [p. 232, 14–20, p. 232, 22–p. 234, 3 Potter; vol. 7, pp. 284–6 Littré])

> And when the liver expands more against the diaphragm, he becomes deranged; and in front of his eyes reptiles seem to appear and beasts of every other kind and fighting hoplites, and he seems to be fighting among them himself; he talks as if he is seeing such things and he attacks and withdraws, if someone does not allow him to go outside; ... and when he sleeps, he starts up out of his sleep when he sees scary dreams. We know that he starts up and is afraid due to his dreams thanks to the following: when he is in his right mind again, he relates that he has seen such dreams as correspond to what he did with his body and said with his tongue.

Most intriguing is the verification included in the last sentence of this passage: proof of a direct link between the patient's actions, which are visible to observers, and the things he sees in his dreams, which are of course unobservable to anyone but the patient.[27] Even though most of the images described in the two passages

[27] The only other concrete example of a direct response of the dreamer's body to what he sees in his dreams is the passage from *Generation*, discussed below. A potential additional reference to the concept is found in *Humors* 4, where the author recommends paying attention to a patient's dreams and what he does in sleep: ἐνύπνια οἷα ἂν ὁρῇ, καὶ ἐν τοῖσιν ὕπνοισιν οἷα ἂν πονῇ (*Humors* 4 [p. 68, 19–20 Jones; vol. 5, pp. 480–82 Littré]). Incidentally, it is interesting to note that Potter, in his Loeb edition, has *Diseases* 2.72 describing the symptoms of phrenitis, which is understandable, considering the evidence elsewhere in the Corpus. Cf. *Internal Affections* 10 (vol. 6, p. 218 Littré); *Diseases* 1.30, 34 (vol. 6, p. 200 Littré) and 3.9 (vol. 7, p. 128 Littré). In turn, the similarity of *Internal Affections* 48 to the two other passages is doubly interesting for the following reason: on the one hand, it is very similar to *Diseases* 2.72, which Potter thought to be dealing with phrenitis, while on the other hand, it has a fascinating potential to be linked to *Prorrhetics* 1.5, because it tells us that dreams of those who suffer from phrenitis are vivid (ἐναργής), as will also be discussed below. Phrenitis has the potential to function as the "missing link" here. Elaborate discussion of this topic, however, is beyond the scope of this footnote. For a broader discussion of phrenitis, see G.C. McDonald, "Concepts and Treatments of Phrenitis in Ancient Medicine" (Ph.D. dissertation, Newcastle University, 2009).

Table 2.1 Resemblance of Imagery in *Diseases*, *Internal Affections*, and *Regimen*

Diseases 2.72	*Internal Affections* 48	*Regimen* 4.92–3
distended diaphragm (αἱ φρένες)	pressure on diaphragm (ἀναπτύσσεται πρὸς τὰς φρένας)	
scary dreams (ὀνείρατα φοβερά)	scary dreams (ἐνύπνια φοβερά)	scary dreams (ἐν τοῖσιν ὕπνοισι φοβεῖ)
seeing the dead (τοὺς τεθνηκότας)		seeing the dead (τοὺς ἀποθανόντας)
seeing frightening things (δείματα)	seeing reptiles and other beasts (ἑρπετὰ καὶ ἄλλα πανταδαπὰ θηρία)	strangely shaped, frightening bodies (ἀλλόμορφα σώματα) and strangely shaped monsters (τέρατα ἀλλόμορφα)
fear (φοβεῖται)	fright and fear (ἀΐσσει καὶ φοβεῖται)	fear (φοβεῖ τὸν ἄνθρωπον)
	collection of bile (χολή) in liver and head	bilious flux (χολέραν)
if untreated, deadly	thick disease (that may end in death)/acute diseases (= *Critical Days* 3)	dangerous disease (νοῦσον κινδυνώδεα)
purgative treatment (καθαίρειν)	purgative treatment (hellebore, κλύζειν)	purgative treatment (ἀποκαθαίρεσθαι [92] and ἔμετον ποιήσασθαι [93])
	imagining to be fighting (αὐτὸς δοκέει μάχεσθαι)	to be fighting (μάχεται)
	seeing fighting hoplites (ὁπλῖται μαχόμενοι)	enemy hoplites (ὁπλῖται πολέμιοι)
	derangement (παραφονέει)	madness (μανίην)
pricking (κεντεῖν) sensation in intestines		being pricked (κεντεῖται) by someone

above do not occur in a state of sleep, Table 2.1 illustrates just how many likenesses they display with imagery of *Regimen* 4.92–3.

Although a number of similarities between the three passages is not sufficient grounds for assuming that the authors' views and underlying theories were of a kind, there are other indications that further comparison might prove fruitful.[28] At the very least, they suggest that certain ideas had penetrated wider circles than others; in all cases, for instance, the recommended treatment involves purgation.[29] It makes one wonder what else the three authors may have agreed upon.[30]

From a theoretical point of view, the passage on dreams that displays ideas closest to those formulated in *Regimen* is part of the eighth book of *Epidemics* 6. It is part of a text from a writing tablet that contains things to which a physician should pay attention (σκεπτέα) when treating his patients:

> ἡλίου θάλπος, ψῦχος, τέγξις, ξυρότης· μεταβολὴ διὰ οἷα, ἐξ οἵων, ἐς οἷα [ἔχει]. πόνοι, ἀργίαι, ὕπνοι, ἀγρυπνίαι. τὰ ἐν ὕπνῳ· ἐνύπνια, κοῖται, καὶ ἐν οἷσι, καὶ ὑφ' οἵων. καὶ τῆς γνώμης ξύννοια, αὐτὴ καθ' ἑωυτὴν, χωρὶς τῶν ὀργάνων καὶ τῶν πρηγμάτων, ἄχθεται, καὶ ἥδεται, καὶ φοβεῖται, καὶ θαρσεῖ, καὶ ἐλπίζει, καὶ † ἀδοξέει † οἷον ἡ Ἱπποθόου οἰκουρὸς † τῆς γνώμης αὐτῆς καθ' ἑωυτὴν ἐπίστημος ἐοῦσα † τῶν ἐν τῇ νούσῳ ἐπιγενομένων.[31]

> Heat of the sun, cold, moistness, dryness. Change, due to what, from what to what. Exertion, rest, sleep, insomnia. Things in sleep: dreams, circumstances in which and because of which one goes to bed, and the meditation of the intellect on its own: separate from the sense organs and physical activity it worries, is

---

[28] Joly (*Recherches*, pp. 193–201) has already pointed out that *Diseases* 2, *Internal Affections*, and *Regimen* (mainly Book 3) display remarkable similarities. In addition, J. Jouanna (*Hippocrates* [Baltimore, 1999], p. 395) points out that *Internal Affections* "contains wording similar to that of *Diseases* II." The likeness of *Diseases* 2.72 and *Internal Affections* 48 to Chapters 92 and 93 of *Regimen* has also been noted before: see the text editions by Littré, Joly and Byl, and Jouanna, and by Palm, "Studien," p. 73; however, as far as I know, the three passages have never been subjected to elaborate comparison.

[29] Cf. Joly, *Recherches*, pp. 196, 200; Hoessly, *Katharsis*, pp. 307–9.

[30] If the three passages are indeed complementary, it would, for instance, be easy to fill in the cells of the table that now remain empty. Cf. M.A.A. Hulskamp, "Medical Dreams in the Hippocratic Corpus: How Innovative Was the Author of *De Victu* Really?," in L. Dean Jones (ed.), *What's Hippocratic about the Hippocratics? Papers Read at the XIIIth Hippocrates Colloquium, University of Texas at Austin, August 11th–13th 2008* (Leiden, forthcoming).

[31] *Epidemics* 6.8.9–10 (p. 174, 1–8 Manetti and Roselli; vol. 5, pp. 346–8 Littré). *Epidemics* 6.8.9–10 has been the subject of both ancient and modern scholarly debate, since the shorthand style of the text has always made it difficult to see what these two paragraphs are really about. Based on textual aspects, but most of all on some striking similarities with *Regimen*, I have joined them together in order to enhance our understanding of them. For a more thorough explanation of my reasons for suggesting this, see Hulskamp, "Medical Dreams." Oliver Overwien, in his (forthcoming) *Corpus Medicorum Graecorum* text edition of the Hippocratic *Humors*, sees links with *Humors* 5 and 9.

> happy, does and does not fear, hopes and despairs, like Hippothoos's servant,[32] who, while her intellect was on its own, was aware of the things that happened during her illness.

This passage explains how the things the intellect (γνώμη) experiences in sleep, that is to say dreams, may be pertinent to medical diagnosis. The first σκεπτέα the author mentions are the four primary qualities: hot, cold, wet, and dry. The fact that he specifies the type of heat as that originating from the sun suggests that the other three qualities mentioned are also external influences on the human body.[33] Second, some sort of change is mentioned, followed by two pairs of opposite events: exertion and rest, sleep and insomnia. The two pairs of opposites and the external four qualities appear to be connected through the process of change (μεταβολὴ διὰ οἷα, ἐξ οἵων, ἐς οἷα), a notion that is supported visually by its position between the two groups of words. If we consider that the concept of illness as a result of imbalance of the body's components is quite common in the Corpus[34] and that sleep is facilitated by a moistening of the body and brings with it a drop in body temperature,[35] it is no great leap to assume that the change (μεταβολή) mentioned in the text pertains to the sleeping process—especially since the main topics of the paragraph appear to be sleep and "things in sleep."[36] Third, the pairs exertion (πόνοι) and rest (ἀργίαι), and sleep (ὕπνοι) and insomnia (ἀργυπνίαι), are mentioned: more things that deserve a physician's attention during illness, as they too can influence the balance of the bodily components. Finally, it is explained why one must heed the "things in sleep": at such a time, the intellect can see things pertaining to its owner's illness when it is not distracted

32 Unfortunately, no additional information is available concerning this servant and her condition, or concerning her master.

33 Galen sees it differently: he takes sun and θάλπος to be separate from each other, which leaves him free to interpret the subsequent four qualities as properties of the body and not as external influences. However, Galen seems the only one to read ἥλιος instead of ἡλίου: *Commentary on Hippocrates' "Epidemics"* 6.8 (p. 455 Pfaff); D. Manetti and A. Roselli, *Ippocrate: Epidemie Libro Sesto* (Florence, 1982), p. 174.

34 Cf. Jouanna, *Hippocrates*, pp. 326, 328; see also Nutton, *Ancient Medicine*, pp. 79–81.

35 For a discussion of Hippocratic ideas on sleep and waking, see M.A.A. Hulskamp, "Sleep and Dreams in Ancient Medical Diagnosis and Prognosis" (Ph.D. dissertation, Newcastle University, 2008), pp. 72–93.

36 Galen sees the two pairs of opposites as influenc*ing*, not influenc*ed*: *Commentary on Hippocrates' "Epidemics"* 6.8 (pp. 456–7 Pfaff). It is a possibility; maybe one interpretation does not have to exclude the other, in which case the connection could work both ways. This is defensible, seeing as the processes of sleep and waking can fulfill the role of both result of *and* influence on the qualities in the body.

by waking activities. The entire passage is strongly reminiscent of the first paragraph of *Regimen* 4, where the role of the soul in sleep is explained:

> ὅταν δὲ τὸ σῶμα ἡσυχάσῃ, ἡ ψυχὴ κινεομένη καὶ ἐγρηγορεόουσα διοικεῖ τὸν ἑωυτῆς οἶκον καὶ τὰς τοῦ σώματος πρήξιας ἁπάσας αὐτὴ διαπρήσσεται. τὸ μὲν γὰρ σῶμα καθεῦδον οὐκ αἰσθάνεται, ἡ δ' ἐγρηγορέουσα γινώσκει πάντα, καὶ ὁρῇ τε τὰ ὁρητὰ καὶ ἀκούει τὰ ἀκουστὰ, βαδίζει, ψαύει, λυπεῖται, ἐνθυμεῖται, ἐν ὀλίγῳ ἐοῦσα. (*Regimen* 4.86 [p. 218, 7–11 Joly and Byl; vol. 6, p. 640 Littré])
>
> But when the body is at rest, the soul, being set in motion and awake, manages her own household, and performs all the activities of the body herself. For the sleeping body does not perceive, but she [sc. the soul], since she is awake, knows all, and sees what is visible, hears what is audible, walks, touches, feels pain, ponders, in her limited dwelling space.

While there is a difference in terminology—*Regimen* speaks of the soul (ψυχή), while *Epidemics* refers to the intellect (γνώμη)[37]—it is beyond doubt that in both cases we are dealing with the concept of independent observation of the body and its condition in sleep by some other, conscious part of the same individual.[38]

---

[37] Galen seems to identify the γνώμη with the soul—Pfaff's translation of Galen's commentary reads "Seele"—which brings Chapters 9 and 10 from *Epidemics* 6 and Chapter 86 from *Regimen* 4 even closer. Additionally, Galen mentions that some interpreters have taken the dreams mentioned in the Hippocratic text to be "die Traumbilder, die der Kranke während des Schlafes sich vorstellt" (Pfaff's translation) ("dream-pictures that the patient imagines during sleep"). He further paraphrases these interpreters' views on what was to be done with such dreams as follows: "Man müsse untersuchen, ob sie beunruhigend und beängstigend, ob sie häßlich, widernatürlich oder ob sie gewöhnliche und übliche Visionen sind" ("One must investigate whether the disturbing and alarming visions, or the ugly visions, are unnatural, or whether they are ordinary and customary"). All of these properties we see described in *Regimen* 4, with recommended treatment to boot. Cf. *Commentary on Hippocrates' "Epidemics"* 6.8 (pp. 458–60 Pfaff).

[38] In addition, there is one earlier indication that the author was thinking of mental processes in sleep. *Epidemics* 6.8.5 is closely related to the issues addressed in *Epidemics* 6.8.9–10: Τὰ ἐν τοῖσιν ὕπνοισι παροξυνόμενα, καὶ ὅσοισιν ἄκρεα περιψύχεται καὶ ἡ γνώμη ταράσσεται, καὶ τἄλλα ὅσα περὶ ὕπνον τοιαῦτα, καὶ οἷσι τἀναντία (Affections with paroxysms in sleep, and cases in which extremities become cold and the mind disordered, and all other things concerning sleep, and cases in which the opposite happens: *Epidemics* 6.8.5 [p. 164, 5–7 Manetti and Roselli; vol. 5, p. 344 Littré]). The author mentions a number of symptoms that occur in sleep, among them the cooling of the extremities and the confusion of the γνώμη. From here the step to the actions of the γνώμη in sections 9 and 10 is relatively

Physiology and Dreams

Chapters 14 and 15 of *On the Sacred Disease* are illuminating with regard to its author's views on the physiological processes surrounding a specific type of dream: nightmares. In Chapter 14 (vol. 6, p. 386 Littré), the author first makes it very clear that the brain is the origin of joy and pain, but also the organ responsible for perception, ratiocination, and the process of forming an opinion. If, however, the brain becomes "unwell"—that is, if the brain becomes too hot, cold, moist, or dry, or if it enters a condition in any way different from its normal condition—this can result in madness, delirium, disorientation, and suchlike, but also in fears and anxieties (δείματα καὶ φόβοι) which can manifest themselves both by day and by night:

> Τῷ δὲ αὐτῷ τούτῳ καὶ μαινόμεθα καὶ παραφρονέομεν, καὶ δείματα καὶ φόβοι παρίστανται ἡμῖν τὰ μὲν νύκτωρ, τὰ δὲ καὶ μεθ' ἡμέρην, καὶ ἀγρυπνίαι καὶ πλάνοι ἄκαιροι, καὶ φροντίδες οὐχ ἱκνεύμεναι, καὶ ἀγνωσίαι τῶν καθεστεώτων καὶ ἀηθίαι. Καὶ ταῦτα πάσχομεν ἀπὸ τοῦ ἐγκεφάλου πάντα, ὅταν οὗτος μὴ ὑγιαίνῃ, ἀλλ' ἢ θερμότερος τῆς φύσιος γένηται ἢ ψυχρότερος ἢ ξηρότερος, ἤ τι ἄλλο πεπόνθῃ πάθος παρὰ τὴν φύσιν ὃ μὴ ἐώθει. (*Sacred Disease* 14 [p. 26, 4–14 Jouanna; vol. 6, pp. 386–8 Littré])[39]

> And because of this same thing [sc. the brain] we are mad and delirious, and fears and anxieties come to us—some at night, some in the daytime—and sleeplessness, ill-timed fits of uncertainty, unjustified worries, failure to recognize real things, and a sense of not belonging. And we suffer all these things because of the brain, when it is not healthy, but has become warmer than normal, or colder, or moister, or dryer, or suffers from some other unnatural affliction to which it is not accustomed.

The cause of such changes in the brain lies with the humors. The author explains that two humors in particular have an effect that can be discerned at night: bile and blood. Both heat up the brain when they enter the head in too great a quantity. When bile rises up to the head through the veins in large

---

small. Manetti and Roselli (*Ippocrate*, p. 165) notice the connection as well. In addition, there is the potential link to *Epidemics* 6.43, where the author refers to a patient's ability to know things "in other ways," which may well include (medical) dreams.

[39] I adopt the use of ἀγρυπνίαι in line 3 from Grensemann's 1968 text edition. For an explanation of the reasons for my adaptation, see Hulskamp, "Sleep and Dreams," pp. 182–3.

quantities,[40] the effects are clearly noticeable: it causes screaming and shouting at night. The observer can deduce that bile is the culprit here, because it is this humor that causes frightening dreams.[41] The effect of too much blood in the brain is somewhat more subtle: the patient is in distress, there is a reddening of the face, and the eyes are bloodshot—the latter of which would, for obvious reasons, be easy to miss during sleep. In this case, however, the fearful dream is what draws blood to the brain in the first place; it is not an effect of the heating of the brain, as is the case with bile.[42]

For the author of *On the Sacred Disease*, the medical relevance of dreams seems minimal—at least as far as we can tell from this treatise—and his own interest in the content of dreams appears to be limited to their general nature. He finds dreams relevant only when they disturb the patient's sleep in the form of nightmares and make him cry out or become red in the face, for in such cases there are a number of things he can infer with regard to the condition of the brain and the types of humors and qualities at work there. We could imagine that, based on these findings, the physician can draw conclusions about the rest of the body as well, seeing as there must be something wrong with humor management if excess bile and phlegm exist in the first place; however, such must remain a matter of conjecture.[43] Besides, we must remember that *On the Sacred Disease* was written from an explanatory, not a diagnostic, point of view. This could explain the lack of any apparent interest in the potential significance of dreams with regard to medical diagnosis.

Another type of dream that receives a relatively elaborate physiological explanation is the wet dream. The author of *Generation* describes how semen is

40 J. Jouanna (*Hippocrate: La Maladie Sacrée* [Paris, 2003], p. 115) points out that bile has its seat in the liver; this is the reason why bile has to rise up to the head.

41 The author has explained that bile causes fear and a rowdy kind of madness, because it heats up the brain: *Sacred Disease* 15 (p. 27, 8–p. 28, 4 Jouanna; vol. 6, p. 388 Littré); cf. Jouanna, *Hippocrate: La Maladie Sacrée*, p. 116.

42 *Sacred Disease* 15 (p. 28, 7–p. 29, 3 Jouanna; vol. 6, p. 390 Littré). Grensemann chooses to delete the καὶ before ἐπὴν at *Sacred Disease* 15 (p. 28, 10 Jouanna), thus seeing only one cause for the heating of the brain, namely the influx of blood—a solution of which Jouanna disapproves, and I agree, for there are clearly two different explanations for a rising temperature in the brain. See H. Grensemann, *Die Hippokratische Schrift "Über die Heilige Krankheit"* (Berlin, 1968), p. 100; and Jouanna, *Hippocrate: La Maladie Sacrée*, p. 117. It remains unclear, however, whether the nightmares that draw the blood to the brain are a result of bile in the head—in which case the blood would become a secondary heating factor—or if they are indeed mere happenstance. See also Hulskamp, "Sleep and Dreams," pp. 185–6.

43 In the apocryphal Hippocratic *Letter* 19, the content of *Sacred Disease* 14–15 is paraphrased.

produced in the body and how accordingly wet dreams come to be. When the privy parts are stimulated, all the fluid present in the body becomes hot, liquid, and frothy because of the movement.[44] At this point, the strongest and fattiest part of the fluid separates from the rest and moves to the spinal marrow,[45] from there to the kidneys, then from the kidneys through the testicles to the pudenda. It is not via the urethra that ejaculation occurs, but via another route (*Generation* 1 [p. 44, 14–p. 45, 3 Joly; vol. 7, p. 470 Littré]). The mechanics of the wet dream are of a similar nature:

> καὶ οἱ ἐξονειρώσσοντες διὰ τάδε ἐξονειρώσσουσιν· ἐπὴν τὸ ὑγρὸν ἐν τῷ σώματι διακεχυμένον ᾖ καὶ διάθερμον, εἴτε ὑπὸ ταλαιπωρίης, εἴτε καὶ ὑπὸ ἄλλου τινὸς, ἀφρεῖ· καὶ ἀποκρινομένου ἀπ' αὐτοῦ ὁρᾶν παρίσταταί οἱ ἡ λαγνείη· ἔχει γὰρ τὸ ὑγρὸν τοιοῦτο ὅπερ λαγνεύοντι. (*Generation* 1 [p. 45, 3–8 Joly; vol. 7, pp. 470–72 Littré])

> And those who have wet dreams have them because of the following: when the fluid in the body becomes diffuse and heated through, either because of hard labor or because of something else, it becomes frothy. And ejaculation is accompanied by erotic scenes [sc. in dreams]; for the fluid behaves as it would in coïtus.

In case of a wet dream, then, there is a direct link between the bodily humor and the contents of a person's dreams: it is the state of the fluid in the body—hot and frothy—that leads a person to see erotic dreams and ejaculate in his sleep. However, it remains unclear how these dream images are generated or where they come from. Does the soul perhaps play a role here? The author indicates that he has already dealt with this type of dream elsewhere, but unfortunately the work he is referring to seems to have been lost (*Generation* 1 [p. 45, 8–10

---

[44] *Generation* 1 (p. 44, 10–12 Joly; vol. 7, p. 470 Littré). It is interesting to note that Aristotle's views on the reproductive processes also feature heat and foam: *Generation of Animals* 2.3 ("normal" reproduction), 3.1.11 (spontaneous reproduction).

[45] Two older theories about the origin of sperm are drawn upon here: (1) sperm is derived from all parts of the body (pangenetic theory); and (2) sperm is derived from the brain and the spinal marrow (encephalo-myelogenic theory). Cf. E. Lesky, "Die Samentheorie in der hippokratischen Schriftensammlung," in E. Berghoff (ed.), *Festschrift zum 80. Geburtstag Max Neuburgers: mit 91 internationalen medicohistorischen Beiträgen* (2 vols, Vienna, 1948), vol. 2, pp. 302–7, at pp. 302, 304–5; I.M. Lonie, *The Hippocratic Treatises "On Generation", "On the Nature of the Child", "Diseases IV"* (Berlin and New York, 1981), pp. 101–2; R. Joly, *Hippocrate:De la Génération, De la Nature de l'Enfant, Des Maladies IV, Du Foetus de Huit Mois* (Paris, 1970), p. 44 note 4; J. Jouanna, *Hippocrate: Maladies II* (Paris, 1983), p. 257.

Joly; vol. 7, p. 472 Littré]); we can imagine that it might have contained some answers for us.

Wet dreams also occur in other Hippocratic treatises, where they usually figure as symptoms in disease descriptions and individual case histories.[46] In each case, the patient invariably suffers from some form of heat or fever.[47] It is not unthinkable, then, that the occurrence of wet dreams may immediately have led a Hippocratic physician to conclude that his patient had too much heat in his body.

Dreams as Symptoms

In the Hippocratic Corpus, there are four texts in which dreams are mentioned as a point of diagnostic interest, but without mention of *specific* dream content, although this does not mean that it was considered unimportant or left out of consideration.

In a summation of things that are to be paid heed, *Humors* 4 mentions "the dreams a patient sees" and "what he does in sleep" (ἐνύπνια οἷα ἂν ὁρῇ, καὶ ἐν τοῖσιν ὕπνοισιν οἷα ἂν πονῇ: *Humors* 4 [p. 68, 19–20 Jones; vol. 5, pp. 480–82 Littré]). This harks back to what we have seen in *Internal Affections* 48, where the link between actions in sleep and dream imagery was made explicit. *Humors* does not provide any additional information—which in itself is not surprising as this is a summation—and we are left to assume that the meaning of the two nightly symptoms is either already clear enough not to require further explanation or was made clear elsewhere.[48]

---

[46] E.g., *Diseases* 2.51 (p. 188, 9–18 Jouanna; vol. 7, p. 78 Littré) ; *Internal Affections* 43 (p. 216, 17–19 Potter; vol. 7, p. 274 Littré) and 47 (p. 226, 20; p. 228, 11–12; p. 228, 22–3; p. 230, 1–2 Potter; vol. 7, p. 282 Littré); *Epidemics* 4.57 (p. 150, 1–6 Smith; vol. 5, p. 196 Littré) and 6.8.29 (p. 190, 5–p. 192, 3 Manetti and Roselli; vol. 5, p. 354 Littré); *Regimen* 1.35 (p. 156, 4 Joly and Byl; vol. 6, p. 520 Littré). For a discussion of these passages, see Hulskamp, "Sleep and Dreams," pp. 190–92.

[47] A common assumption made by medical authors is the reciprocal causal relation between heat and disturbance or irritation; an example of this is the friction that occurs when the privy parts are rubbed, as discussed above in *Generation* 1; cf. Lonie, *Hippocratic Treatises*, pp. 100–101, 106. On several occasions, there is also mention of the (spinal) marrow, which is a vestige of older generational theories of semen: Lesky, "Samentheorie," p. 302. There is, however, no diagnostic value in this.

[48] It is interesting to note that in *Tub.* Mb 23, a medieval commentary on the Hippocratic *On Humors*, this little phrase is linked to *Regimen* 4.88 (vol. 6, pp. 642–4 Littré). Thus, if "what a patient dreams and what he does in sleep" is unlike reality, this can indicate an excess or deficiency. The commentary also draws on Plato and Galen and rejects Aristotle. See P. Demont, "Le commentaire du chapitre 4 du traité Hippocratique des *Humeurs* dans

Prorrhetic 1.5 informs us that "in phrenitis[49] dreams are vivid" (ἐνύπνια τὰ ἐν φρενιτικοῖς ἐναργέα, p. 75, 10–11 Polack; vol. 5, p. 512 Littré). There is no additional information contained in the aphorism, and the preceding and subsequent aphorisms are not very helpful either. The only meaning that can be extracted from Chapters 3 and 4 is a hint that dryness may play a role here; as it happens, Galen's explanation of the clarity of dreams also features dryness as an important factor, as will be discussed below (*Commentary on Hippocrates' Prorrhetic 1* 1.5 [vol. 16, p. 525, 11–12 Kühn]). That aside, the aphorism is also reminiscent of *Affections* 48, where dreams are apparently so vivid as to rouse someone from his sleep. Perhaps this effect was to be expected in cases of phrenitis?

Ancient Medicine 10–11 links things that happen in digestion to the sort of dreams that will occur in sleep. A simple change to one's regimen will cause the body discomfort, perhaps even illness. Missing lunch may be the cause of many symptoms, such as weakness, hollow eyes, paler and hotter urine, bitter taste in the mouth, hanging bowels, dizziness, depression, and incapacity to work. When, after this, dinner is taken, it will not be digested well and the food goes down accompanied by colic and noise and burns the stomach. In that case, sleep will be bad, and disturbed and turbulent dreams will occur (ἐνυπνιάζονται τεταραγμένα καὶ θορυβώδεα: *Ancient Medicine* 10 [p. 131, 8–9 Jouanna; vol. 1, p. 594 Littré]). All these symptoms together indicate the beginning of illness for many people (*Ancient Medicine* 10 [p. 129, 14–p. 131, 10 Jouanna; vol. 1, pp. 590–94 Littré]). Dreams, then, are merely part of a greater collection of symptoms. Their occurrence seems to be closely related to the state of the stomach, a connection we will also encounter in Galen's theories.

The last passage in which dreams are mentioned is the famous diagnostic checklist in *Epidemics* 1.10. The author mentions that he has taken into account thoughts, sleep, insomnia, and the type and time of dreams (διανοήμασιν, ὕπνοισιν, οὐχ ὕπνοισιν, ἐνυπνίοισι, οἵοισι καὶ ὅτε, p. 199, 16–18 Kühlewein; vol. 2, pp. 668–70 Littré). Not unexpectedly, there is no further explanation, as it would not suit the summation, but the fact that thought, sleep, and dreams are all mentioned in close proximity to one another evokes the passage from *Epidemics* 6 above. Still, even if there is no direct link between these two texts, the author's interest in the content of dreams does indicate an intention to link dreams to the condition of or processes within the dreamer's body, especially

le *Tub*. Mb 23," in V. Boudon-Millot, A. Guardasole, and C. Magdelaine (eds), *La Science Médicale Antique: Nouveaux Regards* (Paris, 2007), pp. 145–88, at pp. 159–60, 181–2.

[49] Usually, phrenitis is loosely translated as "brain fever," although the exact seat of the disease remains unclear. It derives from φρήν, the Greek word for "mind" as the seat of the mental faculties.

because the author mentions not only the importance of the type of dream, but also the time of its occurrence.

Dreams in the Hippocratic Corpus

A number of authors in the Hippocratic Corpus display a marked awareness of the fact that the occurrence and type of dreams can sometimes supply invaluable information regarding their patients' wellbeing. Of the Hippocratics who demonstrate an interest in dreams, the author of *Regimen* provides the clearest evidence of a specific interest in the contents of patients' dreams. His proficiency was the interpretation of dreams—the association of specific dream images with a predetermined meaning—in the course of giving *prodiagnôseis* or, more specifically, uncovering the makings of illness before it had had a chance to manifest itself. Other physicians seem to have had a less systematic interest in the contents of their patients' dreams and appear only to make enquiries in that direction if and when they saw a need for it. Such a need might be prompted by the observation of a dreamer's behavior in sleep, an approach that clearly focuses on dreams per se.

Among the various different Hippocratic views on dreams and their content, and on the use to which dreams were to be put, we may distinguish two different aspects of dreams: dream *imagery*, which, in a medical context, can be interpreted to reveal information about the condition of the body of the dreamer (notably *Regimen* 4 and *Epidemics* 6.8.9–10), and the *character* of dreams, to which a direct meaning is attached, varying from precise (for example, fear indicates bile, while clear dreams indicate phrenitis) to vague (for example, troubled dreams are a bad sign). Outside of *Regimen* 4, imagery and specific dream content appear to be of secondary importance with regard to the character of dreams, and only of interest because of the *effect* they produce on the dreamer, which functions as a symptom on which conclusions are based. Nightmares and otherwise troubled dreams, as well as overly vivid and clear dreams (which were all considered to be unfavorable), could cause a dreamer to display some form of physical activity in their sleep; sometimes it was possible to verify the link between dreams and this physical activity, as is done, for instance, in *Internal Affections* 48. Another type of outwardly recognizable unfavorable dreams were of course wet dreams, which indicated an overabundance of heat in the body. Conversely, a physician's approach may have focused on a pre-existing familiarity with the circumstances of a specific disease, rather than on the symptom of dreams, and thus provide a reason for closer inspection of a patient's dreams. An example of this is phrenitis: in *Prorrhetic* 1, sufferers of this disease are said to experience vivid dreams (the author, though, still has no interest in imagery), and with that information, it was possible, in all likelihood, either to verify an already present suspicion or to achieve a new diagnosis.

It is now clear that a medical interest in dreams is not to be found solely in *Regimen* and that aspects of that author's theories—such as a belief in the independent role of the soul in sleep, the potentially physiological origin of dreams, and most notably the interest in dreams as symptoms within disease processes—are also represented in other Hippocratic treatises. To be sure, the number of treatises is small, but if we consider that in the period of time covered by the Hippocratic Corpus new theories were postulated, and that such new impulses generated new ways of thinking about the causes and symptoms of diseases,[50] this may explain why a relatively new theory like that of medical dream interpretation had not yet been fully integrated, and why Book 4 of *On Regimen* is the only elaboration of how to use dream interpretation in medical diagnosis. In a broad spectrum of views, the author of *Regimen* most strongly emphasized the role of dreams as significant indicators of the dreamer's physical condition and gave dreams a radically prominent position in his (pro)diagnostic theory. As it turns out, this treatise's status is one of less isolation than has been assumed by some scholars,[51] and at the same time is probably less representative of a general tradition than has been presupposed by others.

Galen

As is well known, dreams were of great importance to Galen, both professionally and personally. He might not have become a physician, for instance, had his father not seen a dream that made him send his son away to study medicine.[52] Or perhaps he would have followed Marcus Aurelius into war, with all the potential consequences that this would bring. Or he might not have found a cure for the abscess he once had under his diaphragm, which came to him in a dream (*On Treatment by Bloodletting* 23 [vol. 11, p. 315 Kühn]). Galen, it seems clear, was a firm believer in the potential value of dreams. What, then, was his professional

[50] Cf. V. Langholf, *Medical Theories in Hippocrates: Early Texts and the "Epidemics"* (Berlin and New York, 1990), pp. 74–6.

[51] Cf. F. Kudlien, "Das Göttliche und die Natur im Hippokratischen Prognostikon," *Hermes*, 105 (1977): pp. 268–74, at p. 274; H.W. Nörenberg, *Das Göttliche und die Natur in der Schrift "Über die heilige Krankheit"* (Bonn, 1968), p. 78; Longrigg, *Greek Medicine*, pp. 230–31; van der Eijk, "Divination, Prognosis and Prophylaxis," p. 188.

[52] Greeks "saw" dreams, whereas we "have" them; cf. Dodds, *The Greeks and the Irrational*, p. 105.

view on the interpretation of dreams for diagnostic purposes? Did he regard them in the same way as did the author of *Regimen*? To what extent did he trust dream interpretation as a diagnostic tool?

Galen on Dream Diagnosis

Relatively little evidence of Galen's opinion on the use of dream interpretation for diagnostic purposes has come down to us. The most frequently quoted source is a small independent treatise on dreams called *On Diagnosis from Dreams* (hereinafter *DD*). It has the reputation of being spurious, but Guidorizzi has proven it at least likely to be a compilation or an excerpt from Galen's original work.[53] In addition, an important part of the treatise appears practically verbatim in Galen's commentary on the Hippocratic *Epidemics* 1, which is attributable to Galen with certainty.[54] Guidorizzi, and later Oberhelman, have argued that the treatise is probably a collection of passages on dreams from Galen's oeuvre, most notably from the lost work *On Regimen in Health* (Περὶ διαίτης ὑγιεινῷ), which Galen himself mentions as the treatise in which he has dealt more thoroughly with dreams.[55]

---

[53] Cf. G. Guidorizzi, "L'opusculo di Galeno 'De Dignotione ex Insomniis,'" *Bollettino del Comitato per la Preparazione dell' Edizione Nazionale dei Classici Greci e Latini*, 21 (1973): pp. 81–105.

[54] Cf. S.M. Oberhelman, "Galen, *On Diagnosis from Dreams*," *Journal of the History of Medicine and Allied Sciences*, 38 (1983): pp. 36–47, at p. 40, note 28 and "Dreams in Graeco-Roman Medicine," p. 139; Guidorizzi, "L'opusculo di Galeno," p. 96. Virtually the same passage also appears in the pseudo-Galenic commentary on the Hippocratic *Humors*, which is a Renaissance forgery; cf. K. Kalbfleisch, "Bericht über das Corpus Medicorum Graecorum," *Sitzungsberichte der Königlich Preußischen Akademie der Wissenschaften zu Berlin*, 34(1) (1916): pp. 137–8, at p. 138; G. Demuth, "Ps.-Galeni De Dignotione ex Insomniis: Ausgabe mit Übersetzung und Kommentar" (Ph.D. dissertation, University of Göttingen, 1972), p. 53; Guidorizzi, "L'opusculo di Galeno," p. 96; Oberhelman, "On Diagnosis," p. 40, note 28. R.E. Siegel (*Galen on Psychology, Psychopathology, and Function and Diseases of the Nervous System* [Basel and New York, 1973], p. 169, note 202) mistakes the origin of the *Epidemics* commentary for that of the *Humors* treatise and asserts that the former is a forgery.

[55] *Commentary on Hippocrates' "Epidemics* 1.3.1 (p. 108, 2–3 Wenkebach; vol. 17a, p. 214 Kühn). Wenkebach suspected *DD* to be a compilation from the passage in the commentary on *Epidemics* I: "Fragmentum quod adhuc in editionibus circumfertur libelli qui inscribitur Περὶ τῆς ἐξ ἐνυπνίων διαγνώσεως (VI 832sqq. Kühn) ex hoc commentario Epidemiarum I.1 compilatum esse videtur." Cf. E. Wenkebach and F. Pfaff (eds), *Galeni In Hippocratis Epidemiarum librum I commentaria III, In Hippocratis Epidemiarum librum II commentaria V*, *Corpus Medicorum Graecorum*, 10, 1 (Leipzig and Berlin, 1934), p. 108. However, Guidorizzi ("L'opusculo di Galeno," p. 98) has convincingly proven this not to

In *DD*, dreams are very clearly presented as an aid to medical diagnosis:

> καὶ ἐνύπνιον δὲ ἡμῖν ἐνδείκνυται διάθεσιν τοῦ σώματος. Πυρκαϊὰν μέν <γάρ> τις ὁρῶν ὄναρ ὑπὸ τῆς ξανθῆς ἐνοχλεῖται χολῆς· εἰ δὲ καπνὸν ἢ ἀχλὺν ἢ βαθὺ σκότος, ὑπὸ τῆς μελαίνης χολῆς· ὄμβρος δὲ ψυχρὰν ὑγρότητα πλεονάζειν ἐνδείκνυται· χιὼν δὲ καὶ κρύσταλλος καὶ χάλαζα, φλέγμα ψυχρόν.[56]

> And a dream shows us the condition of the body. <For> someone seeing a conflagration in a dream is being plagued by yellow bile; if smoke or mist or deep darkness [appear in a dream], [someone is being plagued by] black bile; torrential rain shows an excess of cold moisture; and snow and ice and hail [show an excess of] cold phlegm.

Analogy of the dream images to the qualities of the dominant humor seems to be the key to interpretation: blood is hot and moist, phlegm is cold and moist, yellow bile is dry and hot, and black bile is dry and cold.[57] However, medical dreams—dreams that contain metaphorical representations of dominant humors in the body—are only one type of dream; other dreams have their origin in a person's waking thoughts and actions, while others still may carry some prophetic meaning. To distinguish between medical dreams and dreams that are based on daily experiences is not too difficult: it merely requires filtering out anything that has no connection to reality. However, to distinguish between prophetic dreams and the other two types is so problematic that Galen admits that even those with ample experience in such matters can be deceived. He offers no direct solution to this problem.[58]

---

be the case, as: (1) there are parts in the *DD* text that are not present in the commentary, most notably the theory on dreams and their causation; and (2) Galen himself states that he deals with dreams in another treatise, with which both *DD* and the commentary must be connected. Oberhelman ("Dreams in Graeco-Roman Medicine," pp. 139–41) agrees with Guidorizzi, though he adds his own interpretation: that *DD* is not an extract but a compilation of passages. Either way, this remains a matter of conjecture.

[56] *DD*, p. 103, 1–4 Guidorizzi (vol. 6, p. 832 Kühn). I use the critically edited text provided by Guidorizzi in his 1973 article, to which I have made a few minor changes.

[57] Cf. R.E. Siegel, *Galen's System of Physiology and Medicine: An Analysis of His Doctrines and Observations on Blood Flow, Respiration, Humors and Internal Diseases* (Basel and New York, 1968), p. 218. One might think that the fact that one quality belongs to two different humors could pose a problem, but the difficulty seems to be surmountable: one quality is dominant. See, for example, *Temperaments* 2.2 (vol. 1, p. 584 Kühn).

[58] See his comments at *DD*, p. 103, 13–p. 104, 3; p. 104, 21–2; p. 104, 23–6 Guidorizzi (vol. 6, p. 833 Kühn).

Still, to improve the accuracy of medical dream interpretation, Galen offers some helpful suggestions. It is vital to take into account the dreamer's circumstances (time, physical condition of the dreamer, food intake, course of the disease), since these determine the ultimate meaning of the dream.[59] The mechanics underlying the dream process are also explained. While the soul is responsible for the occurrence of prophetic dreams (unfortunately, it is not explained how exactly this works), it is also responsible for the occurrence of dreams that are linked to the condition and the needs of the body:

> ἔοικε γὰρ ἐν τοῖς ὕπνοις εἰς τὸ βάθος τοῦ σώματος ἡ ψυχὴ εἰσδῦσα καὶ τῶν ἐκτὸς ἀποχωρήσασα αἰσθητῶν τῆς κατὰ τὸ σῶμα διαθέσεως αἰσθάνεσθαι, πάντων τε ὧν ὀρέγεται, τούτων ὡς ἤδη παρόντων λαμβάνειν φαντασίαν. (*DD*, p. 104, 33–6 Guidorizzi; vol. 6, p. 834 Kühn)
>
> For the soul, in sleep having dived into the depth of the body and being severed from outside perception, seems to perceive the situation in the body, and to receive images of all the things it yearns for, as if these things are already present.

This statement harks back to the view of the Hippocratic author of *Regimen*, according to whom the soul acts independently of the body during sleep and perceives the things that happen in the body. But there is a distinct difference between the two authors' respective ways of dealing with dreams:

> ἃ τοίνυν ὁρῶσι οἱ κάμνοντες ἐν τοῖς ἐνυπνίοις καὶ πράττειν δοκοῦσι συνενδείξεται πολλάκις ἡμῖν ἐνδείας τε καὶ πλεονεξίας καὶ ποιότητας χυμῶν. (*DD*, p. 105, 49–50 Guidorizzi; vol. 6, p. 835 Kühn)
>
> The things, now, that sick people see in their dreams and what they seem to be doing together will often indicate to us defects and excesses and qualities of humors.

The key word is κάμνοντες (sick people). It indicates that an interest in dreams from a medical point of view is engendered mainly by a person's poor health. This may seem logical, but we must bear in mind that the author of *Regimen* underscored the importance of studying the dreams of healthy people. His was the art of *prodiagnôsis*: although there may not be any manifestation of

[59] *DD*, p. 103, 5–9 and p. 103, 10–12 Guidorizzi (vol. 6, pp. 832–3 Kühn). See also *Commentary on Hippocrates' "Epidemics"* 6.8 (pp. 458, 28–p. 459, 10 Pfaff), where Galen argues that it is important to monitor, besides dreams, the outward, physical symptoms that are revealed in sleep.

illness, someone could already be on his way to becoming ill, unbeknownst to himself or his physician. The main difference, then, lies in their respective goals. *Regimen*'s goal was clear: dreams are used as a means to "test" (as yet) healthy people for impending trouble, and both "good" and "bad" dreams receive ample attention. In *DD*, on the other hand, we sense a predilection for dreams of those who are already ill. Granted, *DD* does provide two examples of dreams that could come to healthy people: people without any humoral excesses dream that they are flying or running very fast, and people whose bodies do not contain putrid humours or too much fecal matter might think they find themselves in sweet smelling places (*DD*, p. 104, 37–43 Guidorizzi; vol. 6, pp. 834–5 Kühn). Such dreams, however, are mere examples, mentioned to illustrate a point to the contrary; they do not receive any further attention and are clearly not part of the central topic of the text—dreams of sick people.

Let us now consider the passage in Galen's commentary on the Hippocratic *Epidemics* 1.10. It is decidedly shorter and, being a rendering of some of the same information we encounter in the first part of *DD*, much less informative than that treatise.[60] A full translation of the passage in the commentary seems appropriate, as none has yet been published:

> ἀλλὰ καὶ περὶ τῶν ἐνυπνίων προεξήγημαι, τῶν τ᾽ ἄλλων καὶ ὅσα διάθεσίν τινα τοῦ σώματος ἐνδείκνυται, καθάπερ κἀν τῷ Περὶ διαίτης ὑγιεινῷ γέγραπται. πυρκαϊὰς μὲν γάρ τις ὁρῶν ὄναρ ὑπὸ τῆς ξανθῆς <ἐν>οχλεῖται χολῆς, <εἰ[61] δὲ καπνὸν ἢ ἀχλὺν ἢ βαθὺ σκότος, ὑπὸ τῆς μελαίνης χολῆς·> ὄμβρους δὲ ψυχρὰν ὑγρότητα πλεονάζειν ἐνδείκνυται, καθάπερ γε καὶ [εἰ] χιόνα καὶ κρύσταλλον καὶ χάλαζαν, φλέγμα ψυχρόν· ἐν χωρίῳ δ᾽ ὁ δοκῶν εἶναι δυσώδει σηπεδόνα χυμῶν, λόφους δ᾽ ἀλεκτρυόνων ἤ τινα πυρρά, αἷμα πλεονάζειν. ζοφώδη δέ τινα ὁρᾶν ἢ ἐν ζοφώδεσι τόποις ἵστασθαι πνεύματα δηλοῖ <καὶ ἐπὶ τῶν ἄλλων ἀνὰ λόγον.> διὸ καὶ προσέθηκε τῷ ἐνυπνίοισι <τὸ> οἵσισι καὶ ὅτε· τὸ μὲν <οἵ>οισι τὰς διαφορὰς αὐτῶν ἐνδεικνύμενον καὶ μὴ προσθέντος αὐτοῦ πρόδηλον ἦν, τὸ δ᾽ ὅτε τὸν καιρόν, ἐν ᾧ γίνεται τὰ ἐνύπνια, τουτέστιν εἴτε κατὰ τὴν εἰσβολὴν τῶν παροξυσμῶν εἴτε κατὰ τὴν ἀκμὴν εἴτ᾽ ἐν ἄλλῳ τινὶ καιρῷ καὶ εἰ μετὰ τροφὴν καὶ ποίαν γέ τινα τροφὴν εὐθέως ἢ χωρὶς τροφῆς, γίνεται γάρ τις ἔνδειξις ἐκ τούτων. ὁ γοῦν χιονίζεσθαι δοκῶν ἐὰν εἰσβολῇ παροξυσμοῦ μετὰ ῥίγους ἢ φρίκης ἢ καταψύξεως γιγνομένου τοῦτο φαντασθῇ, τῷ καιρῷ τὸ πλέον, οὐ τῇ

60 Guidorizzi ("L'opusculo di Galeno," p. 98) provides a useful juxtaposition of the passage from Galen's commentary on *Epidemics* 1.10 and *DD*.

61 Wenkebach has inserted the entire phrase between brackets. I do not know why Wenkebach has used ὁ, but I think the logical choice here is εἰ, which Guidorizzi also uses in his edition of *DD*, from which, we can assume, Wenkebach copied the inserted phrase.

διαθέσει τοῦ σώματος ἀναφέρειν χρή. κατὰ μέντοι τὴν παρακμὴν <ὁ> τοιοῦτον ὄναρ θεασάμενος βεβαιοτέραν ἡμῖν ἔνδειξιν ἐργάσεται τῆς τῶν ἐπικρατούντων χυμῶν ψυχρότητος· ἔτι δὲ μᾶλλον, ἐὰν μη<δὲν> ἐδηδοκὼς ᾖ τῶν φλεγματικῶν ἐδεσμάτων, ὧν ἐν τῇ γαστρὶ περιεχομένων ἐνδέχεταί τινι τοιαύτην γίνεσθαι φαντασίαν, καίτοι τῆς ἐν ὅλῳ τῷ σώματι διαθέσεως οὐκ οὔσης ὁμοίας.[62]

But about dreams I have also spoken before, especially all those that indicate a certain condition of the body, just as has been written in *On Regimen in Health*. For someone who sees conflagrations in a dream is troubled by yellow bile, <if smoke or mist or deep darkness [appear in a dream], [someone is troubled] by black bile>; [seeing] torrential rains shows an excess of cold moisture, just as [seeing] snow and ice and hail [shows an excess of] cold phlegm. Appearing to be in a smelly place [indicates] a rotten humor, [seeing] cock's combs or something red [indicates] an excess of blood. To see something dark or to stand in dark places indicates breaths <and analogously in other cases.> And that is why he has added "including the kind and time" to "dreams." "The kind" to indicate that there is a difference between them, and if it had not been added, it was clear before; "the time" [to indicate] the moment in time when the dreams occur, that is: either in the beginning of the paroxysm, or in the acme, or at some other moment, and whether directly after food—and especially after some particular food—for some indication comes forth from those things. So when someone appears to be covered in snow, if this is imagined at the onset of a paroxysm combined with shivers or shuddering or chill, it must be attributed more to the moment and not to the condition of the body. But if someone sees such a dream after the acme, it will provide a firmer indication to us of the coldness of the dominant humors; more so, even, if [the dreamer] has not eaten any of the phlegmatic foods, which, when contained in the stomach, allow such an image to occur to someone, even though it is not similar to the condition in the whole of the body.

62 *Commentary on Hippocrates' "Epidemics"* 1.3.1 (p. 108, 1–24 Wenkebach; vol. 17a, pp. 214–15 Kühn). Oberhelman ("Dreams in Graeco-Roman Medicine," p. 140) would rather see "Wenkebach's meddlesome additions, deletions, and emendations" removed. While I do agree with both Guidorizzi and Oberhelman that neither of the two texts can have been a source for the other, I do not think Wenkebach's changes—though made from the standpoint that the *Epidemics* commentary was a model for *DD* and most clearly seen in Guidorizzi's rendering of the text (cf. Guidorizzi, "L'opusculo di Galeno," pp. 96–7)—make much difference to the significance of the passage to Galen's views on medical dream interpretation. This explains my adoption of Wenkebach's text, with only some minor changes.

If nothing else, the passage provides an explanation for, and some instances of the use of, dreams in diagnosis, and gives some helpful hints with regard to the things that need to be factored in to understand the dream's content. On the downside, the passage clearly lacks any explanation of the origin or the mechanics of dreaming, which is emphasized by Galen's reference to his own *On Regimen in Health* for more information on dreams. Of course, since we do not have this treatise, we depend entirely on *DD* for additional information—itself a text whose origin remains obscure. Nowhere else in the Galenic Corpus is there any explanation of how dreams work and from whence they come. The study of some passages with a clear reference to dreams may, however, give us some insight into Galen's views on the matter.

Dreams in Galen's Oeuvre

In his description of the symptoms and treatment of ulcerous fatigue in his *On the Preservation of Health*, Galen declares the following:

> ὡς τὰ πολλὰ μέντοι καὶ τῶν πλεοναζόντων χυμῶν ἐξ ὕπνου τε καὶ ἀγρυπνίας ἔνεστί σοι λαβεῖν διάγνωσιν. ἐπὶ μὲν γὰρ τοῖς ψυχροῖς τά τε κώματα καὶ οἱ μακρότεροι τῶν ὕπνων, ἐπὶ δὲ τοῖς θερμοῖς καὶ δακνώδεσιν ἀγρυπνία, καὶ εἰ καθυπνώσειέ γέ ποτε, φαντασιώδεις τε καὶ θορυβώδεις ὕπνοι ὑποπίπτουσιν, ὡς ἐξανίστασθαι ταχέως αὐτούς. (4.4 [p. 114, 20–25 Koch; vol. 6, p. 259 Kühn])
>
> For the most part, moreover, it is also possible for you to make a diagnosis of the excess fluids from sleep and wakefulness. For with cold fluids, there is coma and longer sleep, but with warm and acrid fluids there is wakefulness, and if he should fall asleep, dreamful and troubled sleep come upon him, and they rouse [him] quickly.

There is indeed mention of dreams, but not even a hint at the possibility of interpreting them for diagnosis. In this case, Galen apparently prefers to rely on his knowledge of what brings about sleep and waking,[63] and on the perceptible

[63] For a more thorough discussion of Galen's views on sleep and waking, see Hulskamp, "Sleep and Dreams," pp. 94–131 and "La Theorie de Galien sur le Sommeil," in V. Leroux, N. Palmieri, and C. Pigné (eds), *Approches Philosophiques et Médicales du Sommeil de l'Antiquité à la Renaissance* (Paris, forthcoming); see also P.J. van der Eijk and M.A.A. Hulskamp, "Stages in the Reception of Aristotle's Works on Sleep and Dreams in Hellenistic and Imperial Philosophy and Medicine," in P.M. Morel (ed.), *La Réception des* Parva Naturalia *d'Aristote* (Paris, 2010), pp. 47–75, at pp. 66–74.

fact that sleep is troubled by dreams, rather than consult the dreams that assail his patient in sleep.[64] Did Galen not care for dream interpretation as part of regular diagnostic activity?

Much the same occurs in Galen's treatise *Art of Medicine*. In his account of compound imbalances of the primary qualities, he describes people in whom there is an excess of heat combined with an excess of moistness:

> ἐὰν δ' ἐπὶ πλεῖστον ὑγρότητός τε καὶ θερμότητος ἥκωσι, νοσώδης τούτοις ἡ κεφαλὴ, καὶ περιττωματικὴ, καὶ ῥᾳδίως ὑπὸ τῶν ὑγραινόντων τε καὶ θερμαινόντων βλαπτομένη. νόστος δ' αὐτοῖς πολέμιος ἀεί. ἄριστα δ' ἐν τοῖς βορείοις διάγουσιν, οὐ μὴν οὐδ' ἐγρηγορέναι δύνανται μέχρι πλείονος, ὕπνῳ τ' ἐπιτρέψαντες ἑαυτοὺς, ἅμα τε κωματώδεις εἰσὶ καὶ ἄγρυπνοι, καὶ φαντασιώδεις τοῖς ὀνείρασιν, καὶ αἱ ὄψεις ἀχλυώδεις, καὶ αἱ αἰσθήσεις οὐκ ἀκριβεῖς. (*Art of Medicine* 8 [vol. 1, p. 327 Kühn])

> And if they arrive at a great quantity of moistness and heat, the head becomes unhealthy, and full of residue, and easily damaged by things that moisten and things that heat. The south wind is always hostile to them. They are best off in the north winds; they cannot stay awake for long, and when they allow themselves to sleep, they are simultaneously comatose and insomniac, and imageful in their dreams, and their vision is misty, and their perception is inaccurate.

Again, there seems to be ample opportunity to include the interpretation of dreams in the description, for instance as a means to determine which humors are involved, but there is no mention of using the dreams, which are "imageful,"[65] to

[64] A little earlier in the same chapter, Galen has pointed out that in case of indigestion in ulcerous fatigue, the correct treatment can be inferred from the patient's behavior during sleep: εἰ δὲ καὶ κατὰ τὴν ἑξῆς ἡμέραν ἔτι παραμένοι, σκεπτέον ἤδη περὶ βοηθήματος ἰσχυροτέρου, καὶ μάλιστ' εἰ διὰ τῆς νυκτὸς ἤτοι κοπώδης ἐπὶ πλέον ἢ ἀσώδης ἢ ἄγρυπνος ἢ ἐν ὕπνοις τισὶ φαντασιώδεσί τε καὶ ταραχώδεσι γένοιτο. τοὺς γὰρ τοιούτους σὺν μὲν ἰσχυρᾷ τῇ δυνάμει δυοῖν θάτερον, ἢ φλεβοτομεῖν ἢ καθαίρειν προσήκει (And if on the sixth day circumstances are still thus, one must now consider stronger measures, and especially if during the night [the patient] becomes either more fatigued, or restless, or insomniac, or has the type of sleep that is dreamful and disturbed. For under such circumstances, with strong *dunamis*, one of two things is indicated: either venesection or purgation: *On the Preservation of Health* 4 [p. 109, 12–17 Koch; vol. 6, pp. 247–8 Kühn]).

[65] It is not entirely clear what Galen means by φαντασιώδης. Based on the occurrences within the Galenic Corpus, I am of the opinion that it means as much as "imageful"—without any positive or negative connotations—and can apply to both waking and sleeping, and both to a state—like the state of sleep—and to people. For instance, in *Art of Medicine* 8 (vol. 1,

such a purpose. Chapter 21 of the same treatise provides a potential explanation: Galen mentions "sleep with more dreams than before" (φαντασιωδέστεροι τῶν ἔμπροσθεν ὕπνοι, *Art of Medicine* 21 [vol. 1, p. 361 Kühn]) as a sign of incipient disease—the operative phrase being "more than before." Deviation from the norm is the main focus of the context, but at the same time it suggests that the occurrence of dreams per se is a completely normal thing, provided that their number lies within the norm. This could be an indication that dreams were only considered if there was a specific *reason* to consider them.

There is one disease in the Galenic Corpus to which dreams and their content are clearly linked, and which has already been discussed briefly in a Hippocratic context: phrenitis. In *On the Affected Parts*, two passages mention a connection between the affliction phrenitis and very vivid dreams. The first passage (4.2 [vol. 8, p. 227 Kühn]) concerns a personal experience of Galen's. He tells us of the time when he was suffering from phrenitis and describes the symptoms he was then displaying. One of his symptoms was dreams so troubled and vivid that he cried out and tried to get out of bed. The treatment administered consisted of the application of wet dressings to the head (4.2 [vol. 8, p. 227 Kühn]), a treatment understandable in light of the second passage (4.4 [vol. 8, pp. 329–30 Kühn]), which is part of an account of the nature of phrenitis. Galen explains that a phrenetic delirium comes on bit by bit and does not manifest itself right away.[66] It is advantageous to diagnose the condition at the earliest possible

p. 327 Kühn), the patient is φαντασιώδης τοῖς ὀνείρασιν, which clearly indicates that his state of *phantasiôdês*-ness occurs in sleep, because it concerns dreams; in *On the Preservation of Health* 4 (vol. 6, pp. 58–9 Kühn), it is sleep that is *phantasiôdês*, which indicates that the sleeper has many dreams. That *phantasiôdês* can definitely refer to dreams, even if these are not mentioned, is clear from *Art of Medicine* 21 (vol. 1, p. 361 Kühn), where Galen clearly states that sleep is more *phantasiôdês* than normal, which indicates that being *phantasiôdês* is not necessarily a sign of (incipient) disease. I believe that roughly the same applies to cognates like *phantasma* and *phantasia*, in that they can be used *in reference to* images seen either in sleep or in waking. For instance, the *phantasiai* mentioned in *Commentary on Hippocrates' "Prognostic"* 1.23 (vol. 18b, pp. 73–4 Kühn), which are a result of cataracts in the eyes, and the *phantasmata* in *On Affected Parts* 1.2 (vol. 8, p. 21 Kühn), which are a result of an accumulation of humors in the stomach, both refer to complaints mainly experienced in waking. On the other hand, in *Commentary on Hippocrates' "Prorrhetics"* 1.1.5 (vol. 16, p. 525 Kühn), Galen speaks of the τὰ κατὰ τοὺς ὕπνους φαντάσματα, and in *Commentary on Hippocrates' "Aphorisms"* 3.24 (vol. 17b, p. 628 Kühn) of ἐν τοῖς ὕπνοις γιγνομένας φαντασίας φοβεράς. Oberhelman ("On Diagnosis," p. 46 note 72) claims that "the word *phantasmata* is significant of bodily disorders according to most ancient writers on dreams," and he cites Aristotle, Artemidorus, and Aristides as sources in support of his claim. While what Oberhelman suggests is of course a possibility, I am not entirely convinced, and I believe such a claim requires a more thorough investigation of the word field.

66 Cf. *On Affected Parts* 5.4 (vol. 8, p. 329 Kühn).

stage, for which a familiarity with the symptoms that precede the condition is necessary.[67] One of the most prominent symptoms is that (future) phrenetics have dreams so clear as to cause a physical reaction. If these vivid dreams coincide with reality, as Galen explains (*Commentary on Hippocrates' "Prorrhetics"* 1.1.5 [p. 20, 15–20 Diels; vol. 16, p. 525 Kühn]), there is no need to interpret them, as that will contribute nothing to prognosis. This line of reasoning recalls the Hippocratic *Regimen*'s rule that similarity to reality is good while dissimilarity to it is bad.[68] If, however, the dreams are so vivid as to provoke a physical reaction in the dreamer, interpretation is useful in the formation of a prognosis:

> εἰ δ' ἐγὼ τὰ προηγούμενα τῶν φρενετικῶν ἐνύπνια λέγω βλέπεσθαι σαφῶς οὕτως, ὡς ἐκθροεῖσθαι τῶν ὕπνων αὐτοὺς ἀναπηδῶντας ἢ φθεγγομένους διὰ τὴν ἐνάργειαν τῶν φαντασμάτων, χρήσιμον εἰς τὴν τοῦ πάθους τούτου πρόγνωσιν· ἡ γὰρ ξηρότης αὐτὴ τῆς ἀγρυπνίας ἐστὶν αἰτία καὶ τῆς τῶν ὀνειράτων ἐμφάσεως. (*Commentary on Hippocrates' "Prorrhetics"* 1.5 [p. 20, 20–24 Diels; vol. 16, p. 525 Kühn])[69]

> But if I say that the previously mentioned dreams of phrenetics are seen so clearly, they are startled from their sleep and jump up and call out because of the clarity of the images, then it is useful [to interpret them] for the purpose of the prognosis of the illness. For dryness itself is the cause of insomnia and of the appearance[70] of dreams.

This is the first explicit mention of interpretation of dreams for the purpose of prognosis outside of the well-known texts of *DD* and the commentary on *Epidemics* 1. Sadly, nothing is said or explained regarding the interpretation of dreams per se; one might have hoped for some suggestions for application, or an example, but it is likely that at this point Galen saw no need to repeat what

---

67 Galen also warns that other afflictions cause a delirium (παραφροσύνη) very similar to a phrenetic delirium; these are not caused by an inflammation of the diaphragm (φρήν), but by an inflammation of the brain. It is useful to know the symptoms that precede real phrenitis in order to distinguish it from these other afflictions; cf. *On Affected Parts* 5.4 (vol. 8, pp. 329–30 Kühn).

68 Galen revered Hippocrates as the single greatest medical authority and was intimately familiar with his works, be they spurious or not. Galen already suspected that not all Hippocratic treatises were authored by the master himself; *Regimen* was one of these. Cf. Nutton, *Ancient Medicine*, p. 219; and W.D. Smith, *The Hippocratic Tradition* (Philadelphia, 2002; electronic revised version of the 1979 edn), p. 59.

69 Cf. also *On Affected Parts* 5.4 (vol. 8, pp. 329–30 Kühn).

70 This does not mean that dryness is the cause of the appearance of dreams per se; it means that because of dryness, dreams will be memorable and will not fade away.

he had already explained elsewhere (probably in the lost treatise *On Regimen in Health*). He does explain that phrenetic people dream so vividly owing to the excessive dryness in their bodies. This makes sense: people with much dryness or a dry constitution—like melancholics, because black bile is dry and cold—always have very clear and vivid dreams,[71] and phrenitis is caused by yellow bile—hot and also dry (*On Affected Parts* 3.9 [vol. 8, p. 178 Kühn]). This also accounts for the treatment of wet dressings applied to the head: in phrenetics, dry is the dominant quality, one that needs to be balanced out. Galen, then, believed that vivid dreams can be an indication of (imminent) phrenitis, even when no observable signs of the disease itself appear yet in the person who has the dreams.[72] He summarizes as follows:

---

[71] Cf. *Commentary on Hippocrates' "Prorrhetics"* 1.1.5 (p. 20, 24–p. 21, 2 Diels; vol. 16, pp. 525–6 Kühn): οὕτω γοῦν καὶ τοῖς μελαγχολικοῖς διὰ τὴν ξηρότητα πάντως ἐναργῆ φαίνεται τὰ κατὰ τοὺς ὕπνους φαντάσματα. καὶ τῶν ὑγιαινόντων δὲ τοῖς μὲν ἐνδεῶς διαιτηθεῖσιν ἐναργεῖς οἱ ὄνειροι γίγονται, τοῖς δ' ἐμπεπλησμένοις ἢ μεθύουσιν οὕτως, ὡς ἀφάνταστοι δοκεῖν εἶναι διαρρεόντων αὐτοῖς τῶν φαντασμάτων ὑπ' ἀμυδρότητος, ὡς μηδὲ ἴχνος αὐτῶν καταλιπεῖν εἰς μνήμην. οὕτω καὶ τῶν παθῶν, ὅσα μεθ' ὑγρότητος ἐγκεφάλου γίνεται, κωματώδη τέ ἐστι καὶ ὑπνώδη καὶ ἀφάνταστα (At least, this is how for melancholics through dryness images in sleep always appear so vivid. And of the healthy people, for those who abide by a strict regimen dreams become vivid, but for those who are full or drunk, it is so that they seem to be without dreams/images as the images fade because of their [sc. these people's] numbness, without leaving a trace of themselves in memory. So it is also for those of the diseases that are caused by wetness of the brain, those are comatose and sleepy and without images). It is interesting to note that Aristotle, too, reasoned that melancholics were more receptive to (prophetic) dreams, albeit for entirely different reasons; see Aristotle, *On Divination through Dreams* 464a32ff.

[72] Galen (*Commentary on Hippocrates' "Prorrhetics"* 1.1.5 [p. 21, 3–10 Diels; vol. 16, p. 526 Kühn]) realizes that not everyone sees it his way, but people who are of a different opinion and believe that it is not possible to diagnose phrenitis by the occurrence of clear dreams are evidently mistaken: μοχθηρὸς οὖν ἐστιν ὁ λόγος τῶν οἰομένων οὐδ' ἐνύπνιον ὁρᾶσθαι τοῖς φρενιτικοῖς ἐναργές, εἴ γέ φασιν, ὡς μηδ' ὅλως ὁρῶσιν ἐνύπνιον ὡς ἂν μὴ κοιμώμενοι. πρῶτον μὲν γὰρ ἑτοίμως λαμβάνουσι τὸ τὰ συμπεπληρωμένα σὺν τοῖς οἰκείοις μεγέθεσι πάθη μόνα καλεῖσθαι ταῖς ἰδίαις προσηγορίαις, ὑπεριδόντες οὐ σμικροῦ λόγου τοῦ κατ' ἀρχὰς ἡμῖν ῥηθέντος, ὡς οὐδὲ προγινώσκεταί τι τοῖς ἰατροῖς μέλλον πάθημα τῶν ἤδη μὲν ἀρχὴν γενέσεως ἐχόντων, οὐδέπω δὲ τοῖς πολλοῖς διὰ τὴν σμικρότητα γνωριζομένων (So the reasoning of those who think that phrenetics do not see vivid dreams is wrong, if they say that they cannot see dreams at all because they do not sleep. First of all, overlooking a not unimportant argument made by us in the beginning, they willingly accept the fact that only diseases that have reached their proper magnitude completely are called by their proper names, assuming that, of those [diseases] which are only at the onset of their coming into being but which are not yet recognized by most because of their smallness, no future/impending disease is predicted by physicians). Cf. also Hippocrates, *Regimen* 1.2 (p. 124, 28–p. 126, 3 Joly and Byl; vol. 6, p. 472 Littré).

ἔπειτα δέ, εἰ καὶ μὴ συγχωρεῖ τις ὀναμάζειν φρενιτικοὺς ἤδη τοὺς μηδέπω σαφῶς παρακόπτοντας, ἀλλ' ὅτι γε φρενιτικοὶ γενήσονται, προγνῶναι δυνατόν ἐστι ἐκ τῶν ἐνυπνίων, ὡς κατὰ τὴν προκειμένην ῥῆσιν ἐγχωρεῖ λελέχθαι τὰ ἐν τοῖς φρενιτικοῖς ἐσομένοις ἐνύπνια προηγούμενα πᾶσιν αὐτοῖς ἐναργῶς ὁρᾶσθαι. (*Commentary on Hippocrates' "Prorrhetics"* 1.1.5 [p. 21, 13–18 Diels; vol. 16, pp. 526–7 Kühn])

And so, if someone does not agree to call those who are not yet clearly mad phrenetics, it is still possible to know beforehand from their dreams that they will become phrenetics; for the passage in question is likely to mean that in those who will become phrenetics antecedent dreams are seen vividly by all of them.

Dreams and Bad Humors

In his discussion of the potential harmfulness of sleep, Galen suggests there is a link between the accumulated humors in the stomach—more specifically at the stomach mouth—and the things we see in sleep. He explains the occurrence of frightful dream images in his *Commentary on Hippocrates' "Aphorisms"* 3.24 (vol. 17b, p. 628 Kühn):

οἱ φόβοι δὲ τοῖς παιδίοις γίνονται κατὰ τοὺς ὕπνους καὶ μάλιστα ἐξ αὐτῶν τοῖς ἀδηφάγοις, ὅταν εὐαίσθητα μὲν ᾖ, ἀσθενῆ δ' ὑπάρχῃ φύσει τὰ κατὰ τὴν γαστέρα χωρία, διαφθείρεται δὲ ἡ τροφή. παρεφυλάξαμεν γὰρ οὐκ ἐπὶ τῶν τηλικούτων μόνον, ἀλλὰ καὶ ἐπὶ τῶν ἤδη τελείων ἐν τοῖς ὕπνοις γιγνομένας φαντασίας φοβερὰς, ὅταν πολλοί τε ἅμα καὶ μοχθηροὶ χυμοὶ βαρύνουσι καὶ δάκνουσι τὰ κατὰ τὴν γαστέρα, καὶ μάλιστα αὐτῆς τὸ στόμα, τοῦτο γὰρ αὐτῆς ἐστι τὸ αἰσθητικώτατον.

But for children, fears occur in sleep, and mostly among the gluttonous ones among them, when they are sensitive [sc. physically], when the area in the stomach is naturally weak, and when the food [in the stomach] decays. For not only when young, but also when adult we pay close attention to frightening images in sleep, when many bad humors simultaneously weigh down and corrode the stomach's surroundings, and especially its mouth—for that part of it is most sensitive.

When there is an accumulation of one or more bad humors at the stomach mouth, this usually causes dreams and troubled sleep (*On Affected Parts* 5.6 [vol. 8, p. 342 Kühn]); on waking, delirium (παράνοια) may ensue as a result of detrimental activity at the orifice (*On Affected Parts* 5.4 [vol. 8, p. 329 Kühn]). The explanation Galen gives is that an accumulation of humors in the stomach may cause images that disturb vision (1.2 [vol. 8, p. 21 Kühn]). These images are a result of vapors that rise from the humors contained within the stomach; these affect the eyes in a way similar to the way cataracts affect the eyes.[73] Although this explanation does not seem to refer to *what* people see in their dreams, but only to the general character of these dreams, the information is still pertinent, especially with regard to the material aspect of this explanation of dream occurrence. Based on the above evidence, it is reasonable to assume that Galen thought, as did the ancient Greeks, that dreams were actually *seen* and that this process actively involved the eyes. One wonders if this process is similar to the generation of the medical dreams Galen mentions in *DD*, but unfortunately that question has to remain unanswered.

Galen and Medical Dream Diagnosis

Galen's views on dreams and their interpretation are reminiscent of *Regimen* on several counts. First, in his commentary on the Hippocratic *Epidemics* 1, just as in the probably spurious *On Diagnosis from Dreams*, Galen presents dreams as a potential diagnostic tool. Second, not all dreams are medical, as some dreams are prophetic and others are merely a representation of the dreamer's diurnal thoughts and actions. Third, if we assume that *On Diagnosis from Dreams* is a correct representation of Galen's views, he also believed that the soul is the generator of (medical) dreams. And, lastly, in his commentary on *Epidemics* 6, Galen applies the interpretive principle that similarity to reality is good, and dissimilarity is bad. However, it should be noted that Galen's interpretation of dream images is much more direct than that employed in *Regimen*. The dream images Galen mentions have qualities that are directly attributable to the specific humors they represent, while on the whole *Regimen* takes the far more metaphorical *microkosmos/macrokosmos* approach.

There are also several ways in which Galen's approach to dreams differs from that in *Regimen*. He admits, for instance, that it is difficult to distinguish medical dreams from prophetic dreams or from dreams that reflect a person's daily thoughts and actions. In addition to that uncertainty, there is even a possibility that dreams occur as a result of vapors that rise upward from the humors in the stomach (though these are usually nightmares). Galen also appears to be interested specifically in dreams of sick people, and not

---

[73] *On the Composition of Drugs according to Places* 2.3 (vol. 12, pp. 540, 642 Kühn); *On Affected Parts* 1.6 (vol. 8, p. 52 Kühn); *Commentary on Hippocrates' "Prognostic"* 1.23 (vol. 18b, pp. 73–4 Kühn). This is a matter of sympathy (see *On Affected Parts* 1.3, 3.1 [vol. 8, pp. 30–31, 137 Kühn]) of the eyes as a consequence of the condition of the stomach, and not a primary affection of the eyes. If the latter were the case, the images would not present themselves to both eyes at the same time; cf. *On Affected Parts* 4.2 (vol. 8, p. 221 Kühn).

so much in dreams of healthy people, while the author of *Regimen*, with the objective of *prodiagnôsis*, saw a necessity to interpret dreams of healthy and sick people alike. As was the case with the majority of the Hippocratic authors, Galen needed a reason to look at dreams or dream content, for example, in case of the vivid dreams of phrenetics (to be) or when there are more dreams than normal (in itself a symptom of incipient disease).[74] An important aspect of Galen's method was his practice of strongly basing his interpretations on factors outside of the dream, such as the dreamer's surroundings, habits, and regimen, and any other available information regarding the patient's physical condition. Unlike the dreams described in *Regimen*, these factors determine the ultimate interpretation of the dream and thus any conclusions regarding the condition of the patient. This is a strong indication that dreams are unlikely to have been the first thing Galen considered in a new case.

If we consider Galen's overall attitude toward dream interpretation, he does not seem overly enthused, although we have to be careful in drawing conclusions based solely on the lack of any explicit comments or references on his part. After all, most of what Galen may have had to say about dreams appears to have been lost with *On Regimen in Health*. Still, if indeed he had faith in this diagnostic tool, it is at least curious that in his many case studies he so seldom utilized dream interpretation. In fact, more than a few instances show Galen *not* employing dream interpretation, but instead favoring other, unquestionably more straightforward and tangible diagnostic and prognostic approaches, such as the inspection of urine and the pulse,[75] even when there is ample opportunity and cause to interpret the patient's dreams to gain insight into his condition. When Galen does mention dreams, it is usually as an extra option, or even an afterthought. All this suggests that dream interpretation had a comparatively low priority on Galen's list of diagnostic procedures. Above all, Galen valued concurrence of various diagnostic indicators, which might or might not include dreams. If all evidence pointed in the same direction, he would confidently cast his diagnosis or prognosis. Following this line of reasoning, we can only infer that if Galen were faced with a choice between

---

74 Some unclarity does remain as to what Galen thinks he might learn from phrenetic dreams, since he already knows that clear dreams are caused by excessive dryness.

75 For a more elaborate rendering of Galen's diagnostic practice, see V. Nutton, "Galen at the Bedside: The Methods of a Medical Detective," in W.F. Bynum and R. Porter (eds), *Medicine and the Five Senses* (Cambridge and New York, 1993), pp. 7–16, 275–6; L. García-Ballester, "Galen as a Clinician: His Methods in Diagnosis," in W. Haase and H. Temporini (eds), *Aufstieg und Niedergang der römischen Welt* (Berlin, 1994), part II, vol. 37.2, pp. 1636–71; Hulskamp, "Sleep and Dreams," pp. 50–69.

the interpretation of dreams and the interpretation of more concrete and direct symptoms, he would choose the latter.

Conclusion

Thanks to some unambiguous evidence, there need be no doubt about the existence of ancient medical interest in dreams and their interpretation. Its overall status as a diagnostic or prognostic tool, however, should be assessed with caution. If, on the basis of the evidence, we were to conjecture when dream interpretation was used, it would be when time was not of the essence, that is, in the matter of nonacute cases. A perfect illustration is *Regimen* 4, in which the lack of acuteness of the situation is proven by the fact that the author is bent on *preventing* disease. Dream interpretation may also have been employed in corroboration of a diagnosis or prognosis that was already indicated by other symptoms—an approach that probably suited Galen best.

I believe that matters should be viewed as follows. Owing to their alleged divine origin and their potential in religious matters, dreams had a good reputation to begin with. When, at the time of the Hippocratic Corpus, a more rational approach to dreams came to be, this fitted in well with other new developments, such as regimen treatment as a new branch of the medical *technê* and a theory of humors as components of the human body. What we have discovered in the Hippocratic Corpus are, on the one hand, the foundations of a medical use for dream interpretation in text passages outside *Regimen* and, on the other, *Regimen* itself as an attempt—perhaps even the first of its kind—at making this elusive nightly phenomenon a concrete part of medicine. That the concept was at least somewhat successful is exemplified by the fact that roughly half a millennium later, Galen, intimately familiar with Hippocratic lore and a great believer in the veracity and significance of dreams, still accepted that dreams and their interpretation could be of value in medical practice. However, Galen also realized the enormous difficulty in deciding which dream is relevant and which is not, as well as in correctly interpreting such a dream. For him, a true logician, this probably weakened the position of medical dream interpretation considerably. In conclusion, we may contend that, yes, the potential of medical dream interpretation was recognized by both the Hippocratics and Galen, and, indeed, its usage in medical practice is attested in some few cases. But at the same time, the evidence strongly suggests that in both Hippocratic and Galenic medical diagnostic and prognostic procedures, the status of dream diagnosis was much less prevalent than has hitherto been suggested.

Chapter 3

Dream Healing in Asclepieia in the Mediterranean

Louise Cilliers and François Pieter Retief

Dreams have intrigued humankind since time immemorial, the ancient Greeks and Romans being no exception. While it was from earliest times commonly accepted that dreams have a divine origin and that certain dreams entail messages from the gods to individuals, the author of the Hippocratic treatise *On Dreams* (*Regimen* 4) was arguably the first Greek to distinguish between prophetic dreams sent by the gods and dreams with a purely physical origin which could have a prognostic and diagnostic purpose. In the sanctuaries of Asclepius, these two kinds of dreams have in a way merged, being a message from the god on medical matters. The core of the treatment in these Asclepieia was the incubation or *enkoimêsis*, during which the patients hoped to experience a dream visit from the god who would cure them directly or otherwise give advice on medicaments or treatment.

In this chapter, various aspects of the experience of patients visiting an Asclepieion will be investigated, as far as it can be recovered. The main points are:

1. the sources for this subject;
2. the influence of the site of the Asclepieia on healing;
3. the procedure, culminating in the *enkoimêsis* and epiphany of the god;
4. the content of the dreams;
5. the vexing question how Asclepius actually cured the patients;
6. the opinions of the ancients regarding the healings; and
7. modern views on the healings, also from a clinical and psychotherapeutic perspective.

Sources

There is no lack of Greek and Roman sources on the Asclepian cult. The most important epigraphic testimony is the four stone stelae or slabs in Epidaurus that have survived,[1] dating back to the fifth century BC, on which the names of men and women healed by Asclepius are inscribed, together with their diseases and how they were healed. In total there are 70 inscriptions or *iamata* on the stone slabs recounting miraculous healings following on the dreams.[2] Furthermore, we have visual testimony in the form of statues, coins, and votive offerings consisting of the representation of healed body parts, as well as medical instruments that have been found at some Asclepieia. Archaeological excavations laying bare the foundations of the buildings give us an understanding of the cult and the procedure in the temple precinct. Literary references abound and are found in many different genres, such as comedy, history, philosophy, poetry, and tragedy.[3]

The problem with these sources, however, is that they seldom provide objective information (see below) or a medical history of the patient, which would have helped us to understand the healing. Schäfer correctly states that the testimonies record "Heilmomenten," not the "Heilverläufe."[4]

The Influence of the Site of the Asclepieia on Healing and Their Setup

In popular literature the Asclepieia have been compared with spas and health resorts[5] due to their supposedly favorable location. This view, which is not

[1] Pausanias (2.27) reports that in his day (second century AD), there were six stelae, "though there were more in antiquity"; translation taken from P. Levi, *Pausanias, Guide to Greece,* vol. 1: *Central Greece* (London, 1979), p. 194.

[2] The inscriptions have been collected, interpreted, and published by E.J. Edelstein and L. Edelstein, *Asclepius: Collection and Interpretation of the Testimonies* (2 vols, Baltimore and London, 1998 [1945]), and will in the course of this chapter be referred to as "T xxx" (xxx = testimony number).

[3] Cf. S.M. Oberhelman, "Dreams in Graeco-Roman Medicine," in W. Haase and H. Temporini (eds), *Aufstieg und Niedergang der römischen Welt* (Berlin, 1993), part II, vol. 37.1, pp. 121–56, at pp. 125–49 for detailed information on the literary sources; and D. Schäfer, "Traum und Wunderheilung im Asklepios-Kult in der griechisch-römische Medizin," in A. Karenberg and C. Leitz (eds), *Heilkunde und Hochkultur, I: Geburt, Seuche, und Traumdeutung in den antiken Zivilisation des Mittelmeerraumes* (Hamburg and London, 2000), pp. 268–72.

[4] Schäfer, "Traum und Wunderheilung," p. 260.

[5] Cf. E. Tick, *The Practice of Dream Healing: Bringing Ancient Greek Mysteries into Modern Medicine* (Wheaton, 2001), p. 58. They have also been regarded as the forerunners of hospitals, but L. Cilliers and F.P. Retief ("The Evolution of Hospitals from Antiquity to the Renaissance," *Curationis,* 25(4) [2002]: pp. 60–66) have shown that hospitals only developed in Christian times. Cf. too F.P. Retief and L. Cilliers, "The Influence of Christianity on Greco-Roman Medicine up to the Renaissance," *Akroterion,* 46 (2001): pp. 61–73.

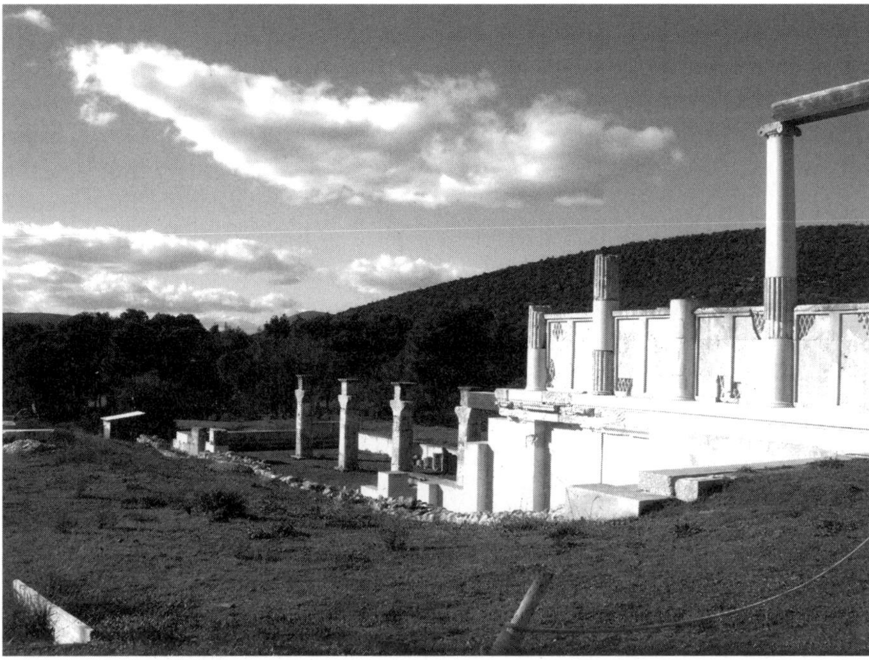

Figure 3.1 Sleeping Chamber for Incubation at Epidaurus. Photograph by S.M. Oberhelman

substantiated by archaeological excavations, can be traced back to the Roman architect Vitruvius (first century BC), who advised that "the most healthy sites be chosen and suitable springs of water in those places in which shrines are to be set up ... for Asclepius in particular."[6]

Some two centuries later, Plutarch expressed the same view as Vitruvius when he stated that the Greeks selected clean and elevated places for the Asclepieia. He furthermore believed that the reason why the sanctuaries were often in remote sites was to isolate the sick from those inside the town.[7] But Plutarch's view also contradicts the facts. Two of the most important sanctuaries, namely those at Epidaurus and Pergamum, are situated in valleys (T 739), while others are on mountain tops (T 762); still others are at some distance from towns, such as Pergamum and Epidaurus. A possible reason why Asclepieia are rarely found within the main religious area of the towns is that Asclepius was a latecomer in comparison with the old Olympian gods

[6] *On Architecture* 1.2.7 (T 707). The reason Vitruvius gives is that during times of epidemics and fevers (possibly malaria, which was endemic in Italy in ancient times), the sick could recover in a salubrious climate.

[7] *Roman Questions* 94, 286D (T 708).

who usually had their temples in the center of a town.[8] Various Asclepieia are, however, within the walls of cities, for instance in Athens[9] and Corinth. In short, they were "in all places which pious reverence considered sacred,"[10] often built over old Apollo temples. The unhealthy, low-lying Tiber Island, for instance, was certainly not an ideal site for the sick to live, nor was the temple of Asclepius in Sparta, as it was in a swamp. In short, the sites of Asclepieia were not chosen with the purpose of benefitting the patients, as is the case with modern health resorts where attention is paid to an ideal location, milieu, and climate.

Although the Asclepieia cannot be equated with modern health resorts, some of them (for instance, those in Epidaurus, Pergamum, Athens, and Kos) developed into huge complexes over the course of time. The architecture of the temple precincts was such that it accommodated the procedure followed in the therapy; it was thus basically the same in most of the approximately 410 Asclepieia in the Mediterranean area, though Pergamum differed in some respects.

In the entrance or porch, numerous *iamata* commemorated the miraculous healing of patients. They were often accompanied by terracotta, marble, or metal votive thank-offerings representing the healed limb or organ (eyes, ears, hands, arms, legs, feet, heads, breast, genitals) and were displayed to impress the pilgrims, to strengthen their minds, and to give them hope.[11] Inside the temple area was the altar where a sacrifice had to be made to Asclepius, and also baths or a well where the patient had to purify himself. The ritual cleansing was followed by the incubation in the sleeping ward or

8 V. Nutton, *Ancient Medicine* (London and New York, 2004), p. 107.

9 The conspicuous site of the sanctuary of the newcomer god Asclepius in Athens (on the southern slope of the Acropolis, under the brow of Athena's Parthenon) and its sheer size (it extended 80 meters across the slope) require comment. No ancient source explains why the cult of Asclepius was imported into Athens in 420 BC. The plague that hit the city in 430–426 BC could not have been the reason, since it had ended six years previously, and plague with its fatalities was outside Asclepius' purview. B.L. Wickkiser (*Asklepios, Medicine and the Politics of Healing in Fifth-Century Greece: Between Craft and Cult* [Baltimore, 2008], pp. 75–93) is of the opinion that the importation of Asclepius and its site in an area so symbolically charged implies a major civic commitment. He ascribes it to the imperialistic ambitions of Athens which led to the Peloponnesian War: Athens' ability to maintain her Empire at this point in time depended on gaining control of the Peloponnese. Forging closer ties with Epidaurus was the key (the harbor at Epidaurus afforded convenient anchorage for the Athenian fleet), hence the importation of the Epidaurian god and the unique location of the temple.

10 Edelstein and Edelstein, *Asclepius*, vol. 2, p. 233.

11 R. Herzog, *Die Wunderheilungen von Epidauros: Ein Beitrag zur Geschichte der Medizin und der Religion* (Leipzig, 1931), p. 60.

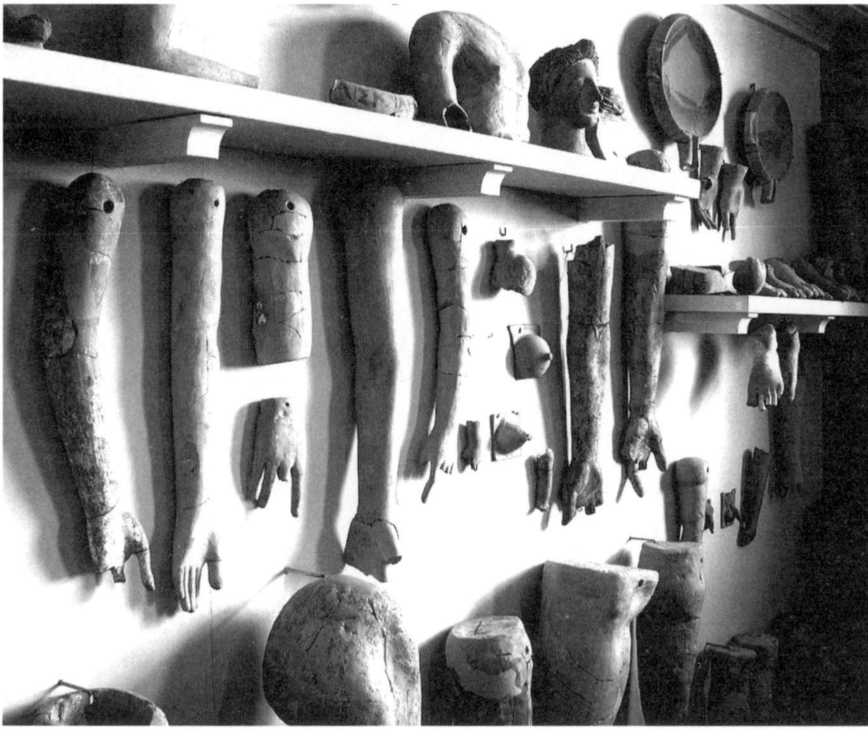

Figure 3.2 Votive Thanksofferings of Healed Body Parts at the Asclepieion at Corinth. Photograph courtesy of www.HolyLandPhotos.org

enkoimêtrion or *abaton*,[12] where the patients slept expecting a visitation of the god. In both Epidaurus and Pergamum there was furthermore a *tholos* or round building of white marble in which some as yet unknown procedures took place (see below).

All Asclepieia housed a temple with a cult statue of Asclepius in the *cella*, and sacred springs were a regular feature. In the inner courtyard, usually surrounded by a marble *stoa* or colonnade, would be the priests' quarters; smaller temples to and statues of related gods could be found in the gardens of the courtyard. Outside the temple area, later additions often included a theater, a stadium, a bath complex, a library, and a *katagôgeion* (hostel) for long-term patients and their relatives.[13] Some Asclepieia, like the one at Kos,

[12] The word *abaton* literally means "the place not to be trodden" and was thus a holy place.

[13] After the institution of the Asclepian festival in the fifth century BC, the hostels would also have been used by those attending the festival. The *katagôgeion* at Epidaurus had two floors and 160 rooms. Pausanias 2.27.6 (T 739) further refers to a building in Epidaurus

were built on terraces with beautiful gardens abounding with wild flowers and oak, cypress, and plane trees.

A Profile of the Patients

Most scholars agree that the most common kind of ailments that caused individuals to visit Asclepian sanctuaries were chronic diseases[14] rather than acute (mostly fever) diseases that were treated by doctors. Wickkiser points out that on many *iamata* the amount of time that the patient had been suffering from an ailment before getting help from Asclepius is recorded.[15] This implies that he or she had previously tried other remedies and consulted physicians but had found them wanting. In fact, many *iamata* record that doctors had despaired, given up, or refused to treat patients with lingering and recurrent conditions (many of which would have been psychosomatic) and that they found help at the Asclepieia.[16]

The question can be asked whether the physicians thought Asclepius to be in competition with them, robbing them of their clients. The answer is no, as the healing practices complemented each other and from the fifth century onwards, physicians gradually began to guard their reputation by not treating hopeless cases (in such instances, the ill would then have visited the Asclepieia). Various Hippocratic authors advised against treating certain ailments,[17] for instance, gout (*Prorrhetic* 2) and certain cases of dropsy and epilepsy (*Regimen, On the Sacred Disease*). Asclepius thus stepped in where the doctors left off. Furthermore, physicians regarded Asclepius as their patron (as the invocation in the Hippocratic Oath shows) and various physicians donated money or their

---

where women could give birth and people could die without desecrating the holiness of the sacred area.

14 Edelstein and Edelstein, *Asclepius*, vol. 2, p. 169; Schäfer, "Traum und Wunderheilung," pp. 264–5; Wickkiser, *Asklepios, Medicine and Politics*, p. 265; Nutton, *Ancient Medicine*, p. 109.

15 Wickkiser, *Asklepios, Medicine and Politics*, p. 58.

16 Cf. *Palatine Anthology* 6.330: "Having despaired of the skill of mortals, but with every hope in the divine, having left Athens with its many offspring, I came to your grove, Asklepios, and in three months was healed of an ulcer that I had on my head for a year"; quotation from Wickkiser, *Asklepios, Medicine and Politics*, p. 134, note 63.

17 Cf. the Hippocratic treatise *Diseases* 1.6: "Correct is ... to treat the diseases that can be treated, but to recognize the ones that cannot be"; translation taken from P. Potter, *Hippocrates: Affections, Diseases I, Diseases II*, Loeb Classical Library, 472 (Cambridge, MA, 1988), p. 113.

medical instruments to the Asclepieia, in addition to the sacrifice they made twice a year on behalf of themselves and those patients whom they had healed.[18]

Procedure

Although there are differences between the various Asclepieia and even at the same sanctuary over time, the procedure and the cures are basically the same. The sick usually visited the Asclepieia themselves, although on rare occasions a proxy could be used.[19]

Preliminary Preparations/Rites

On arrival at the temple area, the patient walked past the inscriptions on stone slabs and the anatomical votives on the walls, which described the successful healings. Few patients would not have been impressed by what they read and saw, the cumulative effect of these preliminaries being to inspire greater trust and confidence in the god and his treatment.[20]

After having entered the sanctuary, the patient began preliminary preparations, which in all the sanctuaries entailed bathing and the offering of sacrifices. The purification not only had a physical function (after all, one had to travel many a mile in the dust) but also a religious function, namely purification of evil thoughts. Porphyry stated that "it is seemly then that those who want to sacrifice go purified in their moral character."[21] At Epidaurus, there were no further ritual preliminaries, as at other Asclepieia, before the incubation, or any religious ceremonies. By purifying body and soul, the supplicants showed their respect to the god. The preliminary rites at the sanctuary of Pergamum, on the other hand, were more complicated. Van Eynde describes a bathing procedure that, according to him, also had a psychological function: the patient would

---

18 Nutton, *Ancient Medicine*, p.111.

19 Cf. T 423.21: "Arata, a woman of Lacedaemon, dropsical. For her, while she remained in Lacedaemon, her mother slept in the temple and sees a dream."

20 A parallel is when one visits a doctor today. While waiting to be admitted to the consulting room (~ *abaton*) for the "epiphany" of the doctor, one often gazes at the medical diplomas (~ votives) of the doctor on the wall, which are intended to assure the patient of his or her training and competence and thus to instill confidence in him or her.

21 *On Abstinence* 2.19 (T 18). Purification with water was important in Greek cults: bathing was considered to purify both body and soul (Plato, *Cratylus* 405B). Oddly, the purification had nothing to do with the disease; Edelstein and Edelstein (*Asclepius*, p. 149 note 16) point out that "disease was never understood as a defilement of the body."

kneel in an empty bath and would then have to pray for the god to provide water for the healing.[22] Priest-physicians would listen to the prayer, and if they thought that the disease was curable, they would in some way or other cause hot water to pour into the bath, which the patient then interpreted as a sign that his prayer was answered. Scholars also relate that fasting (which could last for days) was also required at Pergamum before the incubation.[23]

On the Way to the Abaton

At night, after the purificatory rites and sacrifice, the patient was allowed to enter the sleeping ward or *enkoimêtrion*, also called *abaton* in some sanctuaries.[24] In some Asclepieia the patients could sleep anywhere in the sanctuary, for instance, in the covered stoa, or near the statue of the god as was the case in Athens,[25] or even under the open air.

At Epidaurus, the procedure was once again very simple. The patients would be taken to the *abaton* through the temple area that they had seen during daytime—no secret paths or corridors or horrifying experiences—dressed in ordinary clothes.[26] In the *abaton* they would lie down on the floor on a mere pallet.[27] The lights would then be extinguished shortly thereafter.

At Pergamum, a rather more elaborate procedure followed the purification and sacrifice. An inscription indicates that the patients wore pure white garments, were garlanded with laurel or olive crowns, went barefoot, and wore no rings and belts (T 513).[28] Van Eynde refers to what follows as "the psychotherapeutic phase."[29] The patients now had to reach the round temple or Telesphoreion, where the *enkoimêsis* would take place, via a tunnel of 82 meters under the inner

22 I.E.I.M. Van Eynde, "Het Asklepieion te Pergamon. Een 'therapeutisch centrum' in het teken van Asklepios, Orfeus en Narcissus," *Tijdschrift voor Psychiatrie*, 19(3) (1977): pp. 187–96, at p. 188.

23 E.H. Halbertsma and C. Van Vels-Van Dongen, "Galenus. Arts tussen droom en rede," *Hermeneus*, 61(3) (1989): pp. 170–201, at p. 183.

24 Tick (*The Practice of Dream Healing*, p. 240) refers to it as "the god's consulting room" or "the holiest of the holies."

25 T 427: "Plutarch ... looked at the statue of Asclepius (for he happened to be sleeping in the vestibule of the shrine)."

26 Edelstein and Edelstein, *Asclepius*, vol. 2, p. 149.

27 Aristophanes, *Plutus* 671 (T 421).

28 Edelstein and Edelstein (*Asclepius*, vol. 2, p. 150, note 19) point out that these rules were probably not commonly in force, since Aristophanes in his quite accurate parody of the *enkoimêsis* in the *Plutus* would certainly have mentioned it, and dressing and undressing was a "wonderful topic for a comic poet."

29 Van Eynde, "Het Asklepion te Pergamon," p. 189.

courtyard, with only slots in the roof to provide light during daytime and oil lamps at night.[30] They were brought to this tunnel at about midnight, had to traverse it, and were awaited at the other side by priest-physicians in cloaks covering them from top to toe. The aim, according to Van Eynde, was probably to create a mystical atmosphere that would help to bring the patient into a kind of trance. Here the patients were questioned by the priest-physicians, who would make a diagnosis. After three more days without food, the patient would be susceptible to suggestions.

In the Abaton*: The Dreams*[31]

The incubants' dreams were without exception about the god and their illness. This is understandable. When falling asleep, their minds would be full of all the images they had seen that day: the sanctuary, the temple, the inscriptions, and thank-offerings of patients who had been cured. When they slept, it was with the expectation and hope that they would see the god and that he would bring healing.

Some of the dreams were very simple,[32] while others were long and full of medical detail; patients witnessed operations and heard the god give advice about remedies. This is also understandable since medicine was in some way or other practiced by everybody.[33] Medical knowledge was available to all, as the Edelsteins state: "[I]n antiquity medicine was not yet a science working behind the closed doors of hospitals and universities, unintelligible in its technical detail to the untrained layman."[34] Doctors often gave public lectures on medical problems or openly discussed the situation with the patient. Operations could be attended, and bystanders could watch while the doctor

---

30 Tick (*The Practice of Dream Healing*, p. 30) sees this descent into the "underworld" as the origin of the modern psychotherapeutic method where patients also had to descend into their subconscious and return to the womb where the primal wound occurred and festered, and there they had to await the healing visit of the Self.

31 Regarding the interpretation of dreams in general at the Asclepieia, cf. Oberhelman, "Dreams in Graeco-Roman Medicine," pp. 142–8 and "The Diagnostic Dream in Ancient Medical Theory and Practice," *Bulletin of the History of Medicine*, 61 (1987): pp. 47–60, at pp. 54–60.

32 T 18: "Alcetas of Halieis. This blind man saw a dream. It seemed to him that the god came up to him and with his fingers opened his eyes, and that he first saw the trees in the sanctuary. At daybreak he walked out sound."

33 Oberhelman ("Dreams in Graeco-Roman Medicine," pp. 152–3) remarks that "the reciprocal flow of data exchange and cross-borrowing must have been extensive among physicians, lay people, temple priests and diviners."

34 Edelstein and Edelstein, *Asclepius*, vol. 2, p. 164.

mixed the drugs or applied the bandages. It is thus quite logical that patients could have had such "technical" dreams—they could have experienced a similar procedure before, or watched an operation performed on a kinsman, or the dissection of some animal. The dreams would thus have been reflections of what the patients themselves had experienced or seen. The procedures in real life would have been those executed by human doctors, but if the god performed miracles, well, he was a god after all.

It is interesting to note that the content of the dreams changed over the course of time, always keeping up with the latest medical knowledge. The Edelsteins points out that the god happened to show his prowess as surgeon (T 423.13 and T 412) in the fourth century BC and the first century AD when surgery was greatly in vogue. The god also began advising diets, bathing, and exercise when that became fashionable (T 407).[35] And in Roman times the patients had "'pharmacological dreams' in which they received directions to make potions, poultices and treatments for cleansing, exercise and life-style changes."[36] The reason is not that the god "learned medicine," but that the patients knew (and dreamed) about the latest developments in medicine.

The Epiphany

At night the god revealed himself in a dream to the incubants.[37] The *testimonia* reveal that Asclepius came in the form in which he was portrayed in his statues: as a bearded man, holding a rustic staff (T 850) or as a youth with a beautiful appearance (T 423.1). He spoke with a harmonious voice (T 427) and sometimes even laughed (T 423.35). His expression was benign and compassionate.

Asclepius then approached the patient and made contact with him or her (T 425). At Epidaurus in the early days, the god immediately healed the disease[38] or prescribed the treatment to be followed. The patient thus awoke fully healed the following morning. From Hellenistic times onwards, Asclepius seems to have preferred to act as consulting physician giving advice (T 432), although this was not the end of the miracle cures. Michael Papageorgiou believes that this change in therapy happened because the faith in Asclepius was waning.[39]

---

35 Cf. also ibid., pp. 166–7.

36 Tick, *The Practice of Dream Healing*, p. 109.

37 In T 397 we see that the epiphany was sometimes refused on moral grounds.

38 Cf. Aristophanes' *Plutus*, where the god immediately heals the eyesight of Plutus.

39 "Incubation as a Form of Psychotherapy in the Care of Patients in Ancient and Modern Greece," *Psychotherapy and Psychosomatics*, 26 (1975): pp. 35–8.

What Did the God Actually Do?

There is unfortunately no indication of what happened during the *enkoimêsis* apart from Aristophanes' parody in the *Plutus*, and the dedicatory relief of Archinous.[40] Although Asclepius' procedures remain vague, we can deduce from the *iamata* that surgical procedures were undertaken: Asclepius is said to have used a knife[41] and other instruments; he also made deep incisions into the body (T 423.13, 23, 25 and 27) and yet the patients could get up and walk about the next day without any after-effects. However, to cut open the abdomen, remove the leeches, and stitch the wound up again—as is recorded in T 423.13 and T 423.25—is to steal a march on science: Praxagoras (end of the fourth century BC) was the first to open the bowels of a patient. Herzog refers to such procedures as *adunata* and *apithana*: mere fantasy.[42] The idea could have derived from the dissection of animals or from mummification as performed in Egypt. Even more fantastic are T 423.21 and T 423.23, where patients' heads are cut off and fitted back onto the neck.

Professor Helen Askitopoulou and her team of anesthesiologists at the University of Crete discuss four "case histories" as recorded on the *iamata* at Epidaurus which must have involved actual surgical cures.[43] They were perhaps not very complicated, but could not have been performed without some kind of soporific or narcotic: the opening of an empyema or abscess in the abdomen (T 423.27) and the surgical removals of the point of a spear from the jaw (T 423.12), of an arrow from the lung (T 423.30), and of a spear in the eyes (T 423.32). These patients must have been given some kind of narcotic (most probably opium—see below) before the *enkoimêsis*, since autosuggestion would not have been enough to still the pain of the cutting and the stitching. Askitopoulou concludes: "The physician-priests made sure that the *methods* used during thaumaturgic (miraculous) healings were not made known, but

40 The relief portrays an *enkoimêsis* in a temple in stages. H. Askitopoulou, E. Konsolaki, I.A. Ramoutsaki, and M. Anastassaki ("Surgical Cures under Sleep Induction in the Asclepieion of Epidaurus," in J.C. Diaz et al. [eds], *A History of Anesthesia* [Amsterdam 2002], pp. 11–17, at p. 14) describe it as follows: "It represents the cure of Archinous by the physician Amphiaraos in two stages. On the left, Amphiaraos, standing, cures the shoulder of the young man, while on the right, a sacred snake is licking the shoulder of the sleeping man. Above the man is shown his thankful inscription on a stele."

41 T 423.13: "A man of Torone with leeches. In his sleep he saw a dream. It seemed to him that the god cut open his chest with a knife and took out the leeches, which he gave him into his hands, and then he stitched up his chest again. At daybreak he departed with the leeches in his hands and he had become well."

42 Herzog, *Die Wunderheilungen von Epidauros*, p. 76.

43 Askitopoulou et al., "Surgical Cures under Sleep Induction," pp. 6–9.

made sure that the *results* were recorded on the *iamata*."[44] This view contradicts the Edelsteins' argument that there were no physicians working behind the screens in Epidaurus, but it is difficult to see how such surgical procedures could have taken place without experienced medical personnel on hand (see below for a further discussion).

Asclepius also acted in an advisory capacity, prescribing treatment and salves and drugs (T 421, T 423.9, 17, and 41). This seems to have been the god's preferred way of treatment from Hellenistic times, although it would have been regarded as a lesser miracle. Some of the drugs were mentioned by name, but some were the god's own inventions (T 410 and T 432). The Edelsteins mention some of the "natural remedies": "to apply ashes from his altar (T 438), to take rides or any other kind of exercise (T 435),[45] to go swimming in rivers or the sea, to bathe in the bathhouse or in springs (T 408 and T 432); he also favoured mental gymnastics ranging from the composition of odes to that of comical mimes (T 413)."[46]

The god's advice was often contrary to the mode of conventional healing, for instance, to order the sick, who need rest, to exercise (T 408), to command an patient suffering from asthma to take a walk in the snow, or to instruct a feverish patient to plunge into an ice-cold river. The advice was thus based on the principle of *contraria contrariis*. Aristides' *Sacred Tales* contains many of these paradoxical precepts, which astonished both doctor and patient (T 417, T 405, T 317.8). Galen observed that many of these paradoxical directions were to restore the humoral balance.[47] This is also the view of modern psychologists like Jung, who believe that dreams have as their aim to rectify balance disturbances in the mental equilibrium by producing a content of a complementary or compensatory kind.[48]

Asclepius could also cure by merely touching the patient's body with his hand (T 423.31), stretching forth his hand (T 456), or using a brush to take away the disease (T 423.28). He could remove the disease by the divine kiss (T 423.41) or wipe the disease off with his hand (T 482). The healing thus took place quickly.

The Asclepian cult also included sacred animals that played a role in the healing process. Both the snake and the dog could heal by licking the patient (T 423.17, 26) or by appearing to them in their dreams (T 423.39 and T 421). The

---

44 Ibid., p. 10; emphasis in original.

45 Marcus Aurelius mentioned riding, cold baths, and walking barefoot (*Meditations* 5.8 [T 407]).

46 Edelstein and Edelstein, *Asclepius*, vol. 2, p. 153.

47 *On the Preservation of Health* 1.8.19–21 (T 413).

48 J.A. Hall, *Jungian Dream Interpretation: Handbook of Theory and Practice* (Toronto, 1983), p. 123.

snake in particular was seen as the symbol of the rejuvenation brought about by Asclepius: in the same way that it regenerates itself by shedding its skin, patients would "shed" their disease and become transformed (T 701, T 699, T 692, T 694). Then there was also the cock, the preferred animal of sacrifice to Asclepius, often given as thanksgiving for healing.[49]

Convalescence

Most patients seem to have come for the dream and the treatment and then went home, but some stayed for longer periods (four months, T 64; three months, T 75). Aristides for instance stayed at the Asclepieion at Pergamum for 17 years with some interruptions.[50] As much care was given to this stage as to the foregoing stages: patients could make use of the library, the theater, the bath complexes, attend lectures in the theater, or simply relax with their relatives. An important part of the healing process was also to discuss their ailments and dreams with other patients and the cult personnel, who constituted a kind of healing community in themselves, offering moral support.[51]

Remuneration

No admission fee was required when entering an Asclepieion, but a thank-offering was expected after the treatment (T 423.5). Just as Asclepius decided on the drugs and therapies, he also designated the sacrifices to be made. Fortunately he was satisfied with small dedications. The Edelsteins describe the procedure.[52] At first, the suppliant had to say a prayer thanking the god for the healing (T 482); then the sacrificial animal was given to the sexton, who had to decide whether the offer was acceptable to the god (the god had few predilections, but a cock was the most common sacrifice). If so, the patient addressed the god in another prayer. Then the priest received his share of the offering, and a portion was put into the mouth of the snake as a small tribute to the sacred animal. Finally, a cake was dedicated, the rest being taken home and eaten there. Thank-offerings included not only sacrificed animals but also objects like money, frankincense,

---

49 Tick, *The Practice of Dream Healing*, pp. 25 and 28.

50 H.F.J. Horstmanshoff, "M. Aelius Aristides: A Suitable Case for Treatment," in Barbara Borg (ed.), *Paideia: The World of the Second Sophistic*, Millennium Studies, 27 (Berlin and New York, 2004), pp. 277–92, at p. 286.

51 Horstmanshoff, "Aelius Aristides," p. 290.

52 Edelstein and Edelstein, *Asclepius*, vol. 2, pp. 188–90.

laurel, olive shoots, oak leaves, garlands, songs,[53] poems, brass rings (T 542), candles (T 544), and gold and silver (T 545, T 484).

A Medical Perspective on Dreaming

The phenomena of sleep and dreams have been and still are the subject of numerous research projects headed by neurologists, neurosurgeons, psychiatrists, psychophysiologists, etc. They are still to a greater or lesser extent shrouded in mist. Even today, for example, there is no answer to the question of why we have to sleep,[54] nor is there as yet agreement concerning exactly which parts of the brain are involved in the production of dreams.[55]

The traditional view after the discovery of the stage in the sleep cycle designated as REM (rapid eye movement) in the mid-1950s is that dreaming is closely connected with REM. After about 70 to 100 minutes, the first REM period occurs, followed by a non-REM period. This cycle is repeated at about the same interval four to six times during the night, depending on the total duration of sleep. Ropper states that "most complex dreaming has been found to occur in the REM period," although dreaming also occurs outside the REM periods.[56] Various physiological changes occur during this period: the muscles relax and activity becomes minimal, the EEG (electro-encephalogram) pattern becomes asynchronized, breathing is irregular, and there is a fluctuation of blood pressure, pulse, and respiration.

In 2000, Mark Solms, from the Department of Neurosurgery at the St. Bartholomew's and Royal London School of Medicine, refuted the paradigmatic assumption that REM sleep is the physiological counterpart of dreaming. Although there is a link between REM sleep and dreaming, they are, according to Solms,[57] "doubly dissociable states," are controlled by different brain mechanisms, and probably have different functional purposes. REM can occur without dreaming and dreaming can occur without REM. According to

[53] Plutarch records that Sophocles, who received a healing visit of the god in his house, composed a paean to the god (T 587), which was sung long after his death.

[54] A.H. Ropper and R.H. Brown, *Principles of Neurology*, 8th edn (New York, 2005), p. 333: "Sleep, that familiar, yet inexplicable condition of repose in which consciousness is in abeyance" and "Sleep is a natural repeated unconsciousness that we do not even know the reason for" (p. 337).

[55] Ibid., p. 337.

[56] Ibid., p. 34.

[57] M. Solms, "Dreaming and REM Sleep are Controlled by Different Brain Mechanisms," *Behavioral and Brain Sciences*, 23 (2000): pp. 843–50, at p. 843.

the old model that dominated the field of research for many decades, "dreams are actively generated by the brain stem and passively synthesized by the forebrain ... the dream process is seen as having no primary ideational, volitional or emotional content."[58] Solms, however, shows that dreaming is caused by the forebrain: experiments revealed that patients stopped dreaming after suffering a forebrain lesion, "the region that supports various cognitive processes that are vital for mental imagery."[59] He also pointed out that the visual imagery of dreams is produced by activation during sleep of the same structures that generate visual imagery in waking perception.[60] Dreaming thus appears to be the consequence of various forms of cerebral activation during sleep.

J.A. Hobson and his team of Harvard professors of psychiatry add that during dreams there is a high level of cortical activation which is "a correlate of the mind's ability to access and manipulate significant amounts of stored information"[61] while blocking external sensory input.[62] The brain now turns to internal sources of input, and if these internal signals become unusually strong, "they could come to dominate the system with resulting hallucinosis."[63] These neurophysiological changes alter the mnemonic capacity of the brain-mind, increasing the likelihood of bizarre temporal sequences and associations that are uncritically accepted as reality.

Both Solms and Hobson refer to the fact that dreaming can be artificially generated by the administration of a variety of stimulant drugs, amongst others dopamine agents that "increase the frequency, vivacity and duration of dreaming."[64] Related to this is the following interesting perspective

---

58 Ibid., p. 844.

59 Ibid., p. 846.

60 Ibid., p. 848. Cf. too J.A. Hobson, E.F. Pace-Schott, and R.H. Stickgold, "Dreaming and the Brain: Toward a Cognitive Neuroscience of Conscious States," *Behavioral and Brain Sciences*, 23 (2000): pp. 793–842, who add at p. 824 that "Dreaming is characterized by a deletion of certain circuits active in waking, and, perhaps the accentuation of others."

61 The fact that dreams are a reflection of daytime experiences, the "day's residue" as it were, was already proposed by various authors in antiquity: Aristotle (P.J. van der Eijk, "Aristotle on 'Distinguished Physicians' and on the Medical Significance of Dreams", in P.J. van der Eijk, H.F.J. Horstmanshoff, and P.H. Schrijvers [eds], *Ancient Medicine in Its Socio-Cultural Context: Papers Read at the Congress Held at Leiden University 13–15 April 1992* [Amsterdam, 1995], pp. 447–59, at p. 456) and Galen (Oberhelman, "The Diagnostic Dream," p. 50). Hippocrates already stated that during sleep, the soul's cognitive and sensory processes shift to an internal direction, to the body (Oberhelman, "Dreams in Graeco-Roman Medicine," p. 131).

62 Hobson et al., "Dreaming and the Brain," p. 831.

63 Ibid., p. 838.

64 Solms, "Dreaming and REM Sleep," p. 849.

regarding the possible use of drugs in the Asclepieia, which has been offered by Askitopoulou and her team. They point out that some of the healings described on the *iamata* at Epidaurus involving surgery, even though not very complicated, could not have been carried out without soporific or narcotic substances.[65] They thus suggests that opium could have been used,[66] basing their view on an archaeological finding in the *tholos* at Epidaurus, a building whose function is still uncertain.[67] Pausanias in his travelogue of Greece described the *tholos* as a circular building of white marble and adds: "Inside is a picture by Pausias ... 'Drunkenness' [*Methê*][68] is also there ... drinking out of a wine-glass. You can see a wine-glass in the painting, the crystal cup and a woman's face through it."[69] Some kind of intoxication is suggested here. Considering, too, that the coffered ceiling of this building had panels decorated with very beautiful and lifelike flowers that closely resembled the opium poppy, Askitopoulou suggests that the building was used for some ritual like "the initiation and preparation of the patients before they enter the sacred area of the *abaton*."[70] She supports her view by pointing to the different Greek words for sleeping: the ritual for sleeping in a temple is known as *enkoimêsis*, but in Pausanias 2.27.3 and on the *iamata* the words *katheudô* (to sleep) and *kathupnoô* (to cause someone to sleep completely or to hypnotize someone) are used. She therefore concludes that *enkoimêsis* has the meaning of sleep induced by artificial means: it does not have the meaning of natural sleep, in which case the verb *hypnoô* would have been used.

Three aspects of the medical perspective above might bring us a bit closer to understanding the dreams at the Asclepieia:

(a) The fact that dreaming is activated by the forebrain that supports various cognitive processes and that the mind can during dreaming access significant amounts of stored information could explain why patients dream of their ailments and of the god.

[65] Askitopoulou et al., "Surgical Cures under Sleep Induction," p. 7.

[66] Ibid., p. 5.

[67] S.E. Iakovidis (*Mycenae, Epidaurus: A Complete Guide to the Museums and Archaeological Sites of the Argolid* [Athens, 1999], p. 138) believes that it was most probably a place of worship. Its concentric wall with narrow openings on various axes resembles a labyrinth. It could thus have been related to the chthonic character of the god, and the basement could have been the abode of Asclepius' sacred serpents.

[68] The word *methê* is, according to Askitopoulou ("Surgical Cures under Sleep Induction," p. 14), still used in modern Greek to describe the state of light general anesthesia.

[69] Translation taken from Levi, *Pausanias: Guide to Greece*, vol. 1: *Central Greece*, p. 194.

[70] Askitopoulou et al., "Surgical Cures under Sleep Induction," p. 5.

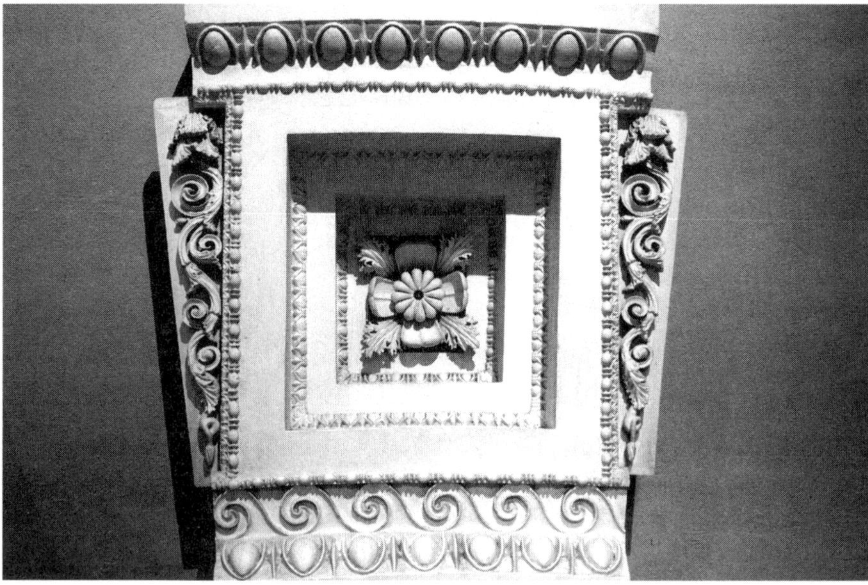

Figure 3.3 Coffered Ceiling of Tholos Building at Epidaurus. Photograph courtesy of www.HolyLandPhotos.org

(b) If these internal sources of input become unusually strong (as would most probably be the case due to the excitement of the patient), it could result in hallucinations, that is, the epiphany of the god.
(c) Furthermore, there is evidence that dreaming can be artificially generated by the administration of stimulants (such as opium) which would increase the vivacity of the dream and would have made the appearance of the god even more realistic and convincing.

In short, the medical perspective helps us to understand *what* the patients would dream about and *how* it would affect them physiologically. However, this perspective still does not explain why patients would wake up healed; we thus have to delve even deeper into dreaming.

A Psychological Perspective on Dreaming

It is possible to explain some of the healings from a psychological perspective, since many of the chronic ailments are psychosomatic (see above). The psychologist Edward Tick believes that a significant transformation can take place in psychosomatic cases through dreams: "Often through transformation the mind can immediately or over time learn to redirect and manage the body's functioning differently, even at cellular level."[71] He explains that if the patients participate in this process, the transformation "belongs" to them and can then more easily be integrated. The readiness and susceptibility of the patients in the Asclepieia when going to sleep have already been pointed out: their preoccupation with their suffering, the sight of the *iamata* and the statue of the god himself in his temple, and their fervent expectation of and belief in their healing —all this would have prepared them emotionally and fine-tuned them, as it were, to react positively on any suggestion.[72]

Askitopoulou confirms this view, stating that the suggestion and expectation of cure would by itself have had a significant curative value.[73] The psychoanalyst Robert Bosnak refers to a recent study where a surgery procedure was compared with a sham placebo surgery in the treatment of osteoarthritis:

> In this study one group received arthroscopic joint surgery while another group was anesthetized, injected with a local anaesthetic, given three stab wounds in the skin with a scalpel, but subsequently no surgery to remove arthritic tissue in the joint was performed. *Both* groups showed comparable levels of improvement with respect to knee pain at six months following their "surgeries."[74]

In another study (also reported by Bosnak), a Dr Leuchter of the University of California in Los Angeles imaged patients with major depression, who had shown positive responses, not to an antidepressant, but to a placebo; his conclusion was that the placebo effect is based on change in the brain function and has the capacity to evoke changes in human physiology. Bosnak further asserts: "Neuro-scientific studies of placebo demonstrate the strong effect imagination has upon the physical body."[75] The patient in the placebo experience is enveloped by the expectation of cure; he thus imagines a quasi-physical environment that presents itself as real, and is in the process accompanied by basic physiological processes.

---

71 Tick, *The Practice of Dream Healing*, p. 248.

72 Tick (ibid., p. 166) refers to this stage when we are flooded with images, perceptions, feelings, and sensations that are of such impact that we are profoundly altered in our body-mind organization as one of "an altered state of consciousness." This could result in a dream, which includes an epiphany and can provoke immediate and radical changes in the body-mind system.

73 Askitopoulou et al., "Surgical Cures under Sleep Induction," pp. 4–5.

74 R. Bosnak, *Embodiment: Creative Imagination in Medicine, Art and Travel* (London and New York 2007), p. 49.

75 Ibid., p. 49.

Evaluations of the Healings

Ancient Reports

The inscriptions are, of course, the "official record" of the god's virtues. But these texts, most probably written by the priests or at least composed under their supervision (T 428, T 438), can hardly be taken at face value as regards their objectivity. There would obviously have been exaggeration of the achievements of the god, and the experiences of disappointed patients who were not cured would certainly not have been made public.

The Edelsteins give a good overview of the views of ancient authors.[76] The Greek comedy writer Aristophanes (fifth/fourth century BC) is our oldest source; his comedy *Plutus* (T 420) is a parody of the procedure of *enkoimêsis* in Athens. It is remarkably correct as far as one's knowledge of the procedure goes, but allowance must of course be made for poetic fantasy and comic license. The same is the case with Plautus (third or second century BC) whose Roman comedy *Curculio* portrays what happened in the Asclepieion at Epidaurus. The second-century AD orator Aristides is our most comprehensive source. His *Sacred Tales* are the orations of this "professional patient" who spent 17 years at the sanctuary at Pergamum. He was an enthusiastic adherent of Asclepius and his work abounds with praise of Asclepius, no matter what unusual treatments the god inflicted on him. Claudius Aelianus (second century AD), an author widely read by Christian writers, reported many cures effected by the god, although without any particulars. According to the Edelsteins,[77] Claudius saw the hand of divine providence in everything and does not hesitate to proclaim the god's achievements.

Two important physicians of the late first and second century AD also commented on the healings, both very positively. Rufus of Ephesus (T 425) and Galen (T 459) both believed in the actuality of the dreams and the reality of the cures. As scientists, their testimonies are important in the assessment of the dreams.

Modern Evaluations

One can understand that the ancients believed in the dreams and the miracles performed by Asclepius, since they did not scrutinize them as critically as we

---

76 Edelstein and Edelstein, *Asclepius*, vol. 2, pp. 145–7.

77 Ibid., p. 146.

do today. The ancients' concept of natural laws was not as rigid as is the case today. Extraordinary and inexplicable events could take place as long as they were supported by good testimonies, even though no rational explanation could account for them. Asclepius' superhuman achievements were thus simply regarded as the result of his divine nature and his cures were "well within the limits of that world which the ancients recognized as real."[78] It is difficult, however, for a person in the twenty-first century to account for the miracles. Some possible explanations will be given below, although of course not all the successful healings can be explained rationally.

One's first reaction when trying to give a rational causation would be to say that the priests played an important role and that some of them at least must have been physicians. The Edelsteins categorically deny that physicians participated in the temple healings in Epidaurus.[79] It must be admitted that there is no mention whatsoever on the *iamata* of physicians; medical instruments were, however, found at Epidaurus, as at other places like Corinth.[80] It therefore becomes possible to explain the surgical procedures mentioned by Askitopoulou et al. (see above). Since Askitopoulou argues that the "operations" were not complicated, it may be that the priests after many years of experience in the sanctuaries could have performed such medical procedures[81] without, however, divulging their methods.

Nevertheless, Pergamum was a different matter. Here priests and physicians worked side by side; Aristides saw no problem in the coexistence of god and physician—in fact, his doctor Theodotus visited him frequently during his stay at the sanctuary. Moreover, on Kos the proximity of the temple of Asclepius and the Hippocratic medical school would have made daily contact inevitable.[82] By the second century AD, the "religious medicine" of the sanctuaries had been

---

78 Ibid., p. 158.

79 Ibid.; cf. also Herzog, *Die Wunderheilungen von Epidauros*, p. 154.

80 See Γ. Καλαντιζής and Ι. Λασκαράτος, "Τα Ασκληπιεία ως νοσηλευτήρια," *Αρχεία Ελληνικής ιατρικής*, 20(1) (2003): pp. 67–75 (especially Figure 7).

81 Cf. Herzog, *Die Wunderheilungen von Epidauros*, p. 157: "Schröpfen, Aderlass, Klystier und ähnliche Allheilmittel konnten in Epidauros von einem halb ärtzlichen Personal ... ausgeführt warden" ("Cupping, bleeding, enemas, and similar panaceas could be carried out by half the medical staff at Epidaurus").

82 Cf. Herzog, *Die Wunderheilungen von Epidauros*, p. 148 regarding Kos: "Es kann danach nicht bezweifelt werden, dass die Ärzte im Asklepieion von Kos, das wie das von Epidauros dem Heilbetreib diente, mitgesprochen, sich am Betrieb beteiligt und ihn durch ärtzliche Beratung und Betreuung in rationelle Bahnen gelenkt haben" ("There can be no doubt hereafter that the physicians at the Asclepieion at Kos, which like the one at Epidaurus was involved in healing activities, joined in and were involved in the procedures, directing these through medical advice and care in rational ways"). He also points out that at Kos

greatly influenced by "rational" (i.e. Hippocratic) medicine, as the medical terminology on thanks-offerings indicates.[83]

Medical Explanations

1. As we saw above, Askitopoulou points out that some of the healings described on the *iamata* at Epidaurus had to be due to surgery done by priest-physicians and that some narcotic (probably opium, deduced from the paintings of the opium poppy on the ceiling of the *tholos*) would have been used in conjunction with it.
2. In an article in the medical journal *The Lancet*, scholars discuss some votive tables found during the excavations at Epidaurus.[84] These inscriptions describe the healing of superficial lesions when licked by certain nonpoisonous snakes (the Elaphe longissima and the Elaphe quattuorlineata) found in Southern Europe.[85] These two large snakes are according to Angelotti quite domesticated (cf. T 692 and T 700) and continued to be associated with religious medicinal beliefs up to the twentieth century. Another example of healing by snakes is the beautifully preserved relief from the Amphiareion, currently in the National Archaeological Museum in Athens, which portrays the patient lying on his bed, with a snake licking his shoulder. Angelotti attributes the snake's curative powers to certain chemicals of the epidermal growth factor (EGF) that has been found in the oral tissues and saliva of these two kinds of snake. It has also been found that when the EGF comes into contact with superficial lesions, it can accelerate the healing. The snake usually encountered the patient as he was sleeping in the *abaton*: Asclepius could visit in serpentine form or, more likely, the sacred snake accompanied a priest. It is also possible that the healing required that the patient enter a sacred cellar (the *tholos*?) where the snakes were kept.

---

there were no miraculous healings. In Pergamum the two fields had merged—incubation and miraculous healings with the help of physicians working on a scientific basis (p. 149).

83 Horstmanshoff, "Aelius Aristides," p. 290.

84 R. Angelotti, U. Agrimini, D. French, C. Curia, and R. Mariani-Constantini, "Healing Rituals and Sacred Serpents," *The Lancet*, 340 (1992): pp. 223–5.

85 The text of one of the *iamata* reads as follows: "A man had his toe healed by a serpent. He, suffering dreadfully from a malignant sore in his toe, during the daytime was taken outside by the servants of the temple and set upon a seat. When sleep came upon him, then a snake issued from the *abaton* and healed the toe with its tongue, and thereafter went back again to the *abaton*" (T 423.17).

Psychotherapeutic Explanations

It has been pointed out that patients who visited the Asclepieia mostly suffered from chronic diseases. Many of these diseases would have been psychosomatic, which would have responded well to the *enkoimêsis* and the dreams. The expectation of and the belief in healing could have brought about a mental transformation that could even have had an influence on the body (see Bosnak above). Askitopoulou and Bosnak (above) also refer to the amazing results of the placebo effect.

Some of the instantaneous healings can be placed in this category. In a detailed discussion, the Edelsteins[86] ascribe them to "nervous disturbances" where patients react positively on an order of the god to do the seemingly impossible:

1. walking though he had been unable to walk before (T 423.35, 37, 38; T 16.8);
2. bringing a large rock to the temple, though he is paralyzed (T 423.15);
3. moving his fingers even though they were stiff before (T 423.3); and
4. speaking after having been mute (T 423.5).

Such "miracles" can perhaps be explained by the shock the patient experienced when he came into direct contact with the supernatural.

Further Explanations

1. The role of the priests in supervising the composition of the *iamata* has been mentioned (see above). The question arises as to whether deceitful priests could not have fabricated descriptions of miracles performed by the god to enhance the reputation of the sanctuary. The Edelsteins[87] categorically deny this and point out that the priests of Epidaurus, Kos, and Pergamum were never accused of fraud. One can imagine quite a bit of exaggeration and underplaying of the role of the priest-physicians, and of telescoping natural cures over a long period into instantaneous miracles to impress readers, but fraud over such a long period would not have been possible. The daily crowds of visitors to the sanctuaries in the Mediterranean came from all classes of society and could not all have been impressionable country bumpkins. In fact, three emperors were

86 Edelstein and Edelstein, *Asclepius*, vol. 2, p. 168.

87 Ibid., pp. 160–61.

treated at Pergamum[88] and the brilliant physician Galen believed in the god's dreams to such an extent that he performed surgeries on that basis. During all those centuries, there was never any doubt that Asclepius appeared to the sick, personally attended to their ailments, and cured them. If most of the attempted cures were failures,[89] the Asclepieia would soon have fallen into disrepute and disuse.

2. Some "miracles" could have been due to nature taking its course or to coincidence (and need not have happened instantaneously):

   i. eyesight that is restored could be ascribed to the fact that the blindness was a passing disorder (T 423.11, 20, 22);[90]
   ii. epilepsy could have been healed by a (timely) fever (T 425); and
   iii. nature could have been the reason for an abscess to open by itself (T 423.27), for an arrow point to come out of a festering sore (T 423.12, 30, 32), and for a stone in the penis to be ejected together with a seminal discharge (T 423.14). And the "miracle" of hair on the head growing again (T 423.19) is explained by the medical expert quoted by Herzog as "*alopecia areata,* die häufig spontan heilt."[91]

3. One should also keep in mind that in antiquity, doctors, due to their lack of knowledge and the lack of modern medicines, could do much less for patients than today, and that patients who were given up as hopeless cases (T 404; T 438; T 582) were perhaps not quite so sick.[92] The number of "hopeless cases" was thus larger and the chances that many would heal spontaneously when turning up at the Asclepieia or that the pains would subside and the symptoms disappear were greater.

---

88 Hadrian in 123 AD, Marcus Aurelius in 162 AD, and Caracalla in 214 AD.

89 Edelstein and Edelstein (*Asclepius*, vol. 2, p. 163) mention some who did not succeed in having visions (T 423.25, 395, 397), but they must have been in the minority.

90 Herzog (*Die Wunderheilungen von Epidauros*, p. 95) quotes a medical expert who explains T 423.4 (Ambrosia who was blind in one eye, but was healed by the god who cut the diseased eyeball and poured in some drug) as follows: "[V]ielleicht mit starker Schwellung der Lider einhergehende einseitige Augenentzündung, die spontaner Heilung fähig ist" ("Perhaps with a strong swelling of the eyelids accompanying unilateral ocular inflammation, spontaneous recovery is possible"). T 423.9 is explained in the same way: since the eyes were so swollen that they were no longer visible, the therapy was to cut the eyelids open.

91 Herzog, *Die Wunderheilungen von Epidauros*, p. 108.

92 Doctors had to guard their reputation and it was considered proper for them not to assume responsibility for what they would be unable to carry through: Edelstein and Edelstein, *Asclepius*, vol. 2, p. 169.

4. The remedies and treatments revealed by the god in the dreams were often the same as the prescriptions of the human physicians. However, because it was the god who had prescribed them, the patients would be much more conscientious in following his orders, with the result that they would regain their health much sooner.
5. Asclepius was popular with women as the multitude of breasts as thank-offerings indicate. In many cases such dedications were made after appeals for fertility (T 39 and 42, where the women dreamt of having sex with a snake) or after the happy outcome of a pregnancy. In the former case, women would sleep in the temple, dream of intercourse with a snake, and then conceive when going home (T 423.4; T 426; T 423.39). Asclepius also treated extended pregnancies, such as those of Kleo (T 423.1), who had been pregnant for five years (a layperson's view, but in reality probably a pseudo-pregnancy, or simply menstruation which did not appear for a number of years); this was also the case with Ithmonike, whose pregnancy lasted three years (T 423.2). One should remember, however, that for the Hippocratic doctors, a pregnancy of up to 12 months was quite natural.[93]
6. In various *iamata* the patients suffered from parasites or worms in the abdomen (T 423.13: leeches; T 423.23: tapeworm; T 423.25: pregnant with worms). Herzog[94] believes that this can be traced back to superstition, which often ascribed pains and cramps in the belly to live creatures (like frogs, snakes, and lizards) in the body which could cause trouble for years before the patients expelled them.

In the long run, however, it is impossible to give a rational explanation for every healing on the *iamata*. The miraculous healings must be seen in context, taking place in the culture in which they occurred more than 2,000 years ago. The belief in the gods never seriously faltered in Graeco-Roman times.[95] Looking at this phenomenon from a modern perspective, it might at first seem irrational and fictitious, but considering that miracles still happen today—it is a common experience that grave illnesses can heal contrary to the expectations of experienced physicians—the healings reported in the Asclepieia should be granted the possibility of really happening.

---

93 Hippocrates, *On the Nature of the Child* 30.

94 Herzog, *Die Wunderheilungen von Epidauros*, pp. 80–81.

95 In fact, well into Christian times there was still the belief that the gods sent the dreams. W.V. Harris (*Dreams and Experience in Classical Antiquity* [Cambridge, MA, 2009], p. 222) points out that in 401 AD, a council was held in Carthage to counteract what was called "a sort of epidemic of dreams." Incubation also still flourished, even among Christians.

Chapter 4

Writing the Medical Dream in the Hippocratic Corpus and at Epidaurus

Lee T. Pearcy

If we ask what constitutes a "medical dream" in classical Greece, we are soon reduced to a tautological statement: a medical dream is a dream that is interpreted as a medical dream. Medical dreams are diagnostic or prognostic, and almost any dream may inform or predict something about the body and its diseases. For the author of *Regimen* 4,[1] dreams of heavenly bodies or weather (4.89); dreams of fields, crops, bodies of water, and other things on the earth (4.90); dreams of everyday objects (4.91); and dreams of the dead, of monsters, or of eating, drinking, fighting, travel, or other daily activities (4.92–3) all may provide clues to a patient's physical state. Content cannot distinguish a medical dream from other kinds. Only the act of interpretation gives a dream informative or predictive character and value.

Interpretation implies an interpreter, and it is striking that in Greece the literature of dream interpretation and the literature of medicine emerge together toward the end of the fifth century BC.[2] In classical and Hellenistic accounts of medical dreams, dreamer and interpreter are never the same person; in fact, apart from epic, drama, and other works of imagination,[3] I know of

[1] The standard edition of Hippocrates is that of Émile Littré, *Oeuvres Completes d'Hippocrate* (10 vols, Paris, 1839–1861). For convenience, I cite where possible from the Loeb volumes of Hippocrates edited by W.H.S. Jones et al. (Cambridge, MA, 1923–). *Regimen* appears in vol. 4 (Cambridge, MA, 1931). All translations are from the Loeb edition, with modifications where necessary.

[2] V. Nutton (*Ancient Medicine* [London, 2004], p. 60) concludes that "the great majority of the [Hippocratic] treatises come from the period 420–350 BC." The earliest Greek dreambook may be Antiphon's *On the Interpretation of Dreams* (*Peri kriseôs oneirôn*), although, as Michael Gagarin (*Antiphon the Athenian* [Austin 2002], p. 99) points out, we have no evidence for the title of such a book until the tenth-century Suda. The author may plausibly be identified with Antiphon the Sophist; see G.J. Pendrick (ed.), *Antiphon the Sophist: Fragments* (Cambridge, 2002), pp. 1–26, 49–53. *Regimen* 4 is not likely to be earlier than c. 370 BC; see R.G.A. van Lieshout, *Greeks on Dreams* (Utrecht, 1980), pp. 187–8.

[3] One of the earliest is Penelope's dream in *Odyssey* 19.535–45.

no first-person account of an actual, or claimed to be actual,[4] dream and its interpretation before Xenophon's description of the dream that motivated him to assume leadership among the Cyreans after Cunaxa (*Anabasis* 3.1, 11–14); Aelius Aristides, long after the period considered in this chapter, may be the first person to record and interpret his own medical dreams.[5] It cannot be the case that no one ever narrated and interpreted his or her own dream; after all, one marker of the bore, according to Theophrastus (*Characters* 3.2), was his eagerness to talk about his own dreams. Nor is it immediately self-evident that all dreams demand interpretation. But until Aelius Aristides, a medical dream is a dream that comes accompanied by its interpretation. Why?

The need for interpretation, I suggest, arose because dreams were one battleground on which the struggle for authority and self-definition was waged as medicine sought to establish and maintain its status as a *tekhnê* in the face of competing paradigms of healing, encroachments from other arts, and a rising class of poorly trained physicians or charlatans posing as *iatroi*.[6] There is reason to believe that the art of medicine encountered increasing competition and criticism during the intellectual ferment of the later fifth and early fourth centuries BC. Earlier references to physicians or the art of medicine are mostly favorable. "A doctor," says a character in the *Iliad* (9.514–15), "is worth many other men" in treating wounds. Aeschylus counts medicine as the greatest of the arts that Prometheus gave to mankind.[7] Democedes of Croton (c. 550–c. 460 BC) earned praise, and ever more lucrative salaries, from the governments of Aegina, Athens, and Samos. When he became a Persian captive after the fall of Samos (522 BC), his status as physician was worth concealing. If his captors had known that they had a Greek physician in their

4 On reasons to be skeptical of many, if not most, ancient reports of dreams, see W.V. Harris, *Dreams and Experience in Classical Antiquity* (Cambridge, MA, 2009), pp. 91–110.

5 On Aristides, with references to earlier literature, see the chapter by Downie in this volume. The first-person dreams recorded in the Ptolemaeus archive from the second century BC lack medical content; see U. Wilcken, *Urkunden der Ptolemäerzeit* (2 vols, Berlin and Leipzig, 1927), vol. 1, pp. 349–50; and G. Shusan, "Greek and Egyptian Dreams in Two Ptolemaic Archives: Individual and Cultural Layers of Meaning," *Dreaming*, 16(1) (June 2006): pp. 129–42.

6 On charlatans, see L. Dean-Jones, "Literacy and the Charlatan in Ancient Greek Medicine," in Harvey Yunis (ed.), *Written Texts and the Rise of Literate Culture in Ancient Greece* (Cambridge, 2003), pp. 97–121.

7 *Prometheus Bound* 478–83; in second place he lists dream interpretation. This is not the place to enter into controversies over the date and authenticity of the play; I am inclined to doubt the conventional attribution to Aeschylus and accept a date between c. 460 and the beginning of the Peloponnesian War; see A. Sommerstein, *Aeschylean Tragedy* (London, 2010), pp. 228–32.

possession, their respect for Greek medicine would have kept Democedes a prisoner forever.[8]

Little more than a century later, however, medicine was an embattled art. In this it was not alone; as the author of the Hippocratic *The Art* 1 put it, "Some there are who have made an art of vilifying the arts." But although many *tekhnai* struggled for definition and authority as the fifth century turned into the fourth—one thinks of rhetoric and philosophy, whose ancient conflict was just getting under way—medicine, precisely because it had been so generally accepted and admired, faced a special burden of self-justification. Many treatises of the Hippocratic Corpus, the earliest of which can be dated to the last quarter of the fifth century, reflect this moment of crisis.

In *Regimen in Acute Diseases*, the Hippocratic author reports that medicine has fallen into ill repute because laymen interpret differences of medical opinion as an indication that medicine is as speculative and imprecise as divination:

> Yet the art as a whole has a very bad name among laymen, so that there is thought to be no art of medicine at all. Accordingly, since among practitioners there will prove to be so much difference of opinion about acute diseases that the remedies which one physician gives in the belief that they are the best are considered by a second to be bad, laymen are likely to object to such that their art resembles divination; for diviners too think that the same bird, which they hold to be a happy omen on the left, is an unlucky one when on the right, while other diviners maintain the opposite. (*Regimen in Acute Diseases* 8)

The Art shows the same concern to counter criticisms of medicine's ineffectiveness and to distinguish it from the operations of chance: "But because not all are healed the art is blamed, and those who malign it, because there are some who succumb to diseases, assert that those who escape do so through luck and not through the art" (4). The same treatise reports other criticisms of medicine: fatal outcomes are always the fault of the physician, never of the patient (7), or physicians refuse to take on intractable cases and take credit for healing patients who would have recovered in any case (8). *The Law* begins: "Medicine is the most distinguished of all the arts, but through the ignorance of those who practice it, and of those who casually judge such practitioners, it is now of all the arts by far the least esteemed." The author of *Prorrhetic* 2 knows from his

[8] Herodotus 3.130–32. For a discussion of Herodotus' account, see M. Michler, "Demokedes von Kroton: Der alteste Vertreter westgriechischen Heilkunde," *Gesnerus*, 23 (1966): pp. 213–29. Skeptical of the account is A. Griffiths, "Democedes of Croton: A Greek Doctor at the Court of Darius," in H. Sancisi-Weerdenburg and A. Kuhrt (eds), *Achaemenid History, II: The Greek Sources* (Leiden, 1987): pp. 37–51.

own experience that "people neither judge correctly what is said and done in medicine, nor report it accurately" (2.2).

The *tekhnê* of medicine depends on diagnosis and prognosis, the ability to foretell what will happen as a patient's disease progresses. In this moment of defining and justifying itself, medicine, *iatrikê*, as reflected in the Hippocratic Corpus, felt a particular need to distinguish itself from another *tekhnê* that depended on knowledge of events to come: divination or *mantikê*. This need surfaces as a suspicion of *mantikê* at several points in the Hippocratic Corpus. The author of *Regimen* 4 allows (4.87) that diviners may be able to interpret such dreams as actually god-sent, but insists that when they attempt to interpret medical dreams, they sometimes get them right and sometimes get them wrong; in neither case do they understand, as a physician does, the true nature of the phenomenon that they attempt to interpret. When physicians offer contradictory advice, says the author of *Regimen in Acute Diseases* (8), laymen are apt to suppose, incorrectly, that their art is no better than *mantikê*.[9]

Prognosis brought the physician's art perilously close to that of the diviner, and so justifying and explaining medical prognosis and distinguishing it from the diviner's forecast became an essential part of defining *iatrikê tekhnê* and establishing its authority. Hippocratic treatises devoted to prognosis give evidence of this concern. *Prognostic* opens by declaring that foresight (*pronoia*) is an excellent thing for a physician because it not only disposes patients to trust their physician, but also enables the physician to provide better treatment. The Hippocratic author implicitly sets medicine against other predictive arts when he observes that "to restore every patient to health is impossible. To do so indeed would have been better even than forecasting the future" (*Prognostic* 1). In the remainder of the treatise, dreams have no part, even as a diagnostic symptom, although the quality of a patient's sleep does figure in prognosis.[10] At *Prorrhetic* 1.5, dreams (*enhupnia*) are important only as a symptom.

Prorrhetic 2.1 provides a window into the anxiety that medical prognosis, which seemed so near to divination, could provoke. The introduction to the work attacks not diviners but physicians who offer showy, excessively detailed predictions (*prorrhêseis*):

---

[9] In *On Girls* (Περὶ παρθένων) (vol. 8, p. 468 Littré), young women who remain without a husband are prone to visions, and when these cease, they "dedicate many different things to Artemis ... being deceived by the bidding of seers [κελευόντων τῶν μάντεων ἐξαπατεώμεναι]."

[10] E.g., *Prognostic* 2: ἐπανερέσθαι χρή, μὴ ἠγρύπνηκεν ὁ ἄνθρωπος, and especially *Prognostic* 10.

> There are reports of physicians making frequent, true, and marvelous predictions, predictions such as I have never made myself, nor ever personally heard anyone else make. Here are some examples. A person seems to be mortally ill both to the physician attending him and to others who see him, but a different physician comes in and says that the patient will not die, but go blind in both eyes. In another case where the person looked in a very poor state, the physician that came in foretold that he would recover, but be disabled in one arm; to another person who was apparently not going to survive, one said that he would recover, but that his toes would become black and gangrenous. Other predictions of this kind are reported in the same form. A different type of predicting is to foretell in merchants and adventurers death to some, madness to others, and other diseases to others; and in making revelations concerning present and past times to be correct in every detail. Another form of prediction is recounted as follows: to discover in athletes and in people that are carrying out exercises and exertions prescribed because of illnesses whether they have failed to eat some of their meal, or have eaten something of a different kind, or have taken too much to drink, or omitted part of their walk, or practiced venery; none of these things escapes their notice, not even if the person disobeys in but little. This is how precise all these kinds of predictions are reported to be.

Two features of this exordium stand out in the light of what has been said about the tension between medical prognosis and popular divination. First, the author claims never to have made "true and marvelous predictions" himself, nor has he heard anyone else do so. Here, as often in the Hippocratic Corpus,[11] an anonymous, perhaps even fictional opponent represents an ideological position. The question at issue is not so much the bedside showmanship of some actual physicians as the line of demarcation between medical prognosis and other kinds of prediction.

This is not to say that we should doubt that any ancient Greek physician ever made the kind of attention-grabbing prediction described in *Prorrhetic* 2.1. Competition between physicians made rhetoric and showmanship a part of a physician's art.[12] The first of *Prorrhetic* 2's three categories of showy prediction describes situations when, after a patient has been diagnosed as mortally ill, another physician declares a different, specific, and (one presumes) accurate prognosis. The medical competition implied here chimes with the statement in *Prognostic* 1 that when a physician can declare "the present, the past, and the

[11] For example, the advocates of *hypotheseis* evoked at the beginning of *Ancient Medicine*.

[12] For remarks on showmanship, physicians lecturing, and competition, see *Precepts* 10–12.

future ... men will confidently entrust themselves to him for treatment." But in the categories of *Prorrhetic* 2, there seems to be a telling slippage between medical prognostic and other kinds of quasi-medical or nonmedical divination. The second category describes predictions addressed to merchants and entrepreneurs, foretelling "death to some, madness to others, and other diseases to others; and in making revelations concerning present and past times to be correct in every detail." Only the inclusion of disease and madness among the predicted outcomes makes this category resemble medical prognosis, and the verb used for this activity, *prophêtizein*, suggests someone claiming to interpret the will of the gods,[13] hardly a usual position for ancient Greek physicians. The third category likewise barely touches on the medical; it seems to describe coaches or trainers who can recognize in athletes or people carrying out an exercise regimen signs of deviation from the assigned program.

In *Prorrhetic* 2, the Hippocratic author firmly sets his theory and practice apart not only from showy, self-serving medical prognoses, but also from other predictions that, because they touch on death, sickness, regimen, and other matters that fall within the remit of a physician, might be confused with medical prognosis: "I, however, shall not prophesy [οὐ μαντεύσομαι] anything like this; rather I record [γράφω] the clinical signs from which one must deduce which persons will become well and which will die, and which will recover or die in a short time." The predictive function of medicine for him has nothing to do with *mantikê* and should not resemble it in any way; instead, it depends on accurate recognition of clinical signs and appropriate reasoning from them.[14]

Enough has been said, I think, to show that in the fifth and fourth centuries BC, at least some physicians were concerned to establish and preserve a demarcation between their kind of prognostication and that of the diviner,

---

13 For the meaning, see H. Liddell and R. Scott, *A Greek-English Lexicon*, revised and augmented by H. Jones, 9th edn (Oxford, 1968), s.v προφητεύω. The author of *Prorrhetics* 2 uses προφητίζω instead of the more usual form.

14 By contrasting his own writing with the diviners' prophesy, the Hippocratic author may be claiming authority through association with the technology of literacy. A full account of the relationship between orality and literacy in the Hippocratic Corpus has yet to be given; in the meantime, see G.L. Miller, "Literacy and the Hippocratic Art: Reading, Writing, and Epistemology in Ancient Greek Medicine," *Journal of the History of Medicine and Allied Sciences*, 45 (1990): pp. 11–40; I.M. Lonie, "Literacy and the Development of Hippocratic Medicine," in F. Lasserre and P. Mudry (eds), *Formes de pensée dans la collection Hippocratique, Actes du IVe Colloque International Hippocratique, Lausanne, 21–26 September 1981* (Geneva, 1983), pp. 145–61; K. Usener, "'Schreiben' im Corpus Hippocraticum," in W. Kullmann and M. Reichel (eds), *Der Übergang von der Mündlichkeit zur Literatur bei den Griechen* (Tübingen, 1990), pp. 291–300.

prophet, or seer. In order to do this, dreams had to be understood and brought into the orbit of medical theory and practice. About a dozen Hippocratic treatises have something to say about dreams,[15] but only *Regimen* 4 offers an explanation of their cause and relationship to health and sickness. The author of *Regimen* 4 was willing to allow that some dreams had divine causation. Those were the province of lay experts, but when it came to interpreting purely physical symptoms caused by the soul's activity during sleep, these same experts were apt to go astray (*Regimen* 4.87). Physiological dreams, the Hippocratic author suggests, arise because in sleep the *psychê* enjoys an autonomous existence and conducts all the acts of perception and movement without input or interference from the organs of sense:

> For when the body is awake the soul is its servant, and is never her own mistress, but divides her attention among many things, assigning a part of it to each faculty of the body—to hearing, to sight, to touch, to walking, and to acts of the whole body; but the mind never enjoys independence. But when the body is at rest, the soul, being set in motion and awake, administers her own household, and of herself performs all the acts of the body. For the body when asleep has no perception; but the soul when awake has cognizance of all things—sees what is visible, hears what is audible, walks, touches, feels pain, ponders. In a word, all the functions of body and of soul are performed by the soul during sleep. (*Regimen* 4.86)

The author of *Regimen* 4 classifies these physiological dreams according to their content: routine daily activities (88), celestial and meteorological phenomena (89), earthly phenomena and activities (90), clothing (91), visions of the dead (92), and a final grouping (93) of monsters (ἀλλόμορφα σώματα), eating and drinking, familiar or fearful objects, fighting, being goaded or bound, travel, crossing rivers, soldiers, enemies, and, once again to close the ring, monsters (τέρατα ἀλλόμορφα). The author also knows that dreams may be caused by anxiety,[16] that they may contain the *Tagesreste* or "remains of the day,"[17] and that

---

[15] To the list at Harris, *Dreams and Experience*, p. 243 and note 75, add perhaps *Sacred Disease* 17, where the brain is said to give rise to δείματα καὶ φόβοι ... τὰ μὲν νύκτωρ, τὰ δὲ καὶ μεθ' ἡμέρην. In what follows I owe much and add little to Harris' exemplary presentation.

[16] *Regimen* 4.89: ὁκόσα δὲ τούτων [sc. celestial bodies] πλανᾶται ἄλλοις ἄλλως, ψυχῆς τάραξίν τινα σημαίνει ὑπὸ μερίμνης.

[17] *Regimen* 4.88: ὁκόσα τῶν ἐνυπνίων τὰς ἡμερινὰς πρήξιας τοῦ ἀνθρώπου ἢ διανοίας ἐς τὴν εὐφρόνην ἀποδίδωσι κατὰ τρόπον γινομένας ὥσπερ τῆς ἡμέρας ἐπρήχθη ἢ ἐβουλεύθη ἐπὶ δικαίῳ.

they can jumble or confuse normal, quotidian events.[18] Over all these categories and descriptions he imposes his master dichotomy, according to which dreams either reflect normal or usual events, in which case they declare a healthy state, or are the opposite, in which case they indicate some unhealthy condition. In such cases, he will recommend a change of diet or exercise to restore health, sometimes adding a conjecture about the somatic cause. The following is a typical example:

> When any one of the heavenly bodies appears to be disfigured, to disappear, or to be arrested in its revolution, if it be through mist or cloud, the malign influence is comparatively weak; if through rain also or hail, the influence is more powerful. In any case it is indicated that a moist and phlegm-like secretion, arising in the body, has fallen to the outer circuit. It is beneficial for this man to make his runs long, wearing his cloak the while, to increase them gradually, that he may perspire as freely as possible, and after exercise to take long walks; luncheon should be left out. Reduce food by one-third, and take five days in gradually resuming the normal quantity. (*Regimen* 4.89)

Although *Regimen* 4 offers the most extensive treatment of diagnostic dreams in the Hippocratic Corpus, its view of them seems to differ from other Hippocratic works in one important respect. Elsewhere in the Corpus, dreams are treated as diagnostic or prognostic signs; when causes are given, they are exclusively somatic. "From the brain and from the brain only," says *Sacred Disease* (17), "arise our pleasures, joys, laughter and jests, as well as our sorrows, pains, griefs and tears ... It is the same thing which makes us mad or delirious, inspires us with dread and fear, whether by night or by day." When the body can no longer cope with a surfeit, according to *Regimen* 3.71, it secretes a substance which disturbs the soul and leads to troubled sleep and dreams, "for as the experiences of the body are, so are the visions of the soul when sight is cut off." *Regimen* 4, however, retreats from this robust materialism to allow that some dreams have supernatural causes. Its author distinguishes god-sent or divine dreams (ὁκόσα τῶν ἐνυπνίων θεῖά ἐστι, 4.87) from those in which the soul reveals maladies of the body (ὁκόσα ἡ ψυχὴ τοῦ σώματος παθήματα προσημαίνει, 4.87). He

[18] *Regimen* 4.88: ὅταν δὲ πρὸς τὰς ἡμερινὰς πρήξιας ὑπεναντιῶται τὰ ἐνύπνια. It may be anachronistic to see in this passage, as Harris (*Dreams and Experience*, p. 245) does, a reference to the "bizarreness" that modern experts view as an essential characteristic of the dream-world; the author is thinking of his fundamental contrast (see above) between dreams that reflect the everyday and dreams that are in some way opposed to it, and the "*tarache* (disorder or confusion)" that Harris cites refers to a somatic condition (σημαίνει τάραχον ἐν τῷ σώματι, 4.88), not a feature of the dream.

is willing to consider the possibility that religious rites and prayer may play a role in healing. If a dream appears to be contrary to some act of the dreamer, he makes no judgment about whether apotropaic rites are in order, but does advise treatment of the body.[19] He recommends prayers to specific deities in certain cases (*Regimen* 4.89) and he ends his work with an acknowledgement that he has finished it with the help of the gods.

No other Hippocratic treatise speaks of dreams as anything other than diagnostic or prognostic signs of physical conditions or mental states. This resolutely secular view should not be passed over without some wonderment. The Hippocratic Corpus, as we have seen, has a good deal to say about dreams and their relationship to the practice of healing. Nowhere in it do we find an example of perhaps the most commonly reported ancient dream: the epiphany or "audio-visual dream-vision proper."[20] Yet surely more than a few people had, or believed that they had had, dreams like the one seen by Eudemus the Cypriot, who dreamed while he was ill that a beautiful young man told him that he would recover.[21] Physicians must have encountered reports of such dreams, and not only as stories out of the shrines of Asclepius. For Hippocratic medicine, though, epiphany dreams and all god-sent visions in sleep belong to a different *tekhnê*, one from which they sought to distance themselves as they struggled to define and defend their own art.

Epiphany dreams about the body, its maladies, and their cures characterized the cult of Asclepius. It is not necessary to imagine, as scholars once did, that the great centers of the cult at Epidaurus, Kos, Lebena, and elsewhere[22] were the homes of a "temple medicine" or that Asclepius and the physicians were locked in a professional rivalry to recognize the tension that led physician and devotee to keep each other at a respectful distance.[23] But because both kinds of practitioner

---

19 *Regimen* 4.88: περὶ μὲν οὖν τῆς πρήξιος εἴτ' ἀποτρέπειν δεῖ εἴτε μή, οὐ κρίνω. His attitude recalls the Greek fisherman's proverb about prayers to keep rats away: "Call the priest—but get a cat."

20 The phrase is from J.S. Hanson, "Dreams and Visions in the Graeco-Roman World and Early Christianity," in W. Haase and H. Temporini (eds), *Aufstieg und Niedergang der römischen Welt* (Berlin, 1980), part II, vol. 23.2, pp. 1395–427.

21 Cicero, *On Divination* 1.53.

22 A recent compendium lists 171 sites where Asclepius was worshiped in mainland Greece and 732 elsewhere in the Mediterranean world: J. Reithmüller, *Asklepios: Heiligtümer und Kulte* (Heidelberg, 2005). On Epidaurus in particular, see R.A. Tomlinson, *Epidauros* (Austin, 1983).

23 For the cooperative relationship between at least some physicians and the worship of Asclepius, and an exploration of the attitude of *Sacred Disease*, see Nutton, *Ancient Medicine,* pp. 111–14; and B. Wickkiser, *Asklepios, Medicine, and the Politics of Healing in Fifth-Century Greece* (Baltimore, 2008), pp. 53–61.

faced the need to look into the future of illness, dreams became a point of uneasy contact between the god and the doctors. Hippocratic authors, as we have seen, say nothing about epiphany dreams and, in at least the case of *Regimen* 4, make a clear distinction between dreams that are useful in medical prognosis and divine dreams that might foretell the future in other ways. For the writers of Asclepius, on the other hand, narrating the wonders of their god meant using some of the techniques and forms of their secular colleagues in healing.

Just as no one knows who wrote any Hippocratic treatise or can be certain when the Corpus was collected in its present form, so the authors and compilers of the most extensive document of Asclepian healing before Aelius Aristides remain anonymous. But at some point, probably before the end of the fourth century BC, someone inscribed four large stelae of grey limestone with a collection of case histories entitled "The Cures of Apollo and Asclepius" and set them up in the sanctuary at Epidaurus.[24] I now turn to these texts, and in particular to what they say about dreams in healing, in the hope of understanding their relationship to the Hippocratics' ideas on the same subject.

There were originally more than four stelae; Pausanias, in the second century AD, saw six but had reason to believe that there had formerly been more.[25] The four that survive contain 70 short narratives. On these stelae are inscribed, as Pausanias says, "the names of both the men and the women who have been healed by Asclepius, the disease also from which each suffered, and how he was healed." Pausanias' itemization requires some qualification. Most of the narratives do indeed begin with a name, but seven of the 20 cases on Stela A are anonymous, as are at least two of the 23 on Stela B. Both men and women are represented, although not equally. Three of the 20 cases on Stela A and eight of the 23 on Stela B are women. Fewer names survive on Stela C, but three of those that do are feminine. Not every miracle involves healing; the god could, for example, mend a broken goblet (*iama* 10) or find a lost boy (*iama* 24).[26]

---

[24] The stelae were published as *Inscriptiones Graecae* IV^2, 1, nos. 121–4, followed by R. Herzog, *Die Wunderheilungen von Epidauros: Ein Beitrag zur Geschichte der Medizin und der Religion* (Leipzig, 1931). For further publication history and textual controversy, see L.R. LiDonnici, "Compositional Background of the Epidaurian IAMATA,'" *American Journal of Philology*, 113 (1992): pp. 25–41, especially p. 25, note 5.

[25] As C. Habicht (*Pausanias' Guide to Ancient Greece* [Berkeley, 1985], p. 155), notes, Pausanias read the tablets carefully.

[26] Did the author think of "healing" the goblet as something that the god would naturally do? The original publication of these texts, *Inscriptiones Graecae* IV^2, 1, nos. 121–4, gave each case history a number, and I will refer to them by this "*iama* number," sometimes with a preceding letter A–D to indicate the stela on which it is found.

The original editor of these texts assumed that they were the work of priests of Asclepius at Epidaurus,[27] and there has never been any cause to challenge that assumption. It seems reasonable to speak of a compiler or compilers rather than an author, and to suppose that the *iamata* were collected during the monumentalizing expansion of the sanctuary in the late fourth century BC.[28] At least some of the narratives drew on earlier votive offerings and inscriptions; *iama* A1, for example, quotes the metrical inscription on a *pinax* set up by a woman named Kleo after an unusually long pregnancy.[29] In one case, *iama* A15, a separate inscription in the first person (*Inscriptiones Graecae* IV^2, 1, no. 125), records the original votive and miraculous healing later summarized on the stele.

The Epidaurian *iamata* reveal many of the same narrative impulses and forms that underlie the case histories of the Hippocratic *Epidemics*. The affinities between the Epidaurian texts and *Epidemics* 5 and 7 seem especially strong and extend to style.[30] In both documents, cases often begin, as Pausanias says, with the name of the sufferer and the complaint presented for healing:

> Aristippus was severely wounded by being shot in the upper belly by an arrow. Terrible pain in the intestine. It was quickly inflamed ... (*Epidemics* 7.98)

> Gorgias of Heracleia with pus. In a battle he had been wounded by an arrow in the lung and for a year and a half had suppurated so badly that he filled sixty-seven basins with pus. (*Inscriptiones Graecae* IV^2, 1, no. 122 [*iama* 30])

Both texts, too, are concerned to establish the validity of their particular mode of healing against skepticism or rival methods. Several of the Epidaurian cases recount the conversion of skeptics by Asclepius:

> A man whose fingers, with the exception of one, were paralyzed, came as a suppliant to the god. While looking at the tablets in the temple he expressed incredulity regarding the cures and scoffed at the inscription. But in his sleep he saw a vision. It seemed to him that, as he was playing at dice below the Temple and was about to cast the dice, the god appeared, sprang upon his hand, and stretched

27 H. von Gaertringen (*Inscriptiones Graecae* IV^2, 1, p. 70) refers to *illas magnas tabulas a sacerdotibus compositas.*

28 LiDonnici, "Compositional Background," p. 29.

29 Οὐ μέγεθος πίνακος θαυμαστέον, ἀλλὰ τὸ θεῖον, / πένθ' ἔτη ὡς ἐκύησε ἐγ γαστρὶ Κλεὼ βάρος, ἔστε / ἐγκατεκοιμάθη καὶ μιν ἔθηκε ὑγιῆ, two hexameters and a pentameter.

30 R. Nehrbass, *Sprache und Stil der Iamata von Epidauros, Philologus* Supplementband 27(4) (1935): pp. 78–9.

> out his [the patient's] fingers. When the god had stepped aside it seemed to him that he bent his hand and stretched out all his fingers one by one. When he had straightened them all, the god asked him if he would still be incredulous of the inscriptions on the tablets in the Temple. He answered that he would not. "Since, therefore, formerly you were incredulous of the cures, though they were not incredible, for the future," he said, "your name shall be 'Incredulous.'" When day dawned he walked out sound. (*Inscriptiones Graecae* IV^2, 1, no. 121 [*iama* 3])

This case occupies a prominent position as the third on Stela A, which bears the introductory formula Θεός/Τύχα ἀγαθά and the title of the whole collection, Ἰάματα τοῦ Ἀπόλλωνος καὶ τοῦ Ἀσκλαπιοῦ. It serves as an introduction to the collection by modeling for readers how to read the texts before them. The anonymous man with paralyzed fingers is prompted to incredulity not by hearing tales of wondrous cures but specifically by reading inscribed narratives like the one in which he appears. The first case, Kleo's five-year pregnancy, incorporates the text of her votive offering; the third case instructs viewers on how to read that text and the other inscriptions with which the sanctuary was littered.[31]

Books 5 and 7 of the Hippocratic *Epidemics* have been less studied than the canonical first and third books. Early editors, eager to distinguish "genuine" works of Hippocrates from later accretions to the corpus, found *Epidemics* 5 and 7 to lack the stylistic unity and scientific bent of 1 and 3; as such, they judged, 5 and 7 must be later works, perhaps by Hippocrates' descendants. *Epidemics* 5 and 7 have seemed rhetorically more elaborate than other books in the collection, and both books show a fondness for circumstantial characterization and a willingness to introduce the author's opinion of other physicians' treatments:

> In Larissa Hipposthenes seemed to the physicians to have peripleumonia. But that was not it. (*Epidemics* 5.14)

> Tychon, at the siege of Datum, was struck in the chest by a catapult, and shortly later there was around him raucous laughter. The physician who removed the wood seemed to me to leave the iron in the diaphragm. (*Epidemics* 7.121)

This latter passage and its counterpart at 5.95 happen to be the only occurrences of the phrase ἐδόκει δέ μοι that I have found in the *Epidemics*, but it is striking that of the 34 occurrences of ἐδόκει in *Epidemics*, 25 are found in Book 7. Book 5 in particular offers a number of judgments on other physicians' treatments,

---

31 On the Epidaurian *iamata* as instructional texts for worshipers, see M.P.J. Dillon, "The Didactic Nature of the Epidaurian Iamata," *Zeitschrift für Papyrologie und Epigraphik*, 101 (1994): pp. 239–60.

often in the form of counterfactual statements like this one from *Epidemics* 5.7 on a patient who suffered as much from repeated bloodlettings and purges as from the infection that they were intended to treat:

> He died a few days after that, from the size and number of the wounds and from weakness of his body. It would appear that, if there had been a single incision adequate for drainage and the pus had been drawn toward the incision and, if another incision had been needed, one adequate for drainage had been cut: if this had been done to him at the right time, it seems that he would have become healthy.

In both the Epidaurian *iamata* and *Epidemics* 5 and 7, then, appear modes of medical discourse typical of the intellectual climate of the fifth and fourth centuries. Both sets of texts collect case histories, often with named patient and diagnosis, and both texts stake out a position against other views, against skepticism in the case of the Epidaurian text and against different modes of treatment in *Epidemics* 5 and 7. I am tempted to add that both seek to uncover the working of general influences on local conditions of healing; what climate and weather are to the *Epidemics*, Apollo and Asclepius are to the Epidaurian texts. The gods are the sacred weather of their places.

This common ground only serves to highlight the differences between the two sets of texts and the way in which they engage each other. Just as the Hippocratic writings on prognosis sought to distance themselves from the other prognostic art of divination, so the Hippocratic case histories take pains to distinguish their methods from those of the miracle texts that resemble them in so many ways. Once again, dreams become a crucial point of distinction.

One or two cases in *Epidemics* 5 seem to respond to the kind of narrative inscribed at Epidaurus. In one, the Epidaurian elements of sleep and a snake combine in an unsettling, and ultimately fatal, way:

> A youth who had drunk much undiluted wine was sleeping on his back in a tent. A shining snake went into his mouth. When he felt it, unable to consider what to do, he ground his teeth together and bit off part of the snake. He was seized by a great pain and brought up his hands as though choking, tossed himself about, and died in convulsions. (*Epidemics* 5.86)

With this may be contrasted *Inscriptiones Graecae* IV^2, 1, no. 121 (*iama* 17):

> A man had his toe healed by a serpent. He, suffering dreadfully from a malignant sore in his toe, during the daytime was taken outside by the servants of the Temple

> and set upon a seat. When sleep came upon him, then a snake issued from the Abaton and healed the toe with its tongue, and thereafter went back again to the Abaton.

It is not necessary to suppose that the author of *Epidemics* 5 was parodying this specific text; serpents figured prominently in the iconography of Asclepius, they appear in other healing narrative and on votive tablets, and, as Pausanias (2.28.1) says, one especially tame kind was peculiar to Epidaurus. Yet there are grounds to suggest that *Epidemics* 5 and 7 are at least in dialogue with the Epidaurian *iamata*, or with similar, perhaps orally transmitted, narratives of Asclepian healing.

Another case from *Epidemics* 5 employs sleep and a sudden cure—elements of the Epidaurian narratives—but in this case there is no dream, no god, and no miracle:

> Eumelus of Larissa grew rigid in his legs, arms, and jaws. He could not extend them or bend them unless someone else extended or bent them, nor open his jaws unless someone else opened them. But no other symptoms. He had no pain and he did not eat, except barley cakes, and he drank honey water. On the twentieth day he fell backwards while sitting and severely struck his head on a stone, and darkness poured over him. Shortly later he stood up and was better. All was relaxed except that when he wakened after sleep his joints were slightly bound. (*Epidemics* 5.23)

Rudolph Nehrbass notes a number of parallels in language between this case and the Epidaurian *iamata*.[32] Some may be due to coincidence of subject matter, but collectively they strengthen a case for dialogue between the texts. Both *Epidemics* 5.23 and 5.86 show the author of *Epidemics* 5 responding to Asclepian case histories in the conflict for authority over healing.[33]

Hippocratic authors, as we have seen, focused on dreams as a point of differentiation between their prognostic art and *mantikê*. Because dreams are

---

32 Nehrbass, *Sprache und Stil*, p. 78.

33 I base this assertion on the assumption that a specialized text for a limited, professional audience, as I take the *Epidemics* to be, is more likely to be reflecting a public document like the Epidaurian texts than the opposite. Uncertainty over the relative dates of *Epidemics* 5 and 7 and the Epidaurian *iamata* makes complete confidence impossible. The *iamata* are usually placed in the second half of the fourth century, following H. von Gaertringen in *Inscriptiones Graecae* IV^2, 1, nos. 121–4. *Epidemics* 7.121 mentions the siege of Daton, assigned by K. Deichgräber, *Die Epidemien und das Corpus Hippocraticum* (Berlin, 1933), p. 145, to Philip of Macedon's Thracian campaigns of 358/357 BC.

characteristic of Asclepian case histories, the authors or compilers of Hippocratic case histories like those in *Epidemics* also used dreams to set their narratives, and thus their *tekhnê*, apart from its alternative. Although sleep, its manner, or its absence is of interest,[34] dreams generally do not figure in the Hippocratic narratives. Dreams are absent from the list of "things from the small tablet, to be observed" at *Epidemics* 6.8, 7 (vol. 5, 345–6 Littré) or the list at *Epidemics* 4.43. When they do appear, they appear as part of a complex of symptoms and play no role in healing or prognosis; at *Epidemics* 4.57, for example, the Hippocratic author carefully disconnects the dream from the fever that is the focus of interest:

> Nicippus had a wet dream [ἐξωνείρασε] in fever, and it made him no worse. The same thing repeatedly occurred and did not harm him. It was predicted that it would end when the fever reached crisis, and so it did. In the same way in a fever, Critias was upset by dreams that cause erections; he, too, stopped at the crisis.

In the sketchy notes at *Epidemics* 4.20, nightmare fevers (ἠπιαλώδεις) are merely listed as one among several symptoms occurring around the setting of the Pleiades. In the fourth century BC, the medical dream, predictive and diagnostic, became one point of distinction between Hippocratic medicine and other predictive *tekhnai*. The Epidaurian *iamata* and *Epidemics* 5 and 7 may reveal the dialogue through which Hippocratic physicians and Asclepian worshippers sharpened their sense of the differences between their healing practices.

[34] For example, *Epidemics* 7.2.

Chapter 5

Dream Hermeneutics in Aelius Aristides' *Hieroi Logoi*

Janet Downie

Introduction

The second-century AD *rhetor* Aelius Aristides is well known for his hypochondria—or, perhaps better, his valetudinarianism—and he was also a great dreamer. In the six discourses known collectively as the *Hieroi Logoi*, or "Sacred Tales," he offers a lengthy first-person account of his illness and divine healing. But the text is also filled with dozens of dream descriptions.[1] For, when he fell ill in the mid-140s AD, Asclepius began to prophesy to him, and Aristides spent two years at the god's sanctuary in Pergamum. This was just the beginning of a long-term relationship with Asclepius, whom he eventually credited with sustaining him over decades of fluctuating health and professional challenges.[2] The primary medium of this relationship, both within the temple and beyond, was dreams.

Aristides' dream narratives in the *Hieroi Logoi* (hereinafter *HL*) should certainly be read in the context of the Asclepian healing cult. At the same time, however, his engagement with dreams goes well beyond the votive conventions that we know from inscriptional evidence. Combining theophany with medical prescription and myriad personal details, Aristides creates complex, shifting

[1] I would like to thank Yelena Baraz, Anton Bierl, Michael Flower, and David Jenkins for reading drafts of this chapter, as well as Christopher Faraone, Shadi Bartsch, and Elizabeth Asmis for feedback on earlier versions of the material. I would also like to thank Steven Oberhelman for his help with the editorial process. The faults that remain, of course, are my own.

See B. Keil (ed.), *Aelii Aristidis Smyrnaei Quae supersunt omnia* (2 vols, Berlin, 1898), vol. 2, pp. 376–466. Of the sixth discourse, only the first 14 lines of text are extant. The *Hieroi Logoi* have been translated into English by C. Behr, *Aelius Aristides: Complete Works* (2 vols, Leiden, 1986), vol. 2, pp. 278–353; cf. C. Behr, *Aelius Aristides and the Sacred Tales* (Amsterdam, 1968).

[2] He offers a synopsis of his debts to the god in the *Lalia to Asclepius* (*Or.* 42) composed in the late 170s AD, some time after the *Hieroi Logoi*.

dreamscapes that expose the hermeneutic challenge and the sense-making power of dream interpretation.[3] Aristides' dream accounts are rhetorically unique in the ancient evidence, and in the *HL*, I suggest, he finds his own use for the medical dream.[4] Therefore, while accepting the premise that Aristides' dreams mattered to him in his real-life pursuit of health and professional success, we should also consider why he gives these narratives the texture they have in this account composed for publication and posterity. Part of the answer, I suggest, is that Aristides was interested in the conjectural process of interpretation and saw profit in appropriating the hermeneutic scenarios of dream divination and medicine for his own self-portrait as an inspired *rhetor*.

In what follows, I begin by examining the language and syntax of Aristides' dream accounts, in order to highlight what sets his dream text apart from other sources on ancient dreaming in the votive context of temple healing. I then consider two episodes of interpretive failure early on in the *HL* that show Aristides' awareness of technical hermeneutic traditions, both medical and divinatory. By describing these episodes of interpretive failure, I suggest that Aristides exposes the uncertainty inherent in conjectural interpretation that is generally obscured by more systematic and theoretical writers on dreams, including his contemporaries Artemidorus and Galen. In the process, he opens up the dream as a space for narrative invention, and so he is able to turn the language of dream theory to his own ends of self-presentation. Doing this under the general aegis of the votive dream, moreover, he can claim divine endorsement for the dreamscapes he elaborates.

Aristides' Dream Language

At the outset of *HL* I, Aristides leads his readers to expect something like an aretalogical account of divine healing oriented toward praise of the god to whom he has entrusted himself "as to a doctor" (1.4). Therefore, when his dreams quickly take over the narrative, it seems natural to place the text within the commemorative tradition of temple incubation.[5] He alludes to places and

---

[3] See the extensive discussion of Behr, *Sacred Tales*, Chapter 8 and Appendix 3, with S.M. Oberhelman, "Dreams in Graeco-Roman Medicine," in W. Haase and H. Temporini (eds), *Aufstieg und Niedergang der Römischen Welt* (Berlin, 1993), part II, vol. 37.1, pp. 121–56, at p. 154.

[4] On the arbitrary nature of the term "medical dream," see Pearcy's chapter in this volume.

[5] See, for example, E.J. Edelstein and L. Edelstein, *Asclepius: A Collection and Interpretation of the Testimonies*, (2 vols, Baltimore, 1945); and A. Petsalis-Diomidis, *Truly*

practices of incubation in the Pergamene Asclepieion,[6] occasionally describes divine epiphanies,[7] and uses the language of divine prescription familiar from ancient votive inscriptions, as Asclepius "commands" and "clearly indicates" various therapeutic actions.[8]

The votive tradition in the temple context brings dreams and medicine into close proximity, but it also simplifies their relationship by eliding hermeneutic activity. Fourth-century BC inscriptions from Epidaurus, for example, present a direct encounter between human and divine that seems to need no interpretation, as dreams themselves are the vehicle for episodes of miraculous healing—sore toes, paralyzed fingers, diseased eyes, and infestations of leeches are reported to have been healed while the patients slept and dreamed their cure.[9] Even when the dream relationship between incubant and god is described in prescriptive rather than miraculous terms, any process of interpretation is omitted as irrelevant to the thanksgiving agenda of the votive context. In a second-century AD votive from Epidaurus, for example, one Marcus Iulius Apellas simply catalogs the god's instructions pertaining to dress, diet, and exercise, along with other direct (if obscure) prescriptions "to take lemon peels, to soak them in water, near the (spot of the) *akoai* in the bath to press against the wall,"[10] and another Imperial-era patient at Pergamum records similarly dietetic injunctions without offering any account of the interpretive process that may have linked divine vision to medical procedure.[11] While styles of commemoration vary over time, and between personal dedications and collective accounts, the emphasis is almost always on successful healing. The closing phrase of Apellas' Imperial-era votive, "full of gratitude, I departed healthy,"[12] echoes the earlier Epidaurian miracle

Beyond Wonders: Aelius Aristides and the Cult of Asklepios (Oxford, 2010), who situates Aristides in the temple complex at Pergamum.

6 At 2.71, for example, he mentions sleeping at the lattice gates of the temple and refers to the sacred well of the temple precinct.

7 He describes three epiphanies of Asclepius (1.71, 2.18, 2.31–3); cf. 2.41 for an epiphany of Athena.

8 Aristides' first contact with Asclepius is by way of a divine command: *epetaxe* (2.7). For other compounds of *tattein*, compare: 1.6, 2.48, 2.59, 2.75, 2.78, 3.9, 3.34, 4.30 (*prostattein*); 1.57, 2.45, 2.47, 2.82, 3.7, 3.27, 4.38, 5.49 (*epitattein*). In the first line of the fragmentary *HL* 6, Aristides writes that the god "directed him" (*diêgen*) and "gave him signs" (*sêmainôn*); cf. 1.66, 2.15, 3.11, 4.39, 4.71, 4.97, 5.1.

9 See L.R. LiDonnici, *The Epidaurian Miracle Inscriptions: Text, Translation and Commentary* (Atlanta, 1995); and B. Wickkiser, *Asclepius, Medicine, and the Politics of Healing in Fifth-Century Greece: Between Craft and Cult* (Baltimore, 2008), Chapter 3.

10 *IG* IV^2, 1, no. 126.

11 H. Müller, "Ein Heilungsbericht aus dem Asklepieion," *Chiron*, 17 (1987): pp. 192–233.

12 *IG* IV^2, 1, no. 126: χάριν εἰδὼς καὶ ὑγιὴς γενόμενος ἀπηλλάγην.

inscriptions and, more generally, the whole tradition of *kat' onar* dedications, which consistently valorize divine agency and positive result, while downplaying human engagement in the process of interpretation and implementation.[13]

Aristides' dream accounts, by contrast, are far from simple. While they convey messages from the god, most of them are so full of detail that the divine message becomes obscure. Much of the first *Logos*, especially, which deals with one of Aristides' recent phases of illness, reads like a sequential dream diary of nighttime visions:[14] "Each of our days, as well as our nights, has a story," he says in the Proemium of *HL* I, "if someone wished either to record the events [*apographein*] one by one or to narrate [*diêgeisthai*] the providence [*pronoia*] of the god ..."[15] But the relationship between record (*apographê*) and narration (*diêgêsis*) is complicated. In the Prooemium of *HL* II, he explains that the present composition (*suggraphê*) is a free-form revision of the original diary record (*apographê*), begun some 27 years earlier at the start of his contact with Asclepius. He now seeks to fill out these bare details with an account of the circumstances and outcomes of his dreams (2.2).[16] Owing to the profusion of the god's deeds, as well as the loss of many of his records, he is compelled to speak "in summary fashion" (*kephalaia legein*, 2.4), in a retrospective account. Whether the diary portion of *HL* I is in fact closer to the elusive *apographê* than other

---

[13] Compare the closing formula common in the Epidaurian accounts, "when day came, he departed healthy" (ἁμέρας δὲ γενομένας ὑγιὴς ἐξῆλθε) at, for example, *stelai* 1.3, 1.4, 1.8, 1.18, 2.28, 2.32 and 2.38 (*IG* IV^2, 1, nos. 121–2). Evidence for the *kat' onar* tradition is surveyed in F.T. van Straten, "Daikrates' Dream: A Votive Relief from Kos and Some Other *Kat'onar* Dedications," *Bulletin Antieke Beschaving*, 51 (1976): pp. 1–26; and G.H. Renberg, "Dream-Narratives and Unnarrated Dreams in Greek and Latin Dedicatory Inscriptions," in E. Scioli and C. Walde (eds), *Sub Imagine Somni: Nighttime Phenomena in Greco-Roman Culture* (Pisa, 2010), pp. 33–62. On the aretalogical agenda of votive inscriptions, see M.P.J. Dillon, "The Didactic Nature of the Epidaurian Iamata," *ZPE*, 104 (1994): pp. 239–60.

[14] The "diary" portion of *HL* I runs from 1.4 to 1.60. Behr dates the oneiric events of the diary to 166 AD, five years prior (cf. 1.59) to the date he hypothesizes for the composition of all six *Logoi* (Behr, *Sacred Tales* and "Studies on the Biography of Aelius Aristides," in W. Haase and H. Temporini [eds], *Aufstieg und Niedergang der Römischen Welt* [Berlin, 1994], part II, vol. 34.2, pp. 1140–233).

[15] 1.3: ἑκάστη γὰρ τῶν ἡμετέρων ἡμερῶν, ὡσαύτως δὲ καὶ νυκτῶν, ἔχει συγγραφὴν, εἴ τις παρ ἓν, ἢ τὰ συμπίπτοντα ἀπογράφειν ἠβούλετο, ἢ τὴν τοῦ θεοῦ πρόνοιαν διηγεῖσθαι ...

[16] By blurring the relationship between the present composition and the original *apographê*, Aristides makes a calculated bid for narrative authority, as discussed by L.T. Pearcy in his "Theme, Dream, and Narrative: Reading the *Sacred Tales* of Aelius Aristides," *Transactions of the American Philological Association*, 118 (1988): pp. 377–91. On the term *suggraphê*, see V. Pirenne-Delforge, *Retour à la Source: Pausanias et la Religion Grecque* (Liège, 2008), pp. 21–40.

parts of the text, we cannot know.[17] Certainly, however, it displays in heightened fashion Aristides' interest in tangling with the hermeneutic problems of dreams in a narrative context.

In *HL* I and the subsequent *Logoi*, Aristides preserves all the hesitations characteristic of attempts to capture the dream world in human language: vacillation of identity; unaccountable shifts in space and time; scenarios that are opaque and can be described only approximately, or in hypothetical terms; and a permeable boundary between account and explanation.[18] Many of these

---

[17] S. Nicosia ("L'Autobiografia onirica di Elio Aristide," in G. Guidorizzi [ed.], *Il Sogno in Grecia* [Rome, 1988], pp. 173–90) suggests that the diary portion of *HL* I (*HL* 1.5–58) has undergone little "secondary elaboration" by comparison with dream narratives in the other *Logoi* (pp. 181–2); compare the similar view of W.V. Harris, *Dreams and Experience in Classical Antiquity* (Cambridge, MA, 2009), pp. 118–22. The "raw" appearance of Aristides' dream narratives is a premise of the psychoanalytic study by G. Michenaud and J. Dierkins, *Les Rêves dans les "Discours Sacrés" d'Aelius Aristide* (Mons, 1972) and of other studies that take a less clinical approach, including D. Gigli, "Stile e linguaggio onirico nei *Discorsi sacri* di Elio Aristide," *Cultura e Scuola*, 61–2 (1977): pp. 214–24; and D. Del Corno, "I sogni e la loro interpretazione nell'età dell'impero," in W. Haase and H. Temporini (eds), *Aufstieg und Niedergang der Römischen Welt* (Berlin, 1978), part II, vol. 16.2, pp. 1605–18. Most radically, T. Dorandi ("Il Diario dei sogni di Elio Aristide: Per una interpretazione del primo *Discorso Sacro* [47 Keil]," *Segno e Testo*, 3 [2005]: pp. 51–69) speculates that *HL* I is closely based on Aristides' actual dream records, written up for publication only later by an unknown imitator. I prefer the hypothesis of M.-H. Quet ("Parler de soi pour louer son dieu: le cas d'Aelius Aristide," in M.-F. Baslez, P. Hoffman, and L. Pernot [eds], *L'invention de l'autobiographie d'Hésiode à saint Augustin* [Paris, 1993], pp. 211–51), who sees Aristides' editorial hand in *HL* I. She maintains that the diary of 166 AD is distinct from the original dream *apographê* and, importantly, was "chosen and perhaps conceived for publication" by Aristides himself (p. 220; my translation).

[18] Vacillation of identity: dreaming that he is at the shrine of Asclepius in the gymnasium in Smyrna, Aristides sees a statue that seems, at one moment, to be a statue of himself and at another moment a statue of Asclepius (1.17). Shifts in space and time: the dream scene shifts abruptly from somewhere near the Warm Springs to the Smyrnean agora (1.22); cf. other examples at *HL* 1.18, 1.43, and 1.44, and see the comments by Del Corno, "I sogni," pp. 1617–18. These features are especially prominent in *HL* I, but they are by no means limited to this part of the text. Gigli ("Stile e linguaggio," pp. 19–20) finds other syntactic markers of dream language in the *HL* more generally: highly paratactic sentence structure with little logical subordination, temporal markers of succession and simultaneity, and expressions ("as if," "as it were") by which Aristides attempts to qualify and define more precisely the scenes he describes. For Harris (*Dreams and Experience*, pp. 65–6, 118–22), Aristides' dreams typify the episodic, as opposed to the epiphanic, dream account. See also W.V. Harris, "Insomnia: The Content of Roman Dreams," in W.V. Harris and E. Lo Cascio (eds), *Noctes Campanae: Studi di storia antica ed archeologia dell'Italia preromana e romana in memoria di Martin W. Frederiksen* (Naples, 2005), pp. 245–61.

narrative and syntactic features are on display in the following example (*HL* 1.26):

> πέμπτῃ ἐφαίνετο μὲν τὸ ἱερὸν τοῦ Ἀπόλλωνος τὸ ἐν τῷ ὄρει τῷ Μιλύᾳ· ἐδόκει δὲ οἰκήματα ἄττα προσγεγενῆσθαι, καὶ ὄνομα εἶναι τῷ χωρίῳ Ἐλεφαντίνη ἀπὸ Ἐλεφαντίνης τῆς ἐν Αἰγύπτῳ· ἔχαιρον δὴ καὶ κατ' αὐτὰ τὰ οἰκήματα καὶ κατὰ τὴν οἰκειότητα τοῦ τόπου τῷ τόπῳ. καὶ δὴ καὶ ἱερέα εἶναι τοῦ θεοῦ τὸν τῆς Ἴσιδος τῆς ἐν Σμύρνῃ ἱερέα, παρ' ᾧπερ καὶ κατάγεσθαι, καὶ ἐνθυμεῖσθαι πρὸς ἐμαυτὸν ὅτι πολλά μοι πρὸς αὐτὸν οἰκεῖα ὑπάρχοι ἐκ πολλοῦ· καί τι καὶ τυγχάνειν παρ' αὐτοῦ πρόσθεν ἐωνημένος, ἔπειτα ὑπόλοιπόν τι ἔχων ἐθέλειν ἀλλάξασθαι. κἀκ τούτου δὴ ἐδόκουν εἰπεῖν τινὰ κοιφὶ μετὰ οἴνου· λαβεῖν τε δὴ εὐθὺς αὐτὸ ὡς ἴαμα καὶ σκοπεῖν εἴτε τῷ προσώπῳ δέοι προσθέσθαι εἴτε καὶ τοῖς ἐντός. καί τινος εἰπόντος ὅτι ἐπικάοι ὅπου ἐπιτεθείη, ἐνθυμηθῆναι ὡς ἐπιτηδείως ἔχοι παντὸς μᾶλλον ψύξεως εἶναι φάρμακον. καί πως ἐκ τούτων εἰπεῖν πρὸς τὸν ἱερέα ὅτι δῆλον ἦν ἐξ ὧν ἀνεγίγνωσκον ὅτι οὐχὶ δεήσοι φαγεῖν. καὶ δῆτα εὐθὺς εἶχον ἐν νῷ ὡς διατελέσων ἄσιτος τὴν ἡμέραν· ἠσίτησα δή.
>
> On the fifth day, the temple of Apollo appeared [in a dream], the one on Mount Milyas. But I dreamed that some buildings had been added, and that the name of the place was Elephantine, from the Elephantine in Egypt. And I rejoiced, indeed, both on account of the buildings themselves and on account of the similarity of the one place to the other. And moreover, [I dreamed] that the priest of the god was the priest of the Isis in Smyrna, with whom [I dreamed] I was staying and [I dreamed] that I thought to myself that I had been very friendly with him for a long time. And that I happened to have bought something from him earlier on, and that since I had something left over, I wanted to make an exchange. And after this I dreamed that someone said "*kuphi* with wine," and that straight away I took it as a remedy and considered whether I should apply it to my face or internally. And when someone said that it would burn where it was placed, [I dreamed] that I thought that it would be especially suitable as a remedy for cold. And somehow after this [I dreamed] I said to the priest that it was clear from what I learned that it would be necessary not to eat. And indeed straight away I had in mind that I would finish the day without eating. And I did.[19]

As is usual in the *HL*, the dream narrative is presented in indirect speech, and Aristides uses standard verbs to introduce the account: the first, ἐφαίνετο (the temple of Apollo appeared), perhaps gives more autonomy to the dreamscape, while the second, ἐδόκει (it seemed), heightens the sense of the dream as an active mental process on the part of the dreamer.[20] Indeed, the dream

19 Translations from the *HL* are my own.

20 The verb *dokeô* is the most common introductory verb for dream accounts, in the *HL* as well as in the ancient evidence more generally. See Behr, *Sacred Tales*, p. 191; J.S. Hanson,

description features a drama of interpretation: in an exchange that resembles a medical consultation, two unidentified interlocutors offer hints about a healing substance—*kuphi* with wine.[21] Extrapolating from the dream-notion that this remedy would best be applied externally, and not consumed, Aristides takes the whole dream as a general injunction against ingesting food and decides to fast. The dream's prescriptive function thus works obliquely and at several levels. For, at another remove, his dream conversation with these unidentified interlocutors is set within the frame of an exchange with a priest, and the whole scene as it unfolds is richly ambiguous: known places of cult in Asia Minor and Egypt merge, furnished with new, imagined buildings and with personnel who reflect the cultural and geographic syncretism of the shifting dreamscape.

The uncertainty of the relationship between dream space and interpretive activity is marked in various ways syntactically. Perhaps the most disorienting feature of this vivid representation of the experience of dreaming is that it is almost impossible to tell where the dream itself begins and ends.[22] The dream appears to be launched with the first introductory expression, "there was a vision," so the second such expression, "it seemed," has a layering effect. Then, no sooner are we inside the space of the dream, but the indirect statement construction is interrupted by another finite verb ἔχαιρον (I rejoiced), which might be either a description of Aristides' affect in the dream (in which case the switch to direct speech marks vividness) or a description of Aristides' waking reflection on what he experienced in the dream. Breaking into direct speech, Aristides seems to blur the boundary between dream and reality.

The complexity of Aristides' Egyptian dream is typical of his accounts in the *HL*, but is unique among the evidence for ancient dreaming, and I suggest that the destabilizing syntax reflects Aristides' interest in problematizing interpretation. He leaves his dream pictures rough-edged and ambiguous, and

---

"Dreams and Visions in the Greco-Roman World and Early Christianity," in W. Haase and H. Temporini (eds), *Aufstieg und Niedergang der Römischen Welt* (Berlin, 1980), part II, vol. 23.2, pp. 1395–427, at p. 1409; and G. Björck, "ONAR IDEIN: De la perception de rêve chez les anciens," *Eranos*, 44 (1964): 306–14.

21 *Kuphi* is a kind of Egyptian incense, traditionally offered to the sun, as Behr explains (*Complete Works*, ad 1.26). See also the discussion in J. Scarborough, "Early Byzantine Pharmacology," *Dumbarton Oaks Papers*, 38 (1984): pp. 213–32, at pp. 229–32.

22 'Εδόκει is reinforced by ἐδόκουν midway through the account, on which subsequent infinitives depend. With the final action of the sentence, ᾐσίτησα δή, we are clearly outside the dream. Behr, in his *Aelius Aristides* and *Complete Works*, italicizes the second-to-last phrase, suggesting (as with ἔχαιρον) that it is part of the dream. This is quite plausible, although perhaps here even more than in the earlier instance, there is the possibility that Aristides reports a waking reflection. In my view, the ambiguity is deliberate. I am grateful to Professor Laurent Pernot for his thoughts on this feature of Aristides' syntax.

portrays dream material and interpretation as inextricably entwined. Thus, while the commemoration of divine healing is an important motivation for his text, Aristides departs from the conventions of aretalogy and commemoration, and instead gives his readers access to hermeneutic uncertainty. Indeed, as we shall see, he goes so far as to depict interpretive failure.

Interpretive Failure

In an oration *To Plato* (*Or.* 2), concerned with defending the art of rhetoric, Aristides draws a parallel between medicine and dream interpretation, as two examples of the conjectural nature of human *technê*. Dream interpreters, and mantic specialists more generally, he says, use reason to make sense of signs that are obscure and ambiguous. Like the physician who faces the challenge of piecing together disparate symptoms to understand his patient's condition and to make a prognosis, so too the mantic interpreter aims at forming a "likely picture" (*eikazein*) in response to whatever issue the enquirer has raised. In any conjectural venture, the question posed is crucial, for it sets the horizon of interpretation, as Aristides explains with reference to the mantic arts (*Or.* 2.167):

> εἰ γὰρ μὴ φράσαις τὸ ἐρώτημα, οὐδὲν ἔχει σοι λέγειν περὶ ὧν εἶδε σημείων ... οὐ γὰρ ἔγκειται τὰ πράγματα αὐτῷ προφαινόμενα, ἀλλὰ τὰς πίστεις τοῖς σημείοις προσάγων εἰκάζει πρὸς τὸν λόγον.

> If you should not state your question, the seer can tell you nothing about the signs he has seen ... For him, matters are not fixed and apparent in advance, but by relating a person's inquiries to the signs he forms a picture (*eikazein*) which has regard for reason [*logos*].[23]

He goes on to suggest that dream interpretation is paradigmatic of the picture-making quality of divination: seers interpret their material, Aristides says, "just like dreams" (*Or.* 2.168). Like mantic phenomena in general, night-visions present a bewildering mass of data, and every interpretive trajectory is crucially conditioned by the choice of a starting point. Only in retrospect can the dreamer and his interpreter collectively decide whether their "likely picture" was the right one.

To narrow the range of possibilities, ancient dreamers needed to determine what kind of dream they thought they had seen: "Is my dream prophetic, or

[23] Translation in Behr, *Complete Works*.

is it the result of poor digestion?" "Does the dream mean what it appears to mean, or was the vision allegorical?" "Are the details of my dream significant or a meaningless reiteration of waking preoccupations?" The temple context of the cult of Asclepius offered one interpretive framework for divine dreams, but outside the cult context, ancient interest in dream interpretation seems to have diverged along two main paths: the mantic and the medical. Oneirocritics, like Aristides' second-century contemporary Artemidorus, were mainly interested in predictive dreams of divine origin (*oneiroi*). Medical practitioners, on the other hand, were interested in just the kind of dream such oneirocritics dismissed: dreams believed to reflect the state of the body's humors and to offer no access to the divine realm of prophecy (*enhypnia*).

Artemidorus presents his *Oneirocritica* as a solution to problems of interpretation that attend specifically the "allegorical" subset of predictive dreams. In this vast taxonomy, he tracks dream symbols across a range of variables, observing how the status of the dreamer—gender, age, trade, state of health, geographical location, social position—appear to affect the meaning of a particular dream-detail.[24] To decode the gods' advice, an interpreter will need to position each dreamer as precisely as possible in relation to the patterns observable in the vast archive of past dreams. Often, however, Artemidorus acknowledges that there is no way of knowing whether an interpretation is correct until one has seen the dream fulfilled (4.24). The fundamentally conjectural nature of the enterprise is the reason for his immense effort of empirical research into "old dreams and their consequences" (1.proemium). His compendium includes some dreams symbolic of illness, but from the outset, he sets aside symptomatic dreams of a physical origin (1.1).

On the other side of the *oneiros/enhypnion* divide, medical writers are concerned precisely with symptomatic dreams that appear to signal the bodily state of the dreamer. The author of the essay on dreams transmitted as the Hippocratic *Regimen* 4 writes that when an individual is asleep, the soul sees and reveals what the body suffers (*Regimen* 3.71) and sets out to offer hermeneutic guidelines for interpreting these visions.[25] While he posits a different origin for dreams, along with a different set of questions to which they may provide answers, this anonymous medical author and others in the Hippocratic tradition nevertheless deploy a symbolic structure that mirrors schemes for interpreting

---

[24] On Artemidorus, see M. Foucault, *The Care of the Self* (New York, 1986), pp. 14–25; and S.R F. Price, "The Future of Dreams: From Freud to Artemidorus," *Past and Present*, 113 (1986): pp. 3–37, especially pp. 13–16.

[25] Ed. Littré, vol. 6, pp. 640–42 (E. Littré [ed.], *Hippocrate, Oeuvres complètes* [10 vols, Paris, 1839–1861]); cf. W.H.S. Jones, *Hippocrates* (4 vols, Cambridge, MA, 1931), vol. 4, pp. 420ff.

divine symbolic dreams.[26] But how does a physician decide that a given dream is prognostic rather than prophetic? Galen, who, like most ancient medical writers, accepted the pertinence of dreams in a variety of contexts, both divinatory and medical, cautions that a doctor can err by interpreting as medical a vision which in fact pertains to a nonmedical aspect of the patient's life:[27]

> The conditions of the body do not account for all of the soul's dream images in sleep. Some dreams come from our daily habits and actions, while others originate in our [waking-state] thoughts. Also, it has been our experience that certain matters are prophetically foreshadowed by the soul. Therefore the diagnosis of the body on the basis of dreams that have their impulse from the body itself becomes no easy task.[28]

Galen goes on to say that it is specifically the prophetic potential of dreams that poses the greatest challenge for physician-interpreters. Dreams that originate in waking thoughts and actions will be easy to recognize and dismiss, but because the future is naturally obscure, it may be difficult to know whether one is dealing with a symbol or a symptom. As an example of just such a category mistake, Galen tells the story of a person who dreamed that his leg had turned to stone. Skilled interpreters, he says, who followed the logic of a common symbolic substitution, took this as a prophetic reference to the man's slaves,[29] so everyone was surprised when the dream turned out to pertain to the man's body: when he

[26] In fact, the bulk of the treatise, after the first few theoretical paragraphs, reads rather like a typical book of dream interpretation. For discussion, see S.M. Oberhelman, "Galen, *On Diagnosis from Dreams*," *Journal of the History of Medicine and Allied Sciences*, 38 (1983): pp. 36–47, at pp. 43–7.

[27] Among medical sects, only the Methodists rejected dreams as a guide to therapy (Oberhelman, "Dreams in Graeco-Roman Medicine," pp. 136–9). In the second century AD, Rufus of Ephesus wrote in his guidelines for physicians interviewing patients that they should ask not just whether, and how, the individual has slept, but also whether he has dreamed, since dreams can convey information about the state of the body's humors. See Rufus of Ephesus, *Corpus medicorum graecorum*, *Supplementum* 4, ed. H. Gärtner (Berlin, 1962), pp. 34–6 (sections 29–33).

[28] Galen, "On Diagnosis through Dreams," p. 103, 13–17 Guidorizzi (G. Guidorizzi, "L'opusculo di Galeno 'De Dignotione ex Insomniis,'" *Bollettino del Comitato per la Preparazione dell'Edizione Nazionale dei Classici Greci e Latini*, 21 [1973]: pp. 81–105) (vol. 6, p. 833 Kühn [C.G.Kühn (ed.), *Claudii Galeni Opera omnia* (20 vols in 22 parts, Leipzig, 1821–1833)]); translation in Oberhelman, "Galen," p. 44.

[29] Cf. Artemidorus 1.47 and 1.48.

suffered paralysis of his leg, it was clear that his advisers had chosen the wrong interpretive framework.[30]

Unlike the technical writers, Aristides is not concerned with the question of a dream's origin. He ascribes all his visions, ultimately, to the god, using the language of divine *oneiros* and symptomatic *enhypnion* interchangeably.[31] Still, he is interested in the problem of arriving at an interpretive framework.[32] Early in the first *Logos*, he is twice derailed by uncertainty about the horizon of interpretation for his dreams—the kind of error that, as the passage from Galen shows, is a persistent hazard of conjectural interpretation. His illness, as the text opens, involves abdominal difficulties, and the episodes of the dream diary center on the issue of bathing. The god has prescribed abstention from baths (*alousia*, 1.6), but Aristides thinks that subsequent dreams may be indicating the opposite.[33] The next dream account describes an interpretive failure, and instead of reporting dream and outcome with retrospective clarity, Aristides depicts hermeneutic confusion (1.7):[34]

> μετὰ δὲ τοῦτο ὄναρ γίγνεται, ἔχον μέν τινα ἔννοιαν λουτροῦ, οὐ μέντοι χωρίς γε ὑπονοίας· ἀλλ' ἐδόκουν τι καὶ μολυνθῆναι· ὅμως δὲ ἔδοξεν λούσασθαι, πάντως δ' εἰ καὶ τῷ ὄντι τοῦτ' ἐπεπόνθειν, ὕδατος δεῖν. εὐθύς τε οὖν οὐχ ὡς ἥδιστα ἔσχον ἐν τῷ βαλανείῳ, καὶ ἐπειδὴ ἐπανῆλθον, ἐδόκει πάντα πλήρη εἶναι, καὶ τὸ πνεῦμα οἷον ἀσθμαίνοντος ἦν· ὥστε ἐπ' ἀρχῇ τῆς

---

30 Galen, "On Diagnosis through Dreams," p. 104, 23–6 Guidorizzi (vol. 6, p.834 Kühn). Cf. Oberhelman, "Galen," p. 45, with notes (63 and 64) on correspondence with Artemidorus' discussion of the symbolism of a paralyzed leg, and dissonance with Hippocratic interpretations of the same.

31 See Artemidorus 4.proemium on the fact that the distinction between *oneiros* and *enhypnion* is a technical one that was understandably disregarded in lay circles.

32 On episodes of interpretive failure, see Behr, *Aelius Aristides*, p. 194, with notes 72–3.

33 Abdominal disorder was understood to result from an excess of moist humors. So, from the Hippocratic writers forward, a "drying" regimen (including abstention from baths) was considered an appropriate corrective; see J. Downie, "Proper Pleasures: Bathing and Oratory in Aelius Aristides' *Hieros Logos* I and *Oration* 33," in W.V. Harris and B. Holmes (eds), *Aelius Aristides between Greece, Rome and the Gods* (Brill, 2008), pp. 115–30, at p. 119, with note 13. In the Hippocratic Corpus, see especially *Regimen* 2.57; *Affections* 53; *Regimen in Acute Diseases* 18. Bathing was believed to help people obtain nourishment from food, so its opposite, *alousia*, was a logical concomitant of fasting: Hippocrates, *Places in Man* 43; and Galen, *Commentary on Hippocrates' On the Nature of Man, Corpus medicorum graecorum*, ed. J. Mewaldt, G. Helmreich, and J. Westenberger (Leipzig and Berlin, 1914), vol. 5, 9, 1, p. 106, 15–21.

34 On this passage, see also Downie, "Proper Pleasures," pp. 119–23.

τροφῆς εὐθὺς ἐπαυσάμην. διαφθορὰ μετὰ τοῦτο ἐκ νυκτὸς καὶ προῆλθεν εἰς τοῦτο, ὥστε μόλις κατέστη πρὸ μεσημβρίας μικρόν.

After this there came a dream [*onar*] that contained some notion [*ennoia*] of bathing—not, however, without a second-order meaning [*hyponoia*] (though I *did* seem [*edokoun*] to be actually defiled [*molunthênai*] in some way), but it seemed [*edoxen*] nevertheless a good idea to bathe, especially because if in fact I had suffered this [defilement], water was necessary. Straightaway, then, I spent some rather unpleasant time in the bathhouse. And when I got out, all [my body] seemed full and my breathing was like an asthmatic's so that, to begin with, I immediately stopped taking nourishment. After this there was corruption [*diaphthora*] from night onwards, and it went on to such an extent that it scarcely let up a little before noon.

Aristides reports neither the details of what he actually saw in his dream (*onar*) nor, indeed, any clear dream symbol. Instead, he refers to a "notion," or "general impression" (*ennoia*) of bathing, and some sense of being defiled (*molunthênai*)—the vagueness of which causes him to hesitate over the dream's "second-order meaning" (*hyponoia*).[35] The convoluted syntax of the description seems to reflect his uncertainty: the first sentence of the passage presents a succession of apparently contradictory qualifications (*mentoi ... alla ... homôs*) that make the account opaque, and as the boundary blurs between "notion" and "second-order meaning," dream appearance (*edokoun*) and interpretive reflection (*edoxen*) intertwine.

Aristides' hesitation reflects uncertainty about the appropriate framework of interpretation for this dream. While he does not offer details about his dream of "defilement," we might imagine an excrement dream—of the sort that Artemidorus and Galen both describe, each offering a very different interpretation. According to Galen, if a person dreams he is standing in excrement or mud, it means either that his humors are disordered or that his bowels are full.[36] According to Artemidorus, on the other hand, a dream involving excrement (animal or human) may portend sickness, particularly if the

35 Aristides' use of these two terms is probably subtechnical, but the distinction between *ennoia* and *hyponoia* seems to be one of dream-picture, or dream-story, versus symbolic, "second-order" meaning. In the *HL*, *ennoia* appears three times (1.28, 1.55, 3.39), but *hyponoia* only appears here (though cf. 1.55, at the end of the diary, for the verbal form). Cf. *Oration* 38.2, where *ennoia* is contrasted with *nous*, which seems to indicate the "message" or "intent" of the dream.

36 Oberhelman, "Galen," p. 46; Galen, "On Diagnosis through Dreams," p. 105, 44–8 Guidorizzi (vol. 6, p. 835 Kühn): "For if a person dreams of passing time in the midst of feces

excrement stains,[37] but as a symbol of impurity it may also pertain to a variety of issues relating to the dreamer's daily life.[38] We can imagine, then, that Aristides' hesitation signals uncertainty about the appropriate hermeneutic framework: within a symbolic framework touching on the social and moral concerns of daily life, "defilement" imposes the requirement of purification—and water is the purifying element par excellence; within a medical framework, on the other hand, "defilement" is likely to mark an intestinal disturbance best treated by keeping the body as dry as possible. If Aristides were to interpret the dream within a medical framework, as an indication of his physical state, he would refrain from bathing, to avoid further indigestion. When he decides, instead, that bathing is the solution to the "defilement" (*molunthênai*), he seems to favor instead an allegorical, Artemidorean interpretive framework: he turns to water as a symbol of purification.

The increased physical discomfort (*diaphthora*) that he suffers as a result seems to indicate that Aristides has chosen the wrong interpretive horizon for this dream, and a second episode of unsuccessful interpretation confirms this (1.8):

> ὄψις δὲ ὀνείρατος οὑτωσί πως εἶχεν, ὡς ἄρα εἴην ἐν ὕδασι θερμοῖς, προκεκυφὼς δὲ εἰς τὸ πρόσθεν ὁρῴην τὰ κάτω τῆς κοιλίας ἀτοπώτερον διακείμενα. ἐβουλευσάμην μὲν δὴ μεῖναι ἐπ' ἀλουσίας, ἔφη δέ τις ὡς οὐκ ἐπ' αὐτοῦ γε τοῦ λουτροῦ τὸ δυσχερὲς ἦν τὸ φαινόμενον, οὐδ' εἰκὸς ὡς αἴτιον φυλάξασθαι. ἐλουσάμην τε εἰς ἑσπέραν καὶ ἅμα τῷ ὄρθρῳ τὸ ἦτρον ἤλγουν, καὶ ἐπεχώρει τὸ ἄλγημα ἐπὶ δεξιὰ καὶ μέχρι βουβῶνος κάτω.

> And the vision of the dream went something like this: that I was in the warm waters, and bending forwards I saw that the lower parts of my intestine were in a disordered state. I thought it was a good idea, therefore, to continue to abstain from bathing. But someone [else] said that the evident difficulty was not on account of the bath per se, and it was not reasonable to guard against it as the cause. So I washed towards evening, and when dawn came I had abdominal pain, and the pain extended on the right all the way down to my groin.

---

and filth, either his humors are bad and foul-smelling and putrid or there is too much feces contained within his bowels."

37 Artemidorus 2.26.3: "[Excrement] indicates despondency and harm, and—when it stains—illness" (δυσθυμίας καὶ βλάβας σημαίνει, μολύνουσα δὲ καὶ νόσον).

38 Artemidorus (2.26) surveys a range of excrement dreams, the significance of which will (as always in Artemidorus) depend upon the identity and personal circumstances of the dreamer, the situation depicted in the dream, and the relative status of anyone else who appears in the dream.

In this second dream, Aristides sees "disorder" (*atopôteron diakeimena*) in his body, and interprets this as a sign that bathing has had (and will have) a negative physical effect. For a symptomatic dream in the medical framework, he is on the right track, until an unidentified interlocutor raises doubts by suggesting that it is not bathing itself that has caused the problem. Since he experiences pain when he eventually does bathe, the process of trial and error confirms his original conjecture that the dream was a symptomatic one, reflecting his physical condition.

In contrast with Galen and Artemidorus, then, Aristides gives his readers an inside view of the conjectural process and the difficulty of determining a dream's horizon of interpretation. As the narrative proceeds, however, he also transcends these early hermeneutic tangles, moving the language and strategies of oneirocriticism inside the divinely sponsored dream and making the dreamscape a space of direct access to divine communication (1.9):[39]

> ἐνάτῃ ἐπὶ δέκα ἔδοξά τινας τῶν βαρβάρων ἐγκρατεῖς γεγενῆσθαί μου, καί τινα αὐτῶν ἐπιέναι μοι καὶ δόξαν παρασχεῖν ὡς στίξοντα· ἔπειτα καθεῖναι τὸν δάκτυλον οὑτωσὶ μέχρι τοῦ λαιμοῦ καί τι ἐγχέαι κατὰ δή τινα ἐπιχώριον νόμον, ὀνομάσαι δὲ αὐτὸ ὀξυσιτίαν· ταῦτα δὲ ὕστερον ὡς ὄναρ διηγεῖσθαι καὶ τοὺς ἀκούοντας θαυμάζειν καὶ λέγειν ὡς ἄρα τοῦτο αἴτιον εἴη τοῦ διψῆν μέν, μὴ δύνασθαι δὲ πιεῖν, τῷ τρέπεσθαι εἰς ὄξος τὰ σιτία. ἐκ δὴ τούτου ἔμετός τε ἐδείκνυτο καὶ προσέταξεν ὁ βάρβαρος λουτροῦ τε ἀποσχέσθαι καὶ διάκονον ἕνα παραστήσασθαι τὸ τήμερον εἶναι. ἀλουσία καὶ ἔμετος μετὰ ῥᾳστώνης.

> On the nineteenth, I dreamed that some of the barbarians had got hold of me, and that one of them approached and made me think he was about to tattoo me. Then [I dreamed] that he put his finger in as far as my throat and poured something in, according to some local custom, and named it "heartburn" [*oxysitian*]. And [I dreamed] that I later recounted [*diêgeisthai*] these things as a dream, and that those listening marveled and said that this was the cause of my being thirsty, yet unable to drink, by virtue of the fact that my food was turning sour. So from this vomiting was indicated, on the one hand, and also the barbarian ordered that I should abstain from bathing and have one servant to assist me that day. Abstention from bathing and vomiting, with a sense of ease.

This dream has two parts: first, Aristides sees himself set upon by barbarians; then, he sees another dream scenario in which he tells the story (*diêgeisthai*)

---

[39] Behr (*Aelius Aristides,* pp. 194–5) catalogs the instances of interpretation within dreams. The most famous classical example of a dream that includes its own interpretation within it is Penelope's dream of the geese at *Odyssey* 19.535–69.

of that attack "as a dream" to an audience who help him to interpret it.[40] In other words, the activity of conjectural interpretation that Aristides might, in the real world, undertake in collaboration with an interpretive community of professional critics, temple staff, or friends and associates is transferred into the dream-space. In this case, the hermeneutic employed is fairly clear: decoding the linguistic components of the name given to the symbolic substance the barbarian has poured down his throat—*oxysitia* (*oxy*, "sharp, acid"; *sitia*, "food")—yields an explanation in medical terms for the conflict between Aristides' desire to drink and his inability to do so: corruption of food in his system. This etymological approach to interpretation appears elsewhere in the *HL*[41] and it was a common technique in ancient dream hermeneutics. However, because the interpretation is placed inside the dream, it is even more forcefully sustained (in theory) by the god's all-knowing power and (in practice) by Aristides' agency as author of this retrospective account. As far as Aristides' narrative presentation is concerned, the dream is self-interpreting.

Aristides' Dream World

As we saw above, when he considers the challenge physicians face in determining whether a particular dream should be considered medically symptomatic, Galen dismisses rather quickly the whole class of dreams that merely reflect the dreamer's daily life. Artemidorus does the same, placing these in the category of *enhypnia*, along with the symptomatic dreams that are beneath his interest.[42] Generally speaking, dreams that appeared simply to reproduce the images and preoccupations of the dreamer's waking life were viewed as nonsignificant and little discussed in ancient literature beyond the tradition of materialist philosophy.[43] But surely the nonsignificant dream lurks at the edge of any interpretive framework: there is always the possibility that a dream means nothing.

---

[40] The infinitives that depend on the introducing verb ἔδοξα (διηγεῖσθαι, θαυμάζειν, λέγειν) make the scene of interpretation part of the dream.

[41] See, for example, *HL* 1.51, where he dreams that he is carrying a volume by Menander and interprets this as a sign from the god that he should "stay" (*menein*).

[42] Artemidorus 1.1. Obviously, Artemidorus differs from Galen in dismissing symptomatic dreams as well.

[43] See A.H.M. Kessels, "Ancient Systems of Dream-Classification," *Mnemosyne*, 22 (1969): pp. 389–424; D. Clay, "An Epicurean Interpretation of Dreams," *American Journal of Philology*, 101 (1980): pp. 342–65; and V. Lev Kenaan, "Delusion and Dream in Apuleius' *Metamorphoses*," *Classical Antiquity*, 23 (2004): pp. 247–82.

While neither Artemidorus nor Galen substantially engages with the problem of the nonmeaningful dream, Aristides does. Problematizing—and ultimately confounding—the distinction between prophetic and symptomatic dreams, he goes a step further by exploiting those dreams typically marginalized as nonmeaningful: investing these kaleidoscopic reconfigurations of waking experience with their own significance, he makes them tools for the creation of personal narrative. For, while he opens the *HL* with a series of dreams oriented quite clearly around questions of illness and healing, as the text progresses, Aristides increasingly includes (perhaps even invents) dream material that is strictly speaking extraneous to his initial prescriptive and prophetic agenda. In the world of dream narrative that he has created from the beginning of the first *Logos*, every detail—whether it speaks meaningfully to the reader or not—is invested with potential meaning by divine sponsorship, and this divine license creates a space for what he calls in *HL* I the "secondary business" (*parergon*) of his dreams—stories that allude to the *realia* of his professional and social life.[44]

An episode from the end of *HL* V illustrates the expansive narrative scope Aristides has claimed for his dreams over the course of the text, and shows also how he uses an interpretive scenario to enhance his professional profile. He relates a dream featuring a pseudo-Hippocratic prescription, which came to him close to the time of the text's composition—so recently, he says, that it was still at the front of his mind (*enaulos*). The account, combining interpretive control with a powerful sense of divine endorsement, proclaims his quasi-heroic persona, even in illness. He reports the god's command (*epitattei*) that he should get up out of bed in spite of his poor health, and we know from the outset that Asclepius "wondrously healed [him] in his customary way," but Aristides also narrates (*diêgeisthai*) at length the dream itself, staging a drama of interpretation in which he is the primary actor, taking the role of the responsible—and surprisingly confident—patient-interpreter (5.49–50):

> ἡκέτην ἰατρὼ δύο καὶ διελεγέσθην ἐν τῷ προθύρῳ ἄλλα τέ μοι δοκεῖν καὶ περὶ ψυχροῦ λουτροῦ. ἠρώτα μὲν ὁ ἕτερος, ὁ δ' ἀπεκρίνετο· 'τί λέγει, ἔφη, Ἱπποκράτης;' 'τί δ' ἄλλο γε ἢ δραμόντα δέκα σταδίους ἐπὶ θάλατταν οὕτως ῥῖψαι;' ταῦτα μὲν δὴ ὡς ὄναρ πεφάνθαι ἐδόκουν. μετὰ δὲ τοῦτο ἐπελθεῖν ὡς ἀληθῶς αὐτοὺς τοὺς ἰατρούς, θαυμάσαι τε δὴ τοῦ ἐνυπνίου τὴν ἀκρίβειαν

44 Quet, "Parler de soi," pp. 220–21: "Comme si sa vie onirique se confondait presque complètement, à cette date, avec la vie éveillée qu'il avait menée antérieurement." Synesius, Aristides' fourth-century AD reader, likewise considered all dreams significant; he was also intrigued by the rhetorical challenge of dream description. See the chapter by Miller in this volume.

> καὶ πρὸς αὐτοὺς εἰπεῖν 'ἄρτι τε ὑμᾶς ἐδόκουν ὁρᾶν καὶ ἄρτι ἥκετε. καὶ δῆτα ὁπότερος μὲν ὑμῶν, ἔφην, ὁ ἐρωτῶν ἦν καὶ ὁπότερος ὁ ἀποκρινόμενος οὐκ ἔχω λέγειν.' ἡ δ' ἀπόκρισις οὕτως εἶχεν, ὡς ἄρα Ἱπποκράτης κελεύοι δέκα σταδίους θεῖν τὸν μέλλοντα λοῦσθαι ψυχρῷ· ἅμα δὲ ἐμαυτῷ μετέλαβον τὸ ἐπὶ θάλατταν, ὡς δηλοῦν † τὴν κατὰ φύσιν τῷ ποταμῷ, καὶ οὕτως εἶπον 'δέκα σταδίους θεῖν τῷ ποταμῷ συμπαραθέοντα.' ἐνεθυμήθην δ' αὐτὸ διὰ τὸ εἶναι ἐν μεσογείᾳ· ἐδόκει σαφὲς εἶναι καὶ χρῆναι οὕτω ποιεῖν.

> Two doctors came and were conversing in the forecourt about various things including—it seemed to me—cold baths. One of them posed a question and the other responded: "What," asked the first doctor, "does Hippocrates say?" "What else but that the patient should run ten stades and immediately jump into the sea?" I dreamed that these things appeared as if in a dream (*hôs onar*). And after that, [I dreamed] that I approached the doctors themselves for real (*hôs alêthôs*), and that I was astonished at the accuracy of the dream and said to them: "Just now I dreamed I saw you, and now you have come. And truly which of you was the questioner and which the respondent I cannot say." But the response was like this, that Hippocrates ordered someone who was about to take a cold bath to run ten stades. But at the same time, I changed for myself the part about "into the sea," as meaning naturally "by the river," and thus I said I was going to "run ten stades going alongside the river." And I thought of this because I was inland. So it seemed clear and necessary to proceed this way.

Naming Hippocrates, the dream doctors evoke medical authority,[45] but what seems at first like a dream scenario of professional consultation and debate soon shifts, turning instead into a kind of oracular moment, in which Hippocrates' response (*apokrisis*) is a divine utterance, a coded, prophetic text that Aristides claims the authority to decipher:[46] "into the sea" really means "alongside the

[45] There is Hippocratic precedent for cold bathing (*Regimen* 2.57), but its combination here with running, and the vigorous nature of the prescription—so at odds with Aristides' weakened condition—are characteristic rather of a pattern of paradoxically athletic cures in the *HL*. For the dream scenario of the medical consultation, compare 1.62–3.

[46] On Aristides' alteration of the dream prescription in this passage (without comment on Hippocrates' cameo appearance), see H. Baumgart, *Aelius Aristides als Repräsentant der sophistischen Rhetorik des zweiten Jahrhunderts der Kaiserzeit* (Leipzig, 1874), pp. 99–100, who compares the episode with other substitutions permitted Aristides by the god: dedication of a ring in place of his finger (2.27); feigned shipwreck in place of real imperilment (2.12). Note, though, that at 5.48–55, Aristides also alters the prescription on his own authority. See recently on this episode H. King, "The Origins of Medicine in the Second Century AD," in S. Goldhill and R. Osborne (eds), *Rethinking Revolutions through Ancient Greece* (Cambridge, 2006), pp. 246–63; and M. Horstmanshoff, "Aelius Aristides: A Suitable Case

river" (as he interprets according to his inland situation). Then, in another discontinuous scene, Aristides dreams that he instructs his companions to fulfill the Hippocratic "prophecy" (*prorrhêsis*), mixing the languages of divine authority and medical tradition (5.51).

Ultimately, this is medical cure as theatrical, or rhetorical, performance—a point underscored by the fact that as preparations are made for Aristides to enact the prophetic prescription, one of the doctors turns to him to ask: "Why don't you entertain us with a declamation [*meletê*] in the meantime?" (5.52). This provides Aristides with the opportunity to record his response: "Because, by Zeus ... it is more important for me to review some of the things I have already written. For I must also converse with men of posterity."[47] The god in turn, he reports, predicts many years of life for Aristides—and, by implication, as Aristides adds, many years of professional engagement as a *rhetor*.[48]

Frequently in the *HL*, Aristides mingles professional assertion with complex scenes of divine dream prescription. The "Hippocratic" dream thus offers an example of what is at stake for him in his engagement with interpretive discourse in the *HL*: having exposed early on the pitfalls that attend upon dream interpretation for ordinary mortals, he strategically integrates its language and procedures into the dream itself, and he elaborates a narrative world saturated with divine significance, over which he has complete hermeneutic control by virtue of his unique relationship with Asclepius. Describing dreams that are intricately layered and full of detail—some of it quite transparently reflecting his most urgent waking concerns—Aristides has found a way to make meaning out of precisely the kind of dream usually dismissed, in the ancient world, as nonsignificant.[49]

---

for Treatment," in Barbara E. Borg (ed.), *Paideia: The World of the Second Sophistic* (Berlin, 2004), pp. 277–90.

47 5.52: ὅτι νὴ Δί', ἔφην ἐγώ, σπουδαιότερόν μοί ἐστιν ἐπελθεῖν τινα τῶν γεγραμμένων· δεῖ γάρ με καὶ τοῖς ὕστερον ἀνθρώποις διαλέγεσθαι.

48 5.52: καὶ ὅς οἰωνίζετο ἔτη πολλά μοι, κἀγὼ εἶπον, 'βουλοίμην ἂν καὶ πολλὰ ἔτη βιῶναι, εἰ μέλλοιμι ἔσεσθαι πρὸς λόγοις.' τὸ μὲν δὴ ὄναρ τοιοῦτον ἐγένετο (He then predicted many years for me, and I said, "I would like to live many years more, if I could be engaged in rhetoric [logoi]." This, then, was the dream as it happened.)

49 For modern readers accustomed to the notion that even the most quotidian dream details may encode truths about the dreamer's psychology, Aristides' desire to imbue his dreams generally with significance seems intuitively right. Still, there is a substantial gap between Aristides' account and this modern sensibility. The Freudian and post-Freudian hermeneutic places the origins of the dream in the realm of the unconscious, and this implies a loss of interpretive control at odds with Aristides' aims in bringing his dreams to an Imperial-era public, where divine visions are frequently socially empowering.

Conclusion

The conjunction of illness and divine dreams is basic to Aristides' personal and professional story in the *HL*, but the texture of his dream accounts makes them more than a simple reflection of the tradition of temple healing and Asclepian cult. In their complexity, his dream narratives depart from the rhetoric of prescriptive clarity and therapeutic success, of aretalogy and commemoration, which is characteristic of the votive tradition. By making the problems of conjectural interpretation highly visible in the *HL*—in the unstable syntax of his accounts, and in the stories elaborated within the dreamscape—Aristides brings into focus a fundamental problem that haunts Greek treatises on dream hermeneutics: the difficulty of determining a dream's horizon of interpretation.

For Aristides, as for many technical writers, the most basic question is whether a dream is symptomatic of his physical condition or whether it pertains symbolically to other aspects of his life, and, as we have seen, in the dream-diary of the first *Logos*, Aristides describes two episodes of hermeneutic failure that highlight precisely this issue. This is, however, only the starting point of the interpretive trajectory of the *HL*, for, as he exposes the limitations of conjectural interpretation, he simultaneously cultivates an expansive sense of divine sponsorship that allows him the freedom to develop wide-ranging, detailed dream stories that serve his own purposes of self-portraiture. As the "Hippocratic" episode from *HL* V illustrates, the conjectural scenario—both mantic and medical—offers a stage for Aristides' claim to an intimate connection with his savior god. By moving the interpretive drama and its consequences inside the dream, he creates a free narrative space for material that would otherwise be extraneous to the prescriptive project: elaborate stories reflecting the preoccupations of his waking life in scenarios that highlight his own agency and interpretive power.

Chapter 6

Illness and Its Metaphors in Artemidorus' *Oneirocritica*: A Negative List

Christine Walde

Artemidorus' *Oneirocritica*, the only extant textbook of ancient Greek professional dream interpretation, seems to open a window to the ancient world, to human beings' fears, wishes, and the daily struggle for existence in the second century AD.[1] Indeed, when reading the *Oneirocritica*, there emerges a world that is colorful, disturbing, uncannily familiar, even fragmented, as every entry in his systematic encyclopedia of dream images sums up a real life's good luck or bad luck in epigrammatic brevity. Since illness, like dreams, is something that all people experience, either personally or by witnessing how it affects someone else, it naturally appears in the imagery and interpretations of the *Oneirocritica*. Moreover, as the body and its wellbeing were the most important economic resource for everybody, especially for the poor and destitute, we may assume that the loss of health and consequently of self-sustenance must have been a constant fear and preoccupation. Indeed, in the veritable *Totentanz* of the *Oneirocritica*, fragility and finality, illness and death are lurking around every corner. For example:

> [A]ll things which can in no ways and under no circumstances get lost, predict, if they get lost in a dream, that the dreamer will die or lose his eyes. Thus somebody dreamt that the heaven had vanished for him. He died; because in the same way as one can no longer make use of lost things, so everything that is no longer used by someone is as good as lost. (1.58)[2]

---

1 On Artemidorus in general, see: G. Weber, "Artemidor von Daldis und sein Publikum," *Gymnasium*, 106 (1999): pp. 209–29; M.A. Holowchak, *Ancient Science and Dreams: Oneirology in Greco-Roman Antiquity* (New York, 2001); and C. Walde, *Antike Traumdeutung und moderne Traumforschung* (Düsseldorf, 2001). The studies of Holowchak and Walde were published independently of each other in the same year. They show striking similarities and even more striking differences in the assessment of the ancient discourses of interpretation. One of the differences is that I am more optimistic concerning the results and progress of Artemidorus.

2 All translations of Artemidorus are my own and are based on the Teubner edition by R.A. Pack: *Artemidori Daldiani Onirocriticon Libri V* (Leipzig, 1963). The most recent

An examination of disease in the *Oneirocritica* is an interesting test case of method, as Artemidorus moves in the twilight zone between professional predictive dream interpretation and various medical approaches to dreams, be it professional scientific medicine, the cult of Asclepius and other gods, or the result of everyday, individual forms of interrelating dreams and bodily functions.[3] These heterogeneous professional and nonprofessional modes of coping with illness are my implicit and explicit coordinates in my treatment here of Artemidorus.

The aim of this chapter, which takes up again the question of how medical and predictive dream interpretation are interrelated, is to provide an overview of how disease figures in the *Oneirocritica* and to describe its associations. Does the imagery of disease form a group of its own? Are medicine and medical treatment reflected in the *Oneirocritica*? What is the position of the *Oneirocritica* in the chorus of dream discourses concerned with the body and health? And what status/function do professional dream interpreters have in the kaleidoscope of medical practitioners and other specialists of *souci de soi*? In what follows, I analyze all the passages in which illness or disease is either mentioned explicitly or can be inferred from the context with relative certainty, although I am aware of the difficulty that all interpretations in which bad outcomes or death are predicted might involve illness too.[4] My methodological focus on images of,

---

English translation is D.E. Harris-McCoy, *Artemidorus' Oneirocritica* (Oxford, 2012), which reproduces Pack's Greek text and contains extensive commentary. I recommend the admirable Italian translation by the late dream scholar D. Del Corno (*Artemidoro, Il libro dei sogni*, 4th edn [Milan, 1993]) or the German translation by K. Brackertz (*Artemidor von Daldis, Das Traumbuch* [Munich, 1979]).

[3] On the several levels of medical professionalism, see the very instructive volume edited by P.J. van der Eijk, H.F.J. Horstmannshoff, and P.H. Schrijvers, *Ancient Medicine in Its Socio-Cultural Context* (Amsterdam and Atlanta, 1995). On medical dream interpretation, see: G. Guidorizzi, "Sogno, diagnosi, guarigione: da Asclepio a Ippocrate," in G. Guidorizzi (ed.), *Il sogno in Grecia* (Bari, 1988), pp. 97–102: S.M. Oberhelman, "The Interpretation of Prescriptive Dreams in Ancient Greek Medicine," *Journal of the History of Medicine*, 36 (1981): pp. 416–24 and "Galen, *On the Diagnosis from Dreams*," *Journal of the History of Medicine*, 38 (1983): pp. 36–47; Holowchak, *Ancient Science and Dreams*; Walde, *Antike Traumdeutung*, pp. 106–26; L.G. Fernández, "La diagnosis onírica en Galeno," *Cuadernos de Filologia Clásica: Estudios griegos e indoeuropeos*, 14 (2004): pp. 139–53; M. Liatsi, "Zur Funktion des Traumes in der antiken Medizin (Hippokrates, de victu IV)," *Antike Naturwissenschaft und ihre Rezeption*, 12 (2002): pp. 7–21.

[4] This is the problem with statistics of frequency. Cf. I. Hahn, who in his *Traumdeutung und gesellschaftliche Wirklichkeit: Artemidorus Daldianus als sozialgeschichtliche Quelle* (Konstanz, 1992) speaks of about 1,400 images being listed in the *Oneirocritica* and about 3,000 interpretations (p. 8); however, his subdivision of the interpretations (p. 9) into those related to economics and society (c. 25–30 percent), to "biology" (illness, health,

and statements on, illness and health has been exaggerated purposely in order to demonstrate in the reverse that dream images that signify illness and health cannot be seen in isolation from the other fields of interpretation.

Definitions of Illness

(1) *General*: Artemidorus' definition of "norms" of waking life is the guideline of all his interpretations (1.3). These norms, presented in "nature, law, customs, art, name, and time," help to assess the distance between waking life and the real/surreal character of the dream images, this distance being *one* of the criteria of his evaluation of dream images. The normalcy of human life includes pain and illness, seen as a non-extractable part of the human condition:

> Therefore, for example, pleasure, pain, hate, love, illness, health, secretions and nutrition, beauty, ugliness, increase, decline, birth, death, and similar terms are according to nature, because they are neither different from nature nor do they form categories of their own; because nature is no empty name, but is named as the circle of all things, that will or will not be ever and everywhere. (4.2)

Even if illness is part of the "normalcy" of life, its occurrence as a dream image is not a positive experience during the dream process ("interior") and so its interpretation is inauspicious and bodes evil ("exterior") (1.5). Even if this is in consonance with certain statements in medical dream treatises where seeing things in harmony with the normal state of things in waking life is an index of good health, Artemidorus in contrast always allows for counterfactual interpretations.[5]

---

birth, death: 20 percent) and family-related issues (marriage, love, children: 10 percent) and to *varia* (e.g., gods and religion) is not convincing, as health is certainly connected with economics, family, and gods too. A searchable database of the *Oneirocritica* is still a *desideratum*. See my own (modest) and preliminary statistics based on chapter frequency in the Appendix. Cf. also the several statistics in this chapter that focus on health (dreams of health by ill dreamers and by healthy dreamers, dream images predicting course of illness, specific disease, etc.). Other useful lists are to be found in E. Ruiz García, "Artemidoro y la arqueología del saber onirocrítico," in R. Teja Casuso (ed.), *Sueños, ensueños y visiones en la Antiguedad pagana y cristiana* (Aquilar de Campóo, 2002), pp. 29–50.

[5] Cf. Artemidorus 4.proemium with Hippocrates, *Regimen* 4.10–14; cf. also Artemidorus' general rule that beautiful, strong, and noble bodies—provided that the beauty is not in excess of human measure—is positive for any dreamer. Instead, to be excessively beautiful has the same meaning as being excessively ugly, for this will bring death to the ill and weakness to the healthy.

(2) *Special*: Artemidorus uses a very broad definition of illness, including every kind of change of the body or frame of mind from a normal, non-attention-demanding status to one where the body or soul requires treatment (any abnormality, discomfort, irritation).[6]

Apparently, Artemidorus' conception of health and illness is oriented at the average male dreamer and therefore has, from our modern perspective, a slightly misogynistic gender bias. Illness as a deviance from an obstacle-free status appears as a temporal or longtime weakening/weakness, as a state of dependency, immobility, and approximation to the female sex or even infancy.[7] Yet, we never find moralistic undertones brandishing illness as justified, self-induced, or as divine vengeance; nor does Artemidorus connect the origin of illness with social status and available means of sustenance (for example, illness caused by malnutrition).

In most cases, beyond the fact that death often results, the severity and the temporal dimension of illness[8] are not defined, but it seems that illness is only mentioned in the *Oneirocritica* when it causes major trouble for the body. In general, this definition—amounting to the simple acknowledgment of illness—is not so distant from contemporary medical definitions, which assess illness as a deviation from a satisfying and normal status and in terms of life expectancy; such assessments lead to further diagnosis and to recommendations of therapy.[9] Nonetheless, the *Oneirocritica* is not a medical treatise, and we should not expect

---

6 Ancient medicine had a holistic approach to illness and health, in that it saw body and soul in constant interaction as one unit; cf. G. Wöhrle, "Aspekte psychosomatischen Denkens in der antiken Medizin und Philosophie," *Gymnasium*, 107 (2000): pp. 383–98.

7 Some dream images are interpreted via characteristics of illness. Immobility: 2.2 (not being able to leave the house); 2.31 (being drafted to the army = losing one's free will); 2.55 (not being able to leave/enter Hades); 3.60 (entering a prison on one's own accord). Femininity: 1.14 (being pregnant; cf. 5.44: an athlete dreaming of being pregnant with twins); 1.14 (having milk in the breasts is bad for athletes and sportsmen as only the weak sex has milk in the breasts); 1.41 (having/seeing a female breast with an ailment). Infancy: 1.16 (wearing diapers and being breastfed, the analogy being that a sick person is as helpless and dependent on nutrition as an infant).

8 E.g., 1.21 (having something woolen on the breast = lengthy consumption); 5.35 (date of ill sister's death predicted by seven black figs, which symbolize seven days of life expectancy).

9 Cf. the very precise chapter by A. Labisch, "Gesundheit," in K.-H. Leven, *Antike Medizin: Ein Lexikon* (Munich, 2005), pp. 350–53, where it is shown that a differentiated concept of health and illness did not exist in classical antiquity, but both were seen relatively, the medium state (being in good and remarkable shape) being viewed as ideal. Indeed, this is, as Labisch (p. 352) mentions, not so removed from the World Health Organization's definition of health.

any more insights from an ancient dream manual than from any ancient treatise. If we take into account Artemidorus' aims and practice, only a very vague notion of illness is needed, namely the fact that some deviance from the normal status of health will occur. This vagueness is not a deficiency of method but a satisfactory enough working-tool in his own professional context.

Enhypnia and Dreams Predicting Illness

Like other writers of advanced ancient dream interpretation, Artemidorus offers a classification of dreams,[10] even if by contrast it is not as pronounced as what we see, for example, in the works of the physician Herophilus (third century BC) and the late antique scholar Macrobius (c. 400 AD). Apart from the *enhypnia* and *oneiroi*, the subcategories are not described in detail; their nature can be reconstructed with some confidence only from discussions of dream classifications in other sources. Whereas Herophilus and Macrobius stressed how the different origins of the dream types impacted their meaning, Artemidorus' most important differentiation is between *enhypnia* and *oneiroi*, that is, between meaningless and meaningful dreams;[11] a dream's origin played a less than secondary role. Apart from their difference in usability and reliability for divination, Artemidorus admits that both *enhypnia* and *oneiroi* may justifiably be called dreams, as the production of their images in sleep is the same (1.1; 4.proemium).

In Artemidorus' fivefold classification, dreams manifesting the current status of body and frame of mind—especially fears, wishes, and digestion—fall into the category of *enhypnia*. In all ancient classifications of dreams, *enhypnia* are a difficult category as they include dreams of different causation—body and soul, psychological and physiological, and "day residues." Their common denominator is "temporal" and "ephemeral," as they show a direct and immediate connection to the dreamer and his waking life. *Oneiroi* differ in that they refer to the *near* past and present, showing nothing hidden to the intelligent and self-conscious dreamer.[12] *Enhypnia* are "meaningless" only in the sense that they have no divinatory nature,[13]

[10] On these classifications, see in general A.H.M. Kessels, "Ancient Systems of Dream-Classification," *Mnemosyne*, 22 (1969): pp. 389–424.

[11] I will come back to this point later below.

[12] But see Artemidorus' observation that *enhypnia* of erudite people who pay attention to their dreams might be encoded as well (4.proemium). This paves the way for a general and monistic theory of dream production.

[13] Artemidorus' classification of dreams of the *enhypnia* as "meaningless" is to be seen under a certain caveat. In general, labeling these dreams as meaningless is a paradoxical act, for if they are an index to the current status of body and soul, this is meaningful too.

Table 6.1 Artemidorus' Typology of Dreams and Interpretative Grids

Meaningless Dreams		Meaningful Dreams			
phantasma/ visum (apparition of ghosts)	*enhypnion/ insomnium* (dreams caused by current status of body and soul; day residues)	*horama/visio* (apparitions of nondivine authorities, with unambiguous advice/orders)	*chrêmatismos/oraculum* (apparition of a divine being, with obvious or slightly oracular/enigmatic advice/order)	*oneiros/somnium*	
				oneiros theôrêmatikos (shows impending future event as it will occur and is fulfilled immediately after waking up)	*oneiros allêgorikos*
No interpretation necessary			Might need an interpretation	Only awareness of event needed	Needs an interpretation

Additional grids of interpretation

(I) Nature, customs, law, time, name, art; this includes the temporal-spatial constellation of the dream images (cf. 1.3; 4.2)

(II) Personal, alien, common, political, cosmic (1.2)

(III) Some dream images predict: (1) many things through many things; (2) few things through few things; (3) many things through few things; or (4) few things through many things (cf. 1.4)

(IV) Special dreams are subdivided in four classes: (1) internally (= while experiencing the dream) and externally (= predicted event) favorable; (2) internally and externally unfavorable; (3) internally favorable and externally unfavorable; and (4) internally unfavorable and externally favorable (cf. 1.5; 4.21)

(V) Social position, culture, lifestyle, sorrows, education, place of residence of the dreamer (1.8 *et passim*)

in contrast to predictive dreams. With the classification of a dream image as an *enhypnion*, the process of interpretation is finished. Illness and other changes of the body with some justification could be (but need not be) subsumed under this category, because if digestion and fears give rise to dreams, illness could use this channel of communication too. However, Artemidorus seems to see a difference, insofar as he explicitly mentions that ill people see *enhypnia* (1.1); since illness is always on their mind, they dream of being cured, consulting doctors, etc., and so these images are a simple wish fulfillment or, in modern terminology again, day residues. Consequently, this dream type is not identical to those dreams used by physicians in medical diagnosis, as *enhypnia* neither indicate the current status of body and soul nor provide a clue of an already present but as yet hidden disease.

The physicians must deal with the reverse problem. In his short treatise *On Diagnosis from Dreams*, Galen, the famous Hippocratean doctor and contemporary of Artemidorus, distinguishes four types of dreams:[14]

a. dreams indicating balance or imbalance of the four humors (origin: body and soul). The dreams normally show a certain distance from the "reality" of waking life, preferably cosmic images, as the human body is seen as a microcosm mirroring the macrocosm. These dreams are the physicians' field of expertise;
b. dreams mirroring things we do everyday;
c. dreams rehearsing things we have thought about;[15] and
d. prophetic dreams, instigated by the gods.

Galen saw no problem in distinguishing health dreams from categories (b) and (c), since they show an obvious connection to the dreamer's reality. But coming to terms with category (d) seems to have been the real challenge, as prophetic dreams and medical dreams might both display the same distance from the quotidian reality of the clients. Artemidorus visualized things differently, however. For him, dreams that indicate illness do not form a category of their own and his *enhypnia* do not comprise the dreams valuable for medical diagnosis.[16] The divine healing advice given at incubation centers or other sites

[14] Cf. the discussion of Galen's *On Diagnosis from Dreams* found in the chapters by Downie, Hulskamp, and Pearcy in this volume; cf. Holowchak, *Ancient Science and Dreams*, p. 140; and Walde, *Antike Traumdeutung*, pp. 121–6.

[15] Holowchak (*Ancient Science and Dreams*, p. 140) reduces (b) and (c) to a single category, "Mirroring Dreams." Even if this makes some sense, I would rather stick to the original fourfold categorization, as thinking and acting seem to me different processes.

[16] In fact, this would be an option too, but it was not taken by any of the ancient dream experts.

is to be included in Artemidorus' *chrêmatismos* (*oraculum/visio*), as several of his entries show.[17]

Is the fact that Artemidorus clearly mentions meaningful dreams, which denote illness, without recourse to an extra category an inconsistency? I would suggest that for practical reasons, Artemidorus has abolished the difference between medical dreams and the prophetic *oneiroi* that predict illness. Compared to the constantly progressing differentiation of dream types that characterize ancient interacting discourses of dream interpretation, this seems to be a step back. But Artemidorus' simplification is better, for this reduction is a milestone on the path to a monistic theory of dream formation and dream interpretation; it accepts that *oneiroi* and *enhypnia* share the quality of being images and experiences that are produced in sleep—their difference lies in their meaning only.[18] If everything can be predicted by an *oneiros*, then illness/health—but one of the spheres where good luck and back luck manifest themselves—is no exception. Artemidorus' *Oneirocritica* aims at a sort of super dream interpretation that integrates all kinds of dream images giving qualified information beyond waking life experience. This is the reason why Artemidorus declines to name an origin/cause for the predictive/divinatory dream—even to the point of stating that, in contrast to philosophers, he is not even interested whether meaningful dreams are produced by the soul or come from outside the dreamer (instilled by an alien agency), as long as the experience proves the dreams to be meaningful (with an obvious inclination to the soul as producer of dreams). This might seem a faulty reduction, but on second glance and in consideration of his cultural and scientific context, this is as good as dream interpretation in antiquity could get; the means to really prove the different origins of the several dream types simply did not exist.[19]

Artemidorus' practical approach did not require a constant theoretical reflection as long as the practice of interpretation—the only verifiable aspect in the whole context—could be maintained. For us moderns it is very difficult to reconstruct this practice, even if we get a glimpse (but no more) of it in the *Oneirocritica*, for we no longer dwell on the theoretical level of dream types, but on the level of individual and supra-individual interpretation and interaction with the clients. Here again, illness is one of the determining factors.

---

17 For example, 5.66, 5.89, 5.92.

18 In this respect, he is the counterpart to the Epicurean Lucretius (first century BC) who in Book 4 of his epic *On the Nature of Things* postulates for dreams a monistic, atomistic origin, but at the same time their utter voidness of meaning. See C. Walde, "Das Theater der Träume: Die Traumtheorie des Lukrez," in R. Heinz and W. Tress (eds), *100 Jahre Freudsche Traumdeutung. Zur Aktualität der Traumforschung Freuds* (Vienna, 2001), pp. 203–24.

19 See my conclusion below on progress in modern dream research.

Illness in Artemidorus: Occurrences and Levels

Illness not only is one of Artemidorus' norms in the process of interpretation; it also figures in several of his interpretative grids/categories and therefore is present on almost every level of his *Oneirocritica*—in the dreamers' classifications, the images, and the interpretations.

(1) Supra-individual Grids: Illness as a Distinguishing Aspect in the Classification of Dreamers

To avoid repetition and enhance the usability of his manual, Artemidorus refers to main groups of dreamers—as if statistically seeing a certain image has a higher recurrence for a certain group of people and is determined by the individual context only to a very small degree.

If an image given is not valid for "everyone," on this first level of classification, Artemidorus operates with simple dichotomies that cover most cases: rich/poor; ill/healthy; free/slave; married/unmarried. Most often the masculine form stands for women too, as the analogy is easily provided. But some images and their interpretation are also modified by "male/female dreamer." As these dichotomies are only the most basic categories, they can occur in combinations (for example, 2.3: poor people also being ill; 5.35: a rich woman who is also sick).

In this inner circle of, or first approach to, interpretation, we find several possible clusters:

a. The dreams concerning health dreamt by *an already ill* person. Here the dreamer is also the one concerned by the interpretation (what I label as personal dreams). The interpretation focuses not on the outbreak but on the course of illness, including therapy, surgery, deterioration, cure, and death. Because the already-manifest illness narrows the focus of interpretation, this is a rather simple task for the professional interpreter of dreams. In rare cases, "ill" is just the dreamer's determining factor, but the dream image is not exclusively interpreted in terms of his own illness. This rarely explained combination is always an option due to the interpretative category of "many things by few signs" (1.4). According to this grid—in anticipation of the Freudian condensation—an image might have more than one meaning. For instance, dreaming of eating onions can be interpreted as personal and/or alien (1.67):

> Eating onions and garlic is inauspicious; possessing them brings luck. Only in regard to ill people does this dream image have a different outcome: Alexander

> of Myndos was in an embarrassing situation, not finding a solution regarding this fact. But I adhere to the following opinion: if someone ill dreams of eating many onions, he himself will recover [a personal interpretation], but will have to mourn the death of somebody else [an alien interpretation]. If he eats only a few onions, he will die [a personal interpretation] as dying people shed but a few tears, in contrast to mourners who shed a lot, as they cry for a long time.[20]

b. The dreams concerning illness dreamt by *a still healthy* person are a more difficult issue, as their possible meaning can be subdivided into two groups: (i) dreams that predict illness of the dreamer *and* the course of illness; if the dream is "personal," this means a dream image concerning the dreamer alone; and (ii) dreams of a healthy person which predict illness/death for someone else, that is, for a different person, if it is an "alien" dream (cf. 4.4). Even if there are a few vicarious dreams among the incubation dreams,[21] the fact that one can have dreams about somebody else's disease/health is certainly the most prominent difference to medical dream interpretation.

If these basic and, as experience shows, rather common interrelations between dreamer, dream images, and their supposed meaning do not lead to a satisfying result, the determining aspects become ever more individual and can be modified by further criteria such as age, profession, and family situation, or paradoxically they become more unspecific—moving from the inner circle of personal dreams to ever wider social contexts of the dreamer to alien dreams (concerning a different person), to dreams that are common (concerning a larger group of people), political (concerning the state), or cosmic dreams (1.2).[22] Certainly, in these wider contexts disease can figure again; for example, a dreamer's profession (physician, midwife, etc.) may be connected to health, or somebody may own an ill slave or relative, or disease may constitute the substance of the dream image.[23]

---

20 This is also a good example for "tradition" in the *Oneirocritica*; cf. below.

21 Cf., e.g., *Inscriptiones Graecae* IV^2, 1, nos. 121–2 (Epidaurus), stele B, XXI (mother dreams about her daughter's health).

22 On this, see M. Foucault, "Einleitung," in L. Binswanger, *Traum und Existenz: Einleitung von Michael Foucault* (Bern and Berlin, 1992), pp. 7–93; and C. Walde, "Dreams in a Prosperous Age: Artemidoros, the Greek Interpreter of Dreams," in D. Shulman and G. Stroumsa (eds), *Dream Cultures* (Oxford, 1999), pp. 121–42.

23 Professional aspects: (1) dream image is favorable/unfavorable to physicians: 1.68: sesame and linseed are favorable; 1.77: thyme and marigold are auspicious; 2.20: vultures are inauspicious; 2.23: eggs are good for physicians, painters, and egg merchants; 2.30: seeing a

(2) Illness as a Result of Interpretation: Certain Image Groups Recurring More Frequently in Connection to Health

In general, as is to be expected, images denoting a process with a certain finality/perspective (of ending, of deprivation) or a change/development to better or worse are observed especially in connection with an auspicious course of illness or with ensuing death (*omina mortis*); however, they can also predict death by other causes, illness being only one of the life risks.

Under the proviso that these images do not exclusively appear in connection with bad health, some recurrent *tropoi* can be observed according to the general characteristics of illness mentioned above:

a. Images of fight, struggle, and controversy: illness is seen as a task, a challenge, as something coming from the outside rather than something produced in/by the dreamer's body. These fights/challenges are visualizations of the hardship and pain inflicted by illness. This challenge can appear in the guise of the following analogies: wrestling and fighting with human beings and gods (1.60: wrestling with a boy, with somebody dead, with somebody unknown; 3.66: being beheaded; 5.61: fighting with Asclepius; 5.87: being raped by Mars); attacking animals (2.11–2.13: various animals; 2.54: wild animals; 3.7: lice); legal suits (2.29); sport contests (1.57: pentathlon; 1.58: short distance running; 1.61: boxing match; 1.62: *pankration*; 1.63: hoplite race; 3.1: throwing dices; 1.59: exclusion from sports contest; cf. 5.13); futile or successful endeavors of another kind (2.26: not being able to leave the house; 2.55: ascent/descent to Hades; 3.60: being retained forcefully).
b. Images of liquids and fire, "elements," mixture, and composition. Foul blood denotes illness for everyone (1.33); vomiting bile or mucus means for everybody, whether ill or in hardship, being liberated from present problems because secreted liquids do not create bodily discomfort any longer (1.33); seeing a water snake announces illness caused by the four humors (2.13); finding a dead fish in one's bed predicts danger arising from the four humors (2.18); images of fountains and sources, if the water is clear, means cure and wellbeing, but if dried up, death (2.27; but

vendor on the market is good; 4.2: the surgeon Apollinides dreams of acting in a performance of Homeric episodes (he performs many surgeries just as actors shed blood without the intention of killing); (2) physicians and midwives as dream image: 2.29: physicians have the same meaning for those dreamers with legal suits as advocates or judges; 4.33: speaking physicians; 4.45: physicians' words generally auspicious; 3.32: midwife. For other examples (seeing other people ill and illness as dream material), see below.

cf. 1.64: swimming in clear seas and sources means illness); seeing Selene predicts death, because she is connected to hydropsy (2.36; cf. 1.80: having intercourse with Selene); seeing clay indicates an imbalanced status of the body as clay is neither water nor earth (3.29); wearing/seeing purple, brightly dried, or multicolored clothes predicts impaired health due to excess of bile and bitter humors (2.3); images involving a cook predict inflammations, deterioration of health, and imbalanced mixture of the humors (3.56).

The underlying disposition to all these images is the balanced or unbalanced mixture of heterogeneous components like heat and cold. In some chapters, the interpretation of images explicitly or implicitly evokes the medical concept of humoral pathology and so offers something like a downgraded medicine, with diagnosis and therapy alike being present. The *Oneirocritica* does not contain enough evidence to prove a direct connection. Rather, oneirocritic imagery—with its parallel to medical dream imagery[24]—might be an index to the popularity of the Hippocratean humoral pathology or be a vague reflection of more general philosophical notions of balanced/imbalanced mixture and conflict of the four elements, which stands behind humoral pathology.

c. Images involving diet/therapy and medicinal plants: cucumber (1.67: salubrious effect); eating onions (1.67) and sea onions (3.50: various interpretations); medical plants (oleander, box-tree, myrtle), which denote a cure (2.25); eating white bread, which signifies illness for poor people (1.69); drinking honey wine, quince wine, quince juice, or myrtle wine, which is a bad omen for poor people because they consume these liquids only when sick (1.66); water and water cures (1.64: bathing with clothes in the *caldarium* denotes illness as only ill people leave their clothes on while bathing; 1.64: an image of a poor man bathing with servants around him predicts illness, as he will need help; 1.64: bathing in warm water, clear sources, or fountains predicts cure for ill people and standstill for negotiations, as only ill or idle people take warm baths; 1.64: swimming in warm waters predicts illness and death for any dreamer; 1.66: drinking warm water announces illness or inactivity in business); purgation of the colon through an enema (5.79); surgery (1.44: cutting the body open);[25] seeing white vegetables (1.67); plants growing from body parts predict surgery if they are plants that are

[24] Cf. Oberhelman, "Prescriptive Dreams," pp. 43–6, who in his notes to his translation of the Galenic treatise lists sundry parallels between Galen's treatise and Artemidorus.

[25] Perhaps this is also a reference to haruspicy.

customarily cut (3.6); surgery as métier of physicians (4.1); a person's dream of Asclepius stabbing him in his abdomen predicts surgery of ulcer of the abdomen and a cure (5.61); a man who dreams of being raped by Mars and feeling pleasure gets relief by undergoing surgery of an abscess of his anus (5.87); a man, about to undergo surgery on his scrotum, dreams of Sarapis advising this surgery as a way to end his pain; he has surgery and dies, consequently having no further problems (5.95).

Whereas in most cases an unspecified illness or the possible course of an already-existing but unspecified disease is predicted, sometimes the type of illness/discomfort is specified, to a certain degree. This is clear from Table 6.2.

(3) Illness as Dream Image: Seeing Oneself or Other People Ill[26]

Changes of one's own body, among them diseases, are also dream material, although they are not necessarily interpreted in terms of future illness:

a. Seeing oneself ill: these images visualize either totally unspecific or visually or haptically obvious forms of illness, mainly skin diseases, fever, paralysis, and blindness. Examples include blindness (1.2: to be blind or become blind means that children will die; etymological interpretation via *pupillai*); deformation/transformation of the eye (1.26; 4.24); to see oneself lying ill (1.5: specifics not given; dream image and its result will both be bad); having foul blood (1.33); having an ulcer in the throat (1.34: a very bad omen); having weak or deformed hips (1.43) and weak or ailing knees (1.47); hernia and venereal diseases (3.45); several skin diseases, including scabies, elephantiasis, and leprosy[27] (3.47); seeing oneself with someone else's illness and handicap means that one will develop the same weaknesses (3.51); vomiting blood and other things (4.26; cf. 5.6); visiting a sickbed (3.22); seeing oneself sleeping in temples (1.81: sleep in general denotes standstill or idleness, but it predicts a cure for people who suffer pain or illness, since sleep heals).
b. Seeing other beings ill: images include humans: seeing an ill mother or wife means less income, wealth, or reputation (1.2); seeing a sickened

[26] At 1.10, Artemidorus lays open the organization and structure of his book. Illness and health as topics of dream imagery are not explicitly mentioned as an extra entry, but are subsumed under body, parts of the body, diet, balneological imagery, etc.

[27] That leprosy is present too shows that Artemidorus is informed about rather recently developed and spread diseases.

Table 6.2 Diseases and Bodily Discomforts Mentioned in the *Oneirocritica*

Disease	Subcategory	Textual Reference
Headache		1.17; 4.22
Unspecific Eye Diseases	General	2.36; 2.39; 4.22
	Bleary Eyes	5.9
	Losing an Eye	5.54
Blindness		1.4; 1.26 (as dream image); 1.48; 2.5; 2.68; 4.58; 5.11; 5.20; 5.44; 5.77; 5.90
Deafness and Muteness	Deafness	1.24
	Deaf-Mute Child	1.76
Consumption		1.21; 1.31; 1.66; 4.54
Symptoms of Poisoning		1.66; 2.14
Discomfort of the Colon/Diarrhea		2.14
Inflammations		2.14; 5.56
Inflammations of the Laryngeal Tract (with Ensuing Death)		5.26
Fever		2.3; 2.11; 4.2
Hydropsy		1.80; 2.36
Ulcers/Abscesses		1.47; 5.61; 5.87
Necrosis of a Bone		5.59
Skin Diseases	Leprosy	3.47
	Elephantiasis	3.47
	Scabies	3.47
Paralysis (Unspecific Handicaps of the *Bewegungsapparat*)	General	1.47; 2.22; 2.47
	Paralyzed Child	4.67
	Broken Hand	5.3
	Weakness of Feet	5.81
	Stroke	5.88

female breast (1.41: inauspicious); visiting a sickbed (3.22: if the patient is known to the dreamer, this means that things will be fulfilled for the ill person [alien dream]; if an unknown person, for the dreamer [personal dream], because seeing oneself or someone unknown makes no difference); seeing people of the same profession (4.1: the rhetorician Philagrus dreamt that the rhetorician Varus was lying ill, and for a long time he could not practice his profession); a master seeing his slave with the same paralysis that he himself has (3.1: he finds out they share the same lover). Animals: dog (2.11: a dog has the same interpretative significance as relatives).

It is remarkable that these images are not exclusively interpreted in terms of illness or as a negative omen, as the chapter on skin diseases (3.37) shows. Scabies, elephantiasis, and leprosy predict for poor people wealth and renown, as these diseases draw the attention of other people; rich and powerful people, on the other hand, will get an important office. To see oneself with the aforementioned diseases is good, but to see others afflicted turns out to be a mainly negative symbol, as the spectator of these diseases will be disgusted. To see family members so affected is even worse: a slave will no longer be of use, a son's lifestyle will not be in accordance with his parent's principles, and a wife will be immoral and cause trouble.

In general, seeing oneself ill is only good for people in fetters or in situations of need, for illness weakens (3.22). For everybody else it denotes great idleness, lack of things necessary for living, and prohibition of travel (sick people do not move around); moreover, the fulfillment of wishes will be denied as a doctor does not allow his patient to have his or her way. Having the same ailments and pains in a dream as some known person denotes that the dreamer will fall prey to the same vices, as bodily diseases are like the irrational passions of the soul (3.51).

Now that we have surveyed how illness occurs in the *Oneirocritica*, let us return to a comparison of medical and predictive dream interpretation.

Prediction and Diagnosis: Differences and Similarities to Medical Dream Interpretation

The binding element of both medical and predictive/divinatory dream interpretation is prognosis, even if the prognosis of each is of a different kind. In his 1988 chapter, Giulio Guidorizzi in his discussion of medical dream interpretation[28] shows how the methods and approaches of divinatory dream interpretation were integrated into medical dream interpretation and highlights some parallels: the physician and the dream interpreter both take the dream as its own semantic system and not as "un vano e caotico affollamento d'immagini nella mente di chi dorme e neppure un' esperienza mistica."[29] They also take for granted the metaphorical (allegorical) nature of dream images[30] and use

[28] Guidorizzi, "Sogno, diagnosi, guarigione"; cf. also for further information Walde, *Antike Traumdeutung* and Holowchak, *Ancient Science and Dreams*.

[29] Guidorizzi, "Sogno, diagnosi, guarigione," p. 96. This means the incubation dream in which divine advice is experienced.

[30] Guidorizzi ("Sogno, diagnosi, guarigione," p. 96), uses the term "simbolico."

the same approach to interpretation, namely deciphering.[31] Both professional groups base their prediction on fragile clues and by thinking in analogies.[32] These parallels may be significant, but we must remember that both groups share the same attitude toward dream interpretation as almost all known methods of dream interpretation, even those on an intercultural level: that dreams, when deemed meaningful, convey these meanings in an indirect, translated form. What separates both the dream-interpreting physician and the divinatory dream interpreter from other methods is that they use dreams in a professional frame.[33] But there still remain crucial differences between Artemidorus and the medical dream interpretation, although we moderns find it difficult to reconstruct what *both* practices constituted.

We have fewer ancient *testimonia* on the medical use of dreams than on divinatory dream interpretation, but the medical treatises of Hippocrates (*Regimen* 4, c. 400 BC), Rufus of Ephesus (*Medical Questions*, early second century AD), and Galen (*On Diagnosis from Dreams*, contemporaneous with Artemidorus) are heterogeneous enough and so offer enough similarities to get a basic idea of this practice. Clients consulted a physician over concerns for their health (either to preserve it or because of problems with it), not because they had had a confusing dream.[34] The doctor not only diagnosed an illness and suggested a therapy that the client hopefully would follow, but, as *Regimen* 4 shows, he also tried to remedy or prevent disharmony of the four humors. Artemidorus' practice, on the other hand, was focused exclusively on dream interpretation: his clients sought his expertise in this field after they had had a dream they could not get out of their mind. The dream professional and his clients alike shared the presupposition that dreams can predict the future. Good or bad things—including illness, its course, and therapy—are *predicted*; therefore, the difference

---

31 Guidorizzi ("Sogno, diagnosi, guarigione," p. 96) draws a parallel with what Freud would call *Chiffriermethode*, but this is inappropriate as Freud characterized fixed symbolism as always recurring in the same way.

32 Cf. also Artemidorus' statements about the perfect interpreter of dreams in 2.25 (most important reference); see also 1.11–12, 4.20, 4.56, 4.67.

33 Cf. Oberhelman, "Prescriptive Dreams"; Holowchak, *Ancient Science and Dreams,* p. 134; Walde, *Antike Traumdeutung*, pp. 106–26; Liatsi, "Zur Funktion des Traumes."

34 One could hypothesize whether a good and obedient patient, trained by his physician, will not start looking out for dreams that might indicate a balance or imbalance of the four humors and then either take measures himself or consult the doctor again. One should also mention that psychoanalytical dream interpretation started with Freud's analyzing his own dreams. The self-analysis after the conclusion of psychoanalysis is always implicit, whereas to my mind Artemidorus could have no interest in his clients' starting to interpret their own dreams. His interpretations are only single episodes in the life of a client, whereas medical dream interpretation and psychoanalysis aim at an integrated view of life and health.

compared to medical dream interpretation lies in the temporal dimension, the time lag between dream and its fulfillment. In the case of already-ill patients, the interpretation serves as a statement on life expectancy; this comes close to what a physician does, but it should not be confused with either the diagnosis or therapy that the physician offers, even if the results for the client may be somewhat similar.

Both physician and dream interpreter faced the same problem of validation and verification, and so they each had to resort to empiricism, intuition, and presupposition of a certain repetition of occurrences. Their interpretations could be validated with certainty only in retrospect. Seen from this perspective, Artemidorus' *Oneirocritica* represents a diligent and constant endeavor to find rules that could be applied *before* the dream's fulfillment. More likely than not, we are following only his steps in this direction, but we can surmise as to where he is heading.

It is interesting that both *Regimen* 4 and Galen experience difficulties with separating health and illness dreams from divinatory/predictive dreams—and not with the separation from the *enhypnia*. Let us take this as a starting point for assessing Artemidorus. To my mind, the physician has the easier part because, in contrast to Artemidorus, he can cling to some (rather) fixed coordinates: his basic assumption is that the balance or the imbalance of the four humors is represented by certain images; the dichotomy of normal (healthy) and pathological states of health is depicted as dreams are produced by the body.[35] The physician conceives the body as a microcosm that is especially represented by images of the macrocosm or by the surplus and deprivation of liquids. But dreams are not his only tools of diagnosis and prevention; they are but one of the traces that illness or health leave behind, and not even the decisive one at that. The physician's difficulties seem to arise from dream classifications and sorting through the several origins of dream images, but this is so only if he relies *exclusively* on dream interpretation. Yet a physician can very well do without it.

Artemidorus, by contrast, deals only with free variables, since he has removed the need for differentiation between predictive dreams and dreams concerned with body and health by classifying both types of dreams as meaningful dreams. Indeed, for him, there remains only the problem of separating *enhypnia* and *oneiroi*, a process that physicians deemed an easy task. Here Artemidorus is more precise: he does not find it amiss to label both *oneiroi* and *enhypnia* as dream images, as both of them are an interior production of sounds, images, and experiences that humans encounter while sleeping. Yet Artemidorus is not really

35 Cf. Liatsi, "Zur Funktion des Traumes," p. 20.

interested in the origins of dreams and especially does not necessarily see health-related dreams as the result of body signals.

Scholars have argued that medical dream interpretation[36] integrated to a degree aspects and dimensions of divinatory dream interpretation. I would rather see it as a "spinoff" of divinatory dream interpretation, a specialization not viable without the master discipline of divinatory oneirocriticism. This integration can only be seen from the perspective of the much wider field of medicine. Artemidorus' *Oneirocritica*, dealing with meanings rather than with origins, brings together different areas and uses of dream interpretation, including those concerned with health and illness. The difficulty of distinguishing health dreams from other dreams only arises in the event of a detailed specialization of dream uses.

At this point, one could argue whether, in case of dreams regarding health, the Artemidorean dream interpreter does not rather function as a lay physician. As he has to define the individual scope of every single interpretation, his first task is as anamnesis with his client (1.9), inquiring among other things about his or her health. At first glance, this seems to be a parody of the medical procedure (cf. Rufus and Galen), but it is actually a standardized procedure applicable to any form of scientific practice concerned with human life. For Artemidorus, the anamnesis is crucial for his division between *enhypnia* (e.g., dreams seen by already ill people) and *oneiroi* concerning the prediction of health and/or other spheres.

In most cases, Artemidorus might have dealt with *enhypnia*, dreams indicating the conditions of the body or mind and sometimes going hand in hand with *oneiroi*. *Enhypnia* can not only be tricky and delusive, but the interpreter is also dependent on the client's narrative talent and truthfulness in order to decipher them. This makes one wonder how the oneirocritic practice was conducted. What happened when Artemidorus classified a client's dream as an *enhypnion* that was solely concerned with a pressing problem or emotional state? The client had to pay anyway, since the classification of a dream as an *enhypnion* is a professional act (and therefore reimbursable). Did Artemidorus offer some advice or consolation? We do not know, but he does admit that a dream interpreter must be prepared to listen to many complaints and sorrows (3.21).

But what about the two types of health-related dreams—those predicting illness and those conveying healing advice? Artemidorus gives us some information about them in 4.22. In this chapter, where he discusses healing advice conveyed in dreams, he chastises those interpreters—physicians, priests, and other interpreters—who construct farfetched, silly, what one

36 Cf. Guidorizzi, "Sogno, diagnosi, guarigione."

could call "Hellenistic" interpretations whose obscurity is not in concordance with the gods' benevolent nature. This passage could certainly be read as a critique of his own method, but more likely than not, Artemidorus is referring to special dream cases of ill people, to either petitionary dreams or dreams introducing a remedy without a special request. It is here where Artemidorus' medical competence becomes apparent: he recommends giving only proven medical advice, such as those certain common diets, baths, and ointments that the gods or good doctors would prescribe (which narrows the horizon of interpretation or rather substitutes the interpretation with medical advice). To apply one's fancy imagination to dream interpretation would be amiss with regard to health, because the gods would never torment human beings with nonsensical things and because the guidelines of a human interpreter should be infused with truth, which in this case means medical experience. This common and sound advice can be judged as a professional attitude, which might be extended to any other realm of competence. We may perceive here a glimpse of why professional dream interpretation was so successful for such a long time and why Artemidorus was especially used and well received by early modern physicians.[37] His practice of interpretation was a sort of super competence, the role of the interpreter including that of a lay physician and/or the distributor to other specialists. Certainly, *rebus sic stantibus*, Artemidorus could not argue with the helpfulness and reliability of healing cults or be a competition to physicians, as they all shared the presupposition of dreams as meaningful regarding matters of health. Not only does he sometimes act as lay physician, but in some cases he tacitly takes over the priests' competence. In Book 5, the exercise part of the *Oneirocritica*, Artemidorus records a remarkable number of dreams figuring/starring Asclepius or Sarapis.[38] Here the line between religious dream interpretation—handed down to us in the form of the inscriptions found at Epidaurus and other incubation sites and in the unique literary *Sacred Tales* of Aelius Aristides—and secular dream interpretation is thin indeed.[39]

---

[37] For an overview of Artemidorus' reception, see C. Walde, s.v. "Artemidorus," in C. Walde (ed.), *Die Rezeption der griechisch-römischen Literatur: Ein kulturhistorisches Werklexikon* (Stuttgart, 2010), pp. 149–58, especially pp. 154–5.

[38] A concise overview of the epigraphic testimony (with an ample bibliography) is to be found in G. Renberg, "Dream-Narratives and Unnarrated Dreams in Greek and Latin Dedicatory Inscriptions," in E. Scioli and C. Walde (eds), *Sub imagine somni: Nighttime Phenomena in Greco-Roman Culture* (Pisa, 2010), pp. 33–61; see also the chapters by Downie and Pearcy in this volume.

[39] Artemidorus tells us that medicine developed out of the incubation practice, with doctors memorizing the god's healing advice (4.22).

In some dream images Asclepius is only used as a code word for health; other images might reflect the practice of petitionary dreams[40] also outside the Asclepian temples in case of bad health, as indeed all of the examples in the *Oneirocritica* are concerned with health.[41] In Artemidorus' classification of dreams, these belong to a subcategory of *oracula* (1.2), although they are requested by the dreamer. Therefore, Artemidorus also advises how to fare with the gods who neither like to be urged nor asked for a specific sign, as they will choose their way of communication (cf. 4.2).

In the case of health-related dreams, especially those seen by already ill people, Artemidorus' practice might have filled a gap for those who could not or would not pay a physician or, for whatever reason, did not want to have recourse to either Asclepius or incubation. The (wandering) interpreter might have been important in villages with a low presence of physicians and was perhaps not as expensive as the medical professional. Under the patronage of Apollo, god of oracles and health, and in good standing with all the other gods, the interpreter acted as a sort of human oracle, helping people to cope with problems of body and mind.[42]

Still unsolved is the question of how our ancient dream interpreter dealt with negative predictions, all the more so as even in non-health-related dreams, life expectancy plays a crucial role too. In the *Oneirocritica*, the approach to other people's health is sober and distanced. Artemidorus is well aware of the dangers and problems arising from a terminal illness, but mirrors only from afar the experiences of the human beings affected; nonetheless, he must have acted accordingly as the messenger of fate. As negative predictions are frequent in the *Oneirocritica,* Istvan Hahn supposes, with little justification, that textbook and practice were two different realms;[43] he devaluates the practice as mere hocus

---

40 On petitionary dreams in the *Oneirocritica*, see, with some reservations, G. Boter and J.-J. Flinterman, "Are Petitionary Dreams Non-Predictive? Observations on Artemidorus' Oneirocritica 1.6 and 4.2," *Mnemosyne*, 60 (2007): pp. 589–607.

41 Asclepius and incubation as points of reference or imagery: Asclepius coming into the house (2.37); sacrifices to Asclepius (2.33; cf. 5.66: a man is asked to sacrifice to Asclepius); petitionary dreams of Asclepius (5.9 and 5.89); Serapis-related dreams (5.92 and 5.95); Asclepius excluding from sport contest. These dream images are rather frequent, but they do not differ in a significant way from dream images featuring other not especially health-related gods (cf. the list of gods perceivable with the senses, among them Asclepius in 2.34, and comments on Helios and Selene in 2.26).

42 *Pace* W.V. Harris, *Dreams and Experience in Classical Antiquity* (Cambridge, 2009), I see this as a legitimate form of *Existenztechnik* in line with Michel Foucault, *Le souci de soi* (Paris, 1984).

43 Hahn, *Traumdeutung und gesellschaftliche Wirklichkeit,* pp. 7–8. Certainly, textbook and practice will differ, as the *Oneirocritica* lays the theoretical foundation and hands down

pocus where the interpreter would have pronounced good tidings only from a love of money, whereas in a textbook he could be "sincere." But the practice of dream interpretation, as with all other *Existenztechniken*, would not have functioned if all interpreters gave only good news, for the deception would have been too obvious. I would rather imagine that a negative prediction coupled with a dramatic fulfillment would have conferred more on the interpreter's fame than a series of positive predictions (even if the latter, used with caution, facilitated client-binding and client-building). We can only guess at the therapeutic effect of visiting a good and proficient dream interpreter, who in his interpretative process offers a kind of talking cure and sets a task to the client, as he has to accept or dismiss its contents.

Aspects of Tradition

Reading the *Oneirocritica* again and again makes oneself wonder about Artemidorus' mode of composition. But on this crucial question, we are left in the dark as well—apart from some remarks by Artemidorus himself in the prefaces of Books 1 and 4 and in scattered passages.[44] Artemidorus writes that he collected (as a first step, noted down on index cards?) dream images and their fulfillment not only by reading and assessing the examples of other dreambooks, but also by questioning other dream interpreters, specialists and laymen alike. He classifies his colleagues into three groups: dream specialists only a bit older than Artemidorus himself; the older venerable specialists (he refers to several colleagues dating back to at least the fourth century BC);[45] and contemporaries he met during his travels. This means that Artemidorus relied on experience (2.70), whether his own or that of others. His own contribution seems to be the system of reference, some entries, and his own systematization of dreams, as he states in the preface to Book 4 as he reflects back to Books 1–3:

> I organized everything that the elder [dream interpreters] had written down only in very sketchy manner and without sufficient explanation, in a subdivided and

interpretations of dream images as the source of knowledge and association, whereas the practice is communicative acting.

44 I do not even think of arguing with extreme positions that see Artemidorus' *Oneirocritica* entirely as a work of fiction.

45 Among these are Alexander of Telmessus and Antiphon. Artemidorus' dominance is felt when reading about the Greek oneirocriticists in D. Del Corno, *Graecorum de re onirocritica scriptorum reliquiae* (Milan, 1969); nearly all of our testimonies about them are based on the *Oneirocritica*.

> totally reliable system, also adding subjects that exhibit new outcomes or that in themselves are new.[46]

But even if Artemidorus emphasizes his own achievement of organizing the material and in certain innovative interpretations, he defines his *Oneirocritica* nonetheless as a tradition-based product. In fact, Artemidorus' integration of a great deal of traditional dream-lore into his advanced dream science is the *Oneirocritica*'s advantage as a comprehensive textbook. This creates a certain tension between the obviously accepted older strata of dream interpretation and his own advanced system. Even if he re-evaluated older material, what were his criteria when selecting examples from other dreambooks? Did he only extract them if their context allowed some assessment of dream image and dreamer?

If we accept that divinatory dream interpretation underwent a constant process of professionalization, this implies that Artemidorus also introduced material of less proficient interpreters who could not have adhered to his strictly standardized method of interpretation and practice. Apart from dream-related matters, Artemidorus' competent interpreter of dreams must have a wide erudition and access to all archives of knowledge (4.4; cf. 4.22)—a claim not only in agreement with the standards of the so-called Second Sophistic and other realms of competence (philosophy, rhetoric, etc.),[47] but a necessary consequence of his concept of dream material and the process of decoding this material. Artemidorus' Aristotelean systematic presentation of his material not only includes basic medicine, but is evident in its details (e.g., biology, geography, literature, and art). Artemidorus examines things (human beings, animals, colors, plants, processes, etc.) from every angle possible. Therefore, very heterogeneous material—residues of multiple disciplines—finds its way into the *Oneirocritica*, which from our perspective can hardly be disentangled again. Certainly, dreaming and health were always connected in some way in the ancient discourses on dreams, and this in the end led to the specialization of professional medical dream interpretation, which was probably never very popular. But I doubt that beyond obvious general parallels the medical practice of dream interpretation can be reconstructed from the *Oneirocritica*, as the material is not specific enough; moreover, references to the interconnection of body and dreams may have infiltrated the interpretation of certain dream images at any time in the tradition of divinatory dream interpretation, especially since divinatory dream interpreters did not adhere to the strict

[46] Cf. 2.44, where Artemidorus distances himself from how his predecessors structured their dream treatises.

[47] Cf. G.W. Bowersock, "Artemidorus and the Second Sophistic," in B.E. Borg (ed.), *Paideia: The World of the Second Sophistic* (Berlin and New York, 2004), pp. 53–63.

division of *enhypnia* and *oneiroi* or of predictive and diagnostic prescriptive dreams.

Metaphors of Illness? A Conclusion

It is difficult not to look for our modern associations of illness or to read ancient texts without certain presuppositions in mind, for example, seeing cancer as a hideously slow-growing enemy or AIDS as a morally tainted disease, as Susan Sontag described in her moving books *Illness as Metaphor* and *AIDS and Its Metaphors.*[48] For Artemidorus, illness has no special metaphors—it is neither a taboo nor is it demonized. It is one of those conditions of bad luck human beings have to come to terms with. Neither ancient physicians nor their patients could rely on our modern tools of diagnosis (looking into the body by X-ray, CT scan, or differentiated blood testing). One could suspect that such a limited "introspection" leads to phantasies going overboard of what illness is doing to a body, but I think it more likely that our modern knowledge enhances our ever-multiplying and multifarious fears and anxieties, whereas the limited approach in antiquity led to equally limited modes of interpreting illness, and ultimately to acceptance.

Artemidorus' interpretations indeed presents us with some contemporary associations, but he does not offer a special imagery for illness/health which would enable us to define what ancient human beings—or even only Artemidorus—thought and felt about illness or how it was perceived as a social phenomenon—no more than we could imagine ourselves. The reason for this is easily found: underlying Artemidorus' interpretation of dreams is the prediction of events in human life in categories of good luck/bad luck and security/danger (*adiaphora* are not as interesting in contrast to medicine, nor are erudition or general satisfaction in life).

Reading secondary literature on other aspects of the *Oneirocritica*—slavery and the body of the master, traveling, sports, etc.[49]—and repeatedly

---

[48] S. Sontag, *Illness as Metaphor* (New York, 1978) and the related book *AIDS and Its Metaphors* (New York, 1988).

[49] For example, A. Filippo, "La simbologia della ricchezza e della povertà nell' 'Onirocriticon' di Artemidoro," *Index*, 13 (1985): pp. 425–38; H. Langenfeld, "Artemidors Traumbuch als sporthistorische Quelle," *Stadion*, 17 (1991): pp. 1–26; M. del Carmen Barrigón Fuentes, "Artemidoro y el mundo del teatro," in F.R. Adrados and A. Martinez Diez (eds), *IX congresso espanol de estudios clasicos* (7 vols, Madrid, 1998), vol. 4, pp. 57–63; M.-T. Olszewski, *Les projections oniriques: une clef de l'iconographie de la 'vita privata' d'époque impériale (à la lumière de l'Onirocriticon d'Artémidore de Daldis)* (Paris, 1998); J. Annequin, "L'autre corps du maitre: Les représentations oniriques dans l'Onirocriticon d'Artémidore

Artemidorus' text demonstrate *ad oculos* that we find always the same images for the several spheres of the *conditio humana*. They follow the same pattern of encoding (part of soul) and decoding (part of interpreter with help of the client). Dream images denoting a future disease are limited neither to images directly connected with health nor to any other distinct group of metaphors. As holds true for Artemidorean imagery in general, they are linked to health/disease by association only and show several grades of analogy:

- *Open/simple analogy*: here disease is indicated by easy decipherable body-images, with only a small difference between the manifest dream image and the contents of interpretation. For example (1.33): vomiting food, blood, or bile, or having foul blood, functions as an image of death and illness. Here the body of the dreamer is used as a projection screen; a negative health status of the dreamer, seen in the dream, stands for any kind of future disease.
- *Complex imagery*: the web of associations is looser and removed from the manifest dream image. For example (1.80): having intercourse with the goddess Selene (in her several manifestations) brings death to almost everyone (with the exception of some professionals, astronomers, travelers, ship-owners, and others), because this image denotes that the dreamer will fall ill with dropsy (the reasoning is that Selene is associated with water and moistness). The basic image of this interpretation is "having intercourse with a god or goddess" (1.80), which, according to the gods' function and the positions of sex, may turn out well or inauspicious. The dream's latent content is not necessarily linked to health only.
- *Deviant imagery*, which needs a special explanation that is not transparent to the (modern?) reader, even on second or third glance.[50] Here the interpreter uses a variety of hermeneutic approaches, very near to the rhetorical practices, including decoding of metaphors and tropes, literary allusions, puns, etymology, and *isopsêphia*.[51] For example (1.67):

de Daldis," in V. Anastasiadis and P.N. Doukellis (eds), *Esclavage antique et discriminations socio-culturelles, Actes du XXVIIIe Colloque International du Groupement International de Recherche sur l' Esclavage Antique (Mytilène, 5–7 décembre 2003)* (Bern, 2005), pp. 305–14; D.E. Harris-McCoy, "The Metaphors and Meanings of Travel in Artemidorus' Dream Book," *New England Classical Journal*, 36(2) (2009): pp. 83–104.

[50] Artemidorus, on the other hand, tells us about his own or other interpreters' difficulty in comprehending the interpretations that previous interpreters had handed down in their books. See, for example, 1.67, 2.proemium, 2.9, 2.66, 2.70.

[51] Cf. Holowchak, *Ancient Science and Dreams*, p. 134; Oberhelman, "Prescriptive Dreams"; Walde, *Antike Traumdeutung*, pp. 154–95. Holowchak states that physicians

> vegetables in general, in context of dry victuals; this chapter serves as a very good example for all three grades of analogy: "Regarding so-called white vegetables, turnips, fodder beets, and pumpkins denote vain hopes, because they have in common that they lie heavy on the stomach and have no nutritious value. To ill people and travelers they predict surgery and wounds inflicted by iron, as these vegetables have to be chopped. Peeled cucumbers are good for ill people, because they stimulate secretion. Watermelons are conducive to friendships and societies, because poets call *pepôn* what is dear to someone; in contrast to this, they prevent the success of commercial transactions, as *pepôn* also means 'limpness.'"

Whereas the general statements on white vegetables and cucumbers and their dietary value (not good for digestion or salubrious) show some reflection of dietary rules and therefore are directly health-related, the special meaning of the image "white vegetable" for ill people and travelers is rather farfetched. Here the analogy runs along the lines of identifying the dreamers' body with the vegetables, and the act of wounding and stabbing the body (with knives, swords, etc., made of iron) with chopping them (as these vegetables need to be chopped when prepared as food). The melons are not seen as vegetables but, in the form of a pun, are harmonized with homophones of their name, *pepôn*.

This one entry also strikingly shows that the same image might have a different meaning for various categories of dreamers: for some, these images are health-related, whereas for others they predict a change in financial respect or a general change in other aspects of life (marriage, death [not the result of illness], etc.).[52] Since health is one of the most important economic resources, the dichotomies ignominy/poverty/illness and reputation/wealth/health share much imagery. Consequently, in the *Oneirocritica*, we can observe several recurrent interpretative gradations (cf. 4.84). In a simple negative gradation, the image *x* is negative:

- for the rich (loss of wealth, reputation);
- for the poor (loss of health);
- for the nonfree (never being freed);
- for the ill (loss of life through death).

---

might have not used these methods, whereas Oberhelman deems it likely that Artemidorus' *Oneirocritica* transmits the methods of medical dream interpretation too. I opt for a mid-position as our testimonies about medical dream interpretation are scarce and the practice of individual physicians who used and decoded dreams may have been idiosyncratic.

[52] Cf. also the very good article on economic aspects of the *Oneirocritica* by Adele Filippo, "La simbologia della ricchezza e della povertà."

Everybody loses the one important issue in his life: the poor have nothing to lose but their health. In a simple positive gradation, on the other hand, image *y* is positive:

- for the ill (regaining health/cure);
- for the nonfree (gaining freedom);
- for the poor (acquiring means of sustenance);
- for the rich (increase in wealth and reputation).

As Artemidorus always allows for counterfactual and more individualized interpretations (based on associations), these two simple gradations can also occur in mixed form, as 1.17 (seeing oneself with a bigger head) shows: this image predicts luck to a rich man without political office, wealth to poor people, victory to athletes, rise of income to bankers, creditors and *enararches* (heads of *symposia*); however, it announces harassment to rich people with an office and to orators and demagogues, headaches to ill people, labors to soldiers, lasting captivity to slaves, and a life in turbulence to idle people.

Artemidorus' interpretation of dreams is not based on a symbolism which consists of mechanical connections between signifier and signified, as some scholars maintain,[53] but relies on a flexible imagery built on associations. Therefore, the images and their interpretations are only starting points. Artemidorus does not explain every connection/interpretation, but leaves room for one's own associations and explanations. In fact, this is not a weak point of his practice, but a rather strong one, as otherwise he would devalue his own focus on the individual dreamer and certain contexts (cf. 4.65). Modifications are always possible as the dream images are determined by a variety of factors (dreamer, tradition of dream interpretation [popular imagery], etc.). To my mind, there must be a strict terminological separation of symbol and image to avoid confusion of Artemidorus' advanced form of text/image interpretation with more simplistic methods of symbolic dream interpretation where something occurring in a dream is equated with the same fact/event/process in waking life—even if sometimes the dreambook seems to suggest a stable analogy (especially in the category "good/bad for everybody"). But Artemidorus himself is very precise in this regard: he asserts that believing in fixed symbols *and* having a great knowledge of dream interpretation will lead

[53] Metaphor and other rhetorical terms are better, as *symbol* has special meaning in rhetorical terminology. In secondary literature, especially of Anglophone provenience, "symbolic" seems to be used indiscriminately for any form of figurative substitute, as if one thing stands for another.

to the mind playing tricks on the dreamer by using imagery in a counterfactual, unexpected way and by enciphering *enhypnia* as well (1.1; 4.proemium).

Artemidorus is unique: probably there was never someone so obsessed with dreams. Certainly, he also has had a great expertise in other divinatory arts, but he deemed the interpretation of dreams as the supreme form of divinatory hermeneutics. Due to his exclusive preoccupation with dreams, he could gain puristic insights into the dream phenomenon: by means of experience and rational reasoning, he discovered what could be recoverable without technology, just short of a monistic explanation of dreams. From the dreamer's perspective, dreams are visual and sensual experiences during sleep which call for an interpretation. The dream narratives and their interpretation, that is, a contextualization of the dream image in the dreamer's waking life, are the only thing humans can have, although they have fallacious access to them. As Artemidorus' experience shows, dreams sometimes predict illness of the dreamer (or of other people), without naming an origin for this evident connection of dreams and health. But even modern (neurophysiological) dream science has so far not been able to identify the causation of dreams. The famous Swiss dream researcher Inge Strauch admits with professional honesty that up to now it is not possible to connect a dream narrative (the dream being a psychic phenomenon) to a body signal; in other words, that the gap between psyche and body cannot be closed scientifically.[54] This is all the more astonishing as the connection between bodily and psychic functions and dream images seems to be obvious and is indeed one of the recurrent approaches in almost every culture, and especially of medical dream interpretation. The modern interpreter of dreams Sigmund Freud was more confident in this regard and tried to sanitize dream interpretation by introducing approaches of natural sciences. But perhaps Artemidorus, in his insistence on interpreting dreams only without looking deeper into their origins, had a more correct intuition about the nature of dreams. Consequently, he developed a comprehensive, repeatable hermeneutic procedure that, next to intuition and capacity of associative thinking, has a highly technical quality in the theoretical background (represented by the textbook) as well as in the practice of interpretation. To my mind, this *technê* is practicable and no more complicated than any other form of hermeneutics.[55] That it seems impractical or even impossible to perform is due to the fact that we modern scholars, struggling with translation and contents alike, are not set in the same cultural

[54] I. Strauch, *Traum* (Frankfurt, 2006), p. 89.

[55] When we classical philologists interpret texts, we use certain implicit and explicit hermeneutical techniques too. The results are not verifiable in every respect, but this is still an accepted practice (at least in the humanities).

and communicative context that defined Artemidorus' procedure. Modern scholars take the easy way out and use the *Oneirocritica* as a means of getting through to the real life of the ancients, but this is fallacious. I would even argue that with no other classical text do we feel so desperately the lack of context and the tradition in which Artemidorus stands. If we were to have been his apprentices for some time or could possess the perspective of his implied and real recipients—being dream interpreters ourselves or at least Artemidorus' erudite contemporaries—the picture would change totally, I suppose, and we would understand better what he was aiming at. A contemporary, accustomed with dream interpretation, might have read the *Oneirocritica* in an amazingly different way, just as Artemidorus himself, who undertook a critical exploration into the landscape of the art of dream interpretation, took a stance vis-à-vis his predecessors. As we are no practitioners of dream interpretation, to us nothing else remains but translating and reading the *Oneirocritica* again and again and, as a result of these constant rereadings, trying to formulate questions. It might very well be that so far we have not posed the right questions, not least because we still cannot define what to expect when we examine and explain the still enigmatic phenomenon of dreams.[56]

Appendix: Statistics

Illness in its different dimensions does not occur in every chapter of the *Oneirocritica*, but it is a rather frequent topic. Often dream images predicting illness or the course of illness are found in clusters in subsequent chapters, perhaps due to Artemidorus' associative manner of composition and organization of his material or because certain image groups have a stronger tendency of denoting bad luck, under which category illness is subsumed.

The five books of the *Oneirocritica* are subdivided into 397 chapters of different length. Sometimes they contain only one image and one interpretation concerning illness, sometimes more. Therefore, two figures are given for every book, the first one indicating the chapter(s) in which the topic is mentioned and the second the occurrences of images and interpretations. These figures may differ.

---

[56] This chapter is dedicated to Ernst Ammann of Basel. I thank Dermot O'Connell of Rome for correcting my English.

Book/ Number of Chapters	I: Ill Dreamers: Any Interpretation except Death (Personal Dreams)	II: Ill Dreamers: Prediction of Death (Personal Dreams)	III: Healthy Dreamers: Prediction of Illness	IV: Alien Dreams Concerning Health	Totals
Book 1: 82	9 / 11	15 / 15	27 / 42	5 / 5	56 / 73
Book 2: 70	18 / 23	15 / 21	18 / 33	4 / 4	55 / 81
Book 3: 66	8 / 8	12 / 12	7 / 9	2 /3	29 / 32
Book 4: 84	2 / 2	6 / 6	8 / 10	6 / 6	22 / 24
Book 5: 95	3 / 3	7 / 7	16 / 16	4 / 4	30 / 30
Total: 397	40 /46	55 / 61	76 / 109	22 /22	193 / 238

I *Ill dreamers: any interpretation except death (personal dreams)*
Book 1: 17, 22, 31, 53, 56, 67 (3), 76, 78, 81
Book 2: 3 (2), 9 (2), 10, 14 (2), 18, 20, 25, 27, 29, 34, 35, 36 (2), 37 (2), 38, 39, 49, 52, 55
Book 3: 5, 7, 9, 42, 50, 56, 60, 66
Book 4: 55, 67
Book 5: 61, 72, 89

II *Ill dreamers: prediction death (personal dreams)*
Book 1: 13, 14, 26, 27, 33, 44, 50, 56, 58, 63, 67, 76, 78, 80, 82
Book 2: 2 (2), 3(2), 13, 20 (2), 27, 29, 30 (3), 31, 33, 36, 37, 39, 49, 65, 68 (2)
Book 3: 1, 5, 6, 13, 32, 41, 49, 50, 56, 57, 58, 66
Book 4: 2, 27, 47, 55, 62, 81
Book 5: 26, 30, 40, 52, 71, 92, 95

III *Healthy dreamers: prediction illness*
Book 1: 2, 4 (2), 14 (2), 16, 21, 24, 26 (4), 32, 33, 40, 41, 43, 47, 48, 50 (2), 57, 60 (3), 64 (3), 66 (4), 67, 68, 69, 71, 76 (2), 77 (2), 78, 80
Book 2: 2, 3 (3), 5, 7, 11, 12 (6), 13 (2), 14, 22, 26 (2), 27, 36 (4), 37 (3), 39, 47, 54, 55, 68 (2)
Book 3: 7, 15, 29, 32, 33, 46 (2), 60
Book 4: 2, 22 (2), 30, 37, 54, 56, 58, 68
Book 5: 3, 6, 9, 11, 44, 51, 52, 54, 59, 60, 66, 77, 81, 88, 89, 90

IV *Alien dreams concerning health*
Book 1: 26, 32, 40, 76, 78
Book 2: 9, 11, 13, 36
Book 3: 23, 66
Book 4: 4, 24, 30, 55, 67, 81
Book 5: 12, 20, 35, 46

PART TWO
Byzantium

Chapter 7
Who Is behind Incubation Stories? The Hagiographers of Byzantine Dream-Healing Miracles

Ildikó Csepregi

As Roland Barthes once warned us, the historical author of a narrative is in no way to be confused with the narrator.[1] In the case of hagiographical writing, caution is even more necessary, for the *narrator of the narrative* often assumes the mask of a previous, even imaginary narrator, who is the creation of his own writing *persona*. A particular case in hagiography is the way in which dream healings are recoded, in that hagiographers tell and reshape someone else's narrative. In the ultimate twist, this narrative mostly retells a dream, seen by the person or by somebody else, which describes a miraculous healing. The dreams of both miracles stories and illness narratives have their own patterns.

In this chapter, I examine who shaped the stories of miraculous healing dreams and how, and the presence of the dreamer/patient and storyteller/narrator/hagiographer (all of whom may be one and the same at times) in examples from Byzantine incubation miracle collections. These include the fifth-century miracles of Saint Thecla, the complex textual tradition that concerns the miracles of Saints Cosmas and Damian, and finally two seventh-century collections: the *Thaumata* of Sophronius, which tells of the healing miracles of Saints Cyrus and John, and the anonymous corpus of the miracles of Saint Artemius.[2] These collections are thematically unified and chronologically

---

[1] This chapter was completed within the framework of the research project "Symbols that bind and break" (European Science Foundation—OTKA Saints Project).

R. Barthes, "Structural Analysis of Narratives," in R. Barthes, *Image, Music, Text* (London, 1977), pp. 79–124, at p. 111.

[2] The editions of the Greek Christian incubation miracle texts are the following: G. Dagron, *Vie et miracles de sainte Thècle: texte grec, traduction et commentaire*, Subsidia Hagiographica, 62 (Brussels, 1978), abbreviated here as *MT*; L. Deubner, *St. Kosmas und Damian: Texte und Einleitung* (Leipzig, 1907), abbreviated as *KDM*; E. Rupprecht (ed.), *Cosmae et Damiani sanctorum medicorum vita et miracula e codice Londoniensi*, Neue

quite close; they also form a small but homogeneous group with respect to their narrative patterning. Christian incubation cults, together with the way in which the miracles were recorded, are heir to the classical and late antique practice of pagan temple sleep and to the pagan incubation healing stories.[3] Even in the seventh century AD, these narratives are closer in many ways to the Asclepian type of miracle narrative than to other works of Byzantine hagiography.[4] In this chapter, I shall outline how the Christian hagiographer put his personal stamp on the miracles and how he created his own hagiographical *persona* within the characteristic patterns of incubation narratives.

The hagiographer, however conscious he may have been as a composer and however seriously he took the demands of literary value, did not rely only on his own literary taste and stylistic repertoire. The formation of the miracle stories was determined by four factors: the figure of the healer saint, the patient or beneficiary of the miracle, the hagiographer, and the traditional generic rules of miracle narrative—in this case, the pattern of the incubation experience.[5]

The saint shaped the miracle with his or her actions, attributes, and gestures, manifestations that were strongly determined by his or her *Vita*, by earlier

---

Deutsche Forschungen, 20 (Berlin, 1935), abbreviated as *CL*; N. Fernandez Marcos, *Los Thaumata de Sofronio: Contribucion al estudio de la incubatio cristiana,* Manuales y anejos de Emerita, 31 (Madrid, 1975), abbreviated as *MCJ*; V.S. Crisafulli and J.W. Nesbitt, *The Miracles of St. Artemios: A Collection of Miracle Stories by an Anonymous Author of Seventh-Century Byzantium*, The Medieval Mediterranean, 13 (Leiden, 1997), abbreviated as *MA*. All of these editions include the Greek texts. See also the French translations of A.-J. Festugière, *Sainte Thècle, Saints Côme et Damien, Saints Cyr et Jean (extraits), Saint Georges,* Collections grecques miracles (Paris, 1971), a partial collection of the miracles of Thecla and of Cyrus and John; and the new complete edition of J. Gascou, *Sophrone de Jérusalem, Miracles des saints Cyr et Jean (BHGF I 477–479)*, Études d'archéologie et d'histoire ancienne (Paris, 2006) for Cyrus and John.

[3] The best analysis of classical incubation miracle patterns is R. LiDonnici, "Tale and Dream: The Text and Compositional History of the Corpus of Epidaurian Miracle Cures" (Ph.D. dissertation, University of Pennsylvania, 1989).

[4] For the comparison of classical and Byzantine incubation stories, see M. Dorati, "Funzioni e motivi nelle stele di Epidauro e nelle raccolte cristiane di miracoli incubatori," *Syngraphé*, 3 (2001): pp. 91–118.

[5] The scheme of incubation stories is the following: name of the sick person, his provenance and profession, his illness, his way to the healer, the dream encounter, miraculous cure or prescribed remedy, and cure obtained. For how these patterns grew out of the requirements of a votive tablet and how they were enlarged, see LiDonnici, "Tale and Dream"; for an ample selection of Asclepian incubation narratives, see M. Girone, *Iamata: Guarigioni miracolose di Asclepio in testi epigrafici* (Bari, 1998). In the Christian incubation stories, the pattern remained the same, along with those additions permitted by the more lengthy format of a miracle collection.

miracles, and by his or her reputation. The saint's customary characteristics were often represented in his or her iconography. The artistic representations that were visible or generally known to the supplicants had an impact on their religious experience and consequently on the narrative itself.

The healer and the patient are important not as individuals but as participants and actors in a cult experience. In the practice of incubation, however, the miracle itself (or the encounter with the healer) takes place in a dream. Unlike other manifestations of Christian saints, the miracle is therefore visible only to the beneficiary of the dream. With the dream being the medium of this religious experience, the dreamer-patient acquires in the formation of the story a greater role than in other fields of Byzantine hagiography. The hagiographer, however much he claims to be an eyewitness, was compelled to rely on the narrative of the dreamer. Dream experiences, and the narrative forms they can assume, were strongly influenced by the dreamer's personality: his faith, fears, expectations, medical and theological knowledge, and the personal elements of his waking world. But the narrative patterns of incubation miracles also influence both the dreamer and the hagiographer. Because the Christian patient, just like the sick pagan supplicant who turned to Asclepius, was conditioned by the stories heard or read about the cult and recorded and listened to in the sanctuary, these narratives fed back into the dream. The hagiographer, on the other hand, hearing a story of a dream cure, located it both consciously as well as involuntarily in the well-tried schemes of incubation narrative.

In this chapter, I will leave aside the role of the healer and the patient in the formation of the story, along with the story patterns characteristic of incubation miracles, and will concentrate on the figure of the narrator, or writer, of the incubation tale. For the reader, the hagiographer is the key figure in the process of molding religious experience into meaningful narrative. In what follows, I shall introduce his role and his person, not only as far as it can be deduced from the stories he wrote but also through his conscious self-presentation. In short, what is the hagiographer to the text?

The Hagiographer as Narrator, Author, Patient, Witness, and Cult Personnel

The above question might be better formulated if we ask in what sense we can regard the hagiographer as an author, narrator, performer, or compiler of the miracle stories. Is he a mere recorder of the text or a creative composer? What is the image he would like to create for himself? What authorial roles (storyteller, collector, or literary virtuoso) and what analogies for such roles can be found in the narratives themselves?[6]

Even as the recording of miracle narratives enjoyed a long and ongoing tradition, the recorder of miracles is certainly familiar from the cultic and literary context of Greek antiquity. But the precise character of his role is difficult to identify, as Vicenzo Longo points out in a learned study.[7] In its original meaning, the Greek word *aretalogos* denoted at the same time a priest recording the wondrous deeds of the god and an official entertainer. The dichotomy implicit in the term reflects the double-faced character of miracle literature itself: its combination of the sacred and the profane.

Apart from their function as propaganda for a cult place or a healer, classical miracle stories, in written and oral form alike, had other important roles. In cases of healing especially, they prepared the pilgrims psychologically, encouraging those who had been waiting for a long time or who had come with those medical problems that might be similar to the ones cured before in the shrine.[8] As the patient's stay in the healing sanctuary could often drag out over months and even years, and because the pilgrim's mood was often heavily determined by his consciousness of sickness, miracle stories also served to entertain, to divert the attention of sufferers, and even to make them laugh, thus alleviating their condition. Furthermore, these tales also equipped visitors to the cult place with a prefabricated story form, telling them how they might expect to witness the miraculous and in what way they were to tell it, in the immediate aftermath of their experience and then also back home, far from the cult site. It was not just the material of the miraculous that pilgrims took away with them but, more significantly, a template for the pilgrim experience in the form of a narrative code or way of describing the circumstances of dreaming, together with the obligatory attributes of the epiphany and the miracle cure.[9]

---

6 On types of narrator, see W.C. Booth, *The Rhetoric of Fiction* (Chicago, 1961), especially Chapters 6–8 for personal versus impersonal narration; and A. Kazhdan, *Authors and Texts in Byzantium*, Variorum Collected Studies Series, 400 (London, 1993).

7 V. Longo, *Aretalogie nel mondo greco*, vol. 1: *Epigrafi e papiri*, Pubblicazioni dell'Istituto di Filologia Classica dell'Università di Genova, 29 (Genoa, 1969), p. 19.

8 For this aspect of miracle stories in the pilgrim experience, see V. Turner and E. Turner, *Image and Pilgrimage in Christian Culture: Anthropological Perspectives,* Lectures on the History of Religions, n.s. 11 (Oxford, 1978).

9 Cf. Dorati, "Funzioni e motivi," p. 98: "Non si trattava solo di convincere i pellegrini presenti nel santuario della validità di una scelta da loro di fatto già compiuta—recarsi in questo piuttosto che in un altro santuario—ma anche di fornire loro gli strumenti necessari per propagare il messagio una volta allontanatisi da Epidauro e ritornati in patria, dove avrebbero potuto portare non solo la propria personale esperienza, ma una 'memoria' più vasta, per così dire, sintetizzata nelle storie esemplari che le stele avevano fatto loro conoscere."

Writing and telling miracles was a double-faceted activity that combined elements of the sacred and the profane, not only in its aspects as religious revelation and entertainment but also because the process itself worked in both directions. As Derek Krueger writes: "[I]n hagiography, authors deployed narrative simultaneously for the improvement of their readers and themselves. These literary acts of the making of saints were doubly generative, producing both the saints and their authors. Composing hagiography made one a hagiographer."[10] Claudia Rapp formulates more markedly the same message: "The hagiographer's function ... parallels that of the saint. Both, as it were, provide perfect models of sanctity, one through his writing, the other through his life."[11]

When writing, the incubation hagiographer had to keep in mind these aspects and functions. His task of collecting and recording the dreams and miraculous cures of the doctor-saints was also closely linked to his relationship to the cult place. He could be a beneficiary of dreams or the saint's miracle, a former patient or a church professional, a priest or a member of a lay sodality formed around the saint. The character of his affiliation to the cult greatly defined the purpose of his narrative (personal thanksgiving for healing, theological propaganda, etc.), while the means he used to gather the miracles, the sources he drew upon, and finally even the conjunction of literary and personal demands all determined how he put his stories together.

Most scholars of the incubation miracle collections[12] are interested primarily in the hagiographer as a historical figure. Thecla's fifth-century hagiographer has been examined as a figure of ecclesiastical politics and as an antagonist of Basil of Seleucia.[13] The extent of the hagiographer's classical education, rhetorical training, and literary and philosophical knowledge, as well as his intimate relationship to the saint and to the cult, has also been addressed.[14]

Our only incubation hagiographer with a name, Sophronius, the seventh-century hagiographer of the miracles of Saints Cyrus and John (who later

---

10 D. Krueger, *Writing and Holyness: The Practice of Authorship in the Early Christian East* (Philadelphia, 2004), p. 2.

11 C. Rapp, "Byzantine Hagiographers as Antiquarians, Seventh to Tenth Centuries," in Stephanos Efthymiadis, Claudia Rapp, and Dimitris Tsougarakis (eds), *Bosphorus: Essays in Honour of Cyril Mango*, Byzantinische Forschungen, 21 (Amsterdam, 1995), pp. 31–44, at p. 41.

12 See the collections listed above in note 2.

13 G. Dagron, "L'auteur des Actes et des Miracles de Sainte Thècle," *Analecta Bollandiana*, 92 (1974): pp. 5–11.

14 Ibid., passim; and S.F. Johnson, *The Life and Miracles of Saint Thekla: A Literary Study*, Hellenic Studies, 13 (Cambridge, MA, 2006), Chapter 4.

became Patriarch of Jerusalem), has also drawn scholars' attention to his own person—mostly because of the role he played in the Arab capture of Jerusalem.[15] As a hagiographer, he was a member of the circle of friends in Alexandria that had formed around John the Almsgiver and included John Moschos and Leotinos of Neapolis.[16] Sophronius wrote the *Laudes* and the *Miracula Cyri et Johanni* partly under this influence and as a result of his stay in Alexandria and Menouthis, where he had a powerful miraculous experience when his eye disease had been cured by the doctor-saints. This personal commitment, just as in the case of Thecla's hagiographer, gives a unique tone to the entire work.

The collections of Thecla and Cyrus and John are the only ones among the incubation corpora that are literary works of art by sole and named authors. The first was transmitted as a work of Basil of Seleucia and the latter, of course, in the oeuvre of Sophronius. They have thus largely escaped the rewriting and interpolation that characterizes other miracle collections.[17] In the material of Saint Artemius, for example, we find that later accretions have greatly transformed the theological message of the miracles. This latter collection, although anonymous, can easily be related to a specific hagiographer-author whose point of view was then adjusted by others, mainly through the straightforward addition of short closing sermons that consist of outbursts against physicians, Jews, pagans, and all sorts of heretics. The hagiographer of Artemius, on the basis of his medical vocabulary and his polemics against doctors, has been regarded by scholars as a physician himself, an ecclesiastical official, or perhaps (and more probably) as a member of a lay sodality attached to the cult; the hagiographer, by the wealth of detail he conveys on the everyday life of the capital and the church building itself, provides a rich source for the social or art historian and attests to a considerable medical knowledge,

---

[15] On Sophronius' person and on the identity of Sophronius the Sophist and Sophronius the Patriarch, see P.S. Vailhé, "Sophrone le sophiste et Sophrone le patriarche," *Revue de l'Orient chrétien*, 7 (1902): pp. 361–85 and 8 (1903): pp. 32–69, 356–87; Fernandez Marcos, *Los Thaumata de Sofronio*, pp. 163–4; and C. Mango, "A Byzantine Hagiographer at Work: Leontinos of Neapolis," in I. Hutter (ed.), *Byzanz und der Westen: Studien zur Kunst des europäischen Mittelalters* (Vienna, 1984), pp. 25–41, at p. 25, with reference to the work of C. von Schönborn, *Sophrone de Jérusalem: vie monastique et confession dogmatique*, Théologie historique, 20 (Paris, 1972) versus I. Ševčenko, "La agiografia bizantina dal IV al IX secolo," in André Guillou (ed.), *La civiltà bizantina dal IV al IX secolo* (Bari, 1977), pp. 87–173.

[16] On this circle of hagiographer-friends and their works, see H. Delehaye, *L'ancienne hagiographie byzantine: Les sources, les premiers modèles, la formation des genres* (Brussels, 1991), pp. 51–68.

[17] It would be interesting to investigate further whether and how a named author contributed to the stability of a miracle text.

which, so it seems, was not necessarily a privilege of the medical practitioners. Two recent hypotheses have found him hidden amongst the characters of the miracles.[18] This approach is the closest to what I attempt to do in my analyses below of passages and narrative situations where the hagiographer puts himself forward. When does he reveal his presence and when does he prefer to remain invisible? According to a recent observation:

> [T]he lives of the saints are also the residuum of a process of authorised self-production, of the making of authors. In generating a Christian authorial *persona*, the author was inevitably the subject of his own creative act. Indeed, the authors of early Christian saints' lives and miracle collections reconceived the production of literature as a highly ritualised technology of the religious self.[19]

During the process by which a hagiographer created his *persona*, reflection on the writing self is manifest in the metaphors he uses to describe or characterize his own activity. His choice of metaphors of authorship is not only based on his temper and the level of his self-esteem, but is also linked to the way he perceives his work as a collector, organizer, and redactor of stories who must struggle to select the best tales from the embarrassment of riches at his disposal.

The Metaphors for Writing Incubation Stories

The author is himself a character in the narrative, portrayed interacting with the saint or with the saint's shrine. Subjecting themselves to a variety of models, hagiographers depicted themselves as participants in the religious system they described and endorsed.[20]

The Hagiographer of Saint Thecla

Thecla's hagiographer calls himself a merchant of precious stones (a *topos* of Byzantine hagiography),[21] which speaks to the value of the saint's narrated deeds. Another image of himself, that of a miner for gold, reflects upon the difficulty of

18 For all these hypotheses, see below.
19 Krueger, *Writing and Holyness*, p. 2.
20 Ibid., p. 9.
21 *MT* 44; for other occurrences, see Dagron, *Vie et miracles de sainte Thècle*, p. 405.

his task in obtaining these treasures, of the chore of carrying off the layers of soil that cover and obscure his precious material.[22]

At the end of the *Vita,* before he embarks upon the saint's miracles, Thecla's hagiographer refers to his hagiographic project and the indispensable help of Thecla. Among his motivations for writing about the miracles, he mentions that he himself was the recipient of the Saint's mercy[23] and, moreover, mentions a request from Thecla communicated through her protégé Achaeus, a friend of the hagiographer (in the words of Dagron, "ami initiateur, sainte inspiratrice"). In the closing section of the corpus, however, the hagiographer addresses a very personal request to Thecla, as if in exchange for his work, that the saint should rescue him from the anger and malevolence of a certain Porphyrius.[24]

Thecla's hagiographer depicts himself as a researcher. He often lets the reader know that he has in fact traveled to the home town of the beneficiary in order to question relatives or living witnesses.[25] In short, he claims to have carried out a form of fieldwork. He draws consciously on Herodotus,[26] and his direct references to the historian are complemented by the impression the hagiographer leaves with us of a researcher, a collector of stories, a man who travels in order to learn.[27] He provides the reader with indications at each step that he is offering the fruits of his own personal research, information he has

---

22 On Thecla's hagiographer as a historiographer (in the *Vita*) versus the researcher and social observer of the *Miracula*, cf. Dagron, *Vie et miracles de sainte Thècle*, pp. 22–3.

23 Ibid., pp. 280–81.

24 Cf. ibid., pp. 16–18.

25 This is the case with the miracles that happened to some inhabitants of Eirênêpolis (*MT* 33–5) where the hagiographer travels to get information. In *MT* 34, he concludes: "All this I have heard from their compatriots themselves who were perhaps even their relatives"; cf. the closing line of *MT* 26: "There are still people who remember this miracle and they are extremely proud to tell it."

26 The hagiographer refers to Herodotus in the introduction to the miracles (Dagron, *Vie et miracles de sainte Thècle*, pp. 286–8), where he tells the story of Croesus and quotes the oracle given to him; he also calls Herodotus ἥδιστον (p. 288, line 64) and attests his knowledge of the historian by hinting at other stories without going into details.

27 Cf. what François Hartog (*Le miroir d'Hérodote: Essai sur la representation de l'autre* [Paris, 1980], pp. 224, 291) writes on Herodotus: "Mais cet travail de repérage et de découpage qui, au mieux, aboutit à un inventaire, plus ou moins complet, de figures inertes, s'il est indispensable, ne suffit pas. Les diverses figures ont, en effet, mises en mouvement par le narrateur, qui intervient de multiples façons, à l'intérieur même de son récit: la lecture doit alors se faire attentive à toutes les marques d'énonciation, qui disposent ces figures et qui, pour le destinataire, les lestent finalment d'un poids spécifique de persuasion. Pour les Histoires, l'affaire se joue, avant tout, entre ces quatre marques, ou ces quatre opérations: *j'ai vu, j'ai entendu*, mai aussi *je dis, j'écris* ... Que l'historiant initial, aventuré dans la narration, ait rencontré en elle la fiction, c'est ne pas un accident fortuit: cela meme appartient au procès

sought out directly. In *MT* 28, in the metaphor of carrying away the layers of soil that cover the stories, he specifies that his task after arriving at the deepest level of miracle stories is to rearrange the memory about them, their order of events, and the place and the way they happened.[28] He often incorporates the narrator of a given miracle into the narrative frame.[29]

Sophronius

Sophronius follows the opposite method in handling his sources. He never mentions them, apart from some general and schematic remarks, such as that the healed patient told everyone about the miracle that had happened to him. His compositional model is different from Thecla's hagiographer, who was so keen to name his sources. Sophronius aims to produce a free-flowing narrative, a chain of dream stories created in accordance with his own editorial principles. He foregrounds his own activity as a writer more than the narrator of Thecla's miracles (who subscribed to another image of the narrator-self, that of the Herodotean researcher). Sophronius is reticent about his sources and presents himself as an omniscient narrator. This image Sophronius has of himself is confirmed by the way in which he introduces himself at the beginning of the work—in a riddle, in question-and-answer form, by giving his name, his hometown, and his profession. Immediately after this quiz, in a short prelude to the miracle collections, he begins with a trope of classical Greek poetry. He lists how other people might praise the saints and concludes: "But for me, for whom words [*logoi*] are dearer than my homeland, I am convinced that the martyrs take their pleasure in words, as they themselves are called witnesses of the Word of God."[30] What is more, as Sophronius continues (incidentally confirming Derek Krueger's analysis),[31] the words that narrate saints' deeds also sanctify the

---

fondamental. Les 'sources' d'Hérdote sont fictives, en dépit de sa volonté historienne d'aller en 's'enformant', parce que la fiction appartient au procès de la narration primitive se faisant."

[28] Dagron, *Vie et miracles de sainte Thècle*, p. 362, lines 7–8: διαδιδράκοντα μνήμην καὶ τάξιν καὶ τόπον καὶ τὸ ὅπως ἐγένετο ...

[29] Cf. the list that Dagron (*Vie et miracles de sainte Thècle*, p. 26) gives for the living beneficiaries of miracles or their descendants. For example, in *MT* 11, someone tells of the miracles that he experienced as a child; in *MT* 19, the son reports the miracle that happened to his mother when she was pregnant.

[30] *Patrologia Graeca*, vol. 87.3, col. 388C: ἡμεῖς δὲ οἷς λόγος ἐστὶν τῶν γηΐνων ὑλῶν τιμαλφέστερος ... ᾧ καὶ χαίρειν τοὺς μάρτυρας πείθομαι, ὡς Λόγου Θεοῦ χρηματίσαντες μάρτυρες.

[31] Most elaborated in his *Writing and Holyness*, Chapter 4 ("Hagiography as Devotion").

writer. The image of the oral composer is foregrounded when he refers to his eye disease as a case of Homeric blindness.

The other metaphor Sophronius uses to describe his endeavors is that of Saint Peter, who foolishly attempted to walk on water. Elsewhere Sophronius, who takes his literary enterprise with the utmost seriousness, compares his role and writing method to the activity of the physician, thus perhaps placing himself closer to the work of the doctor-saints. He claims to work "just as the Asclepiadai do, [who] by mixing painful and useful remedies with honey purge those who need purgatives. I imitate them by adding to the previous sweet miracles these following harsh ones, and attaching these to the more pleasant things and making the end delightful" (*MCJ* 32). Behind the simile there might stand not only the professional claim that conforms to the saints' healing function but also the intellectual fascinations of Byzantine medical science.

The Miracles of Cosmas and Damian: Multiple Authors, Multiple Narrators

The larger and better-known collection of Saints Cosmas and Damian (hereinafter *KDM*) is a compilation and multiple redaction of 36 manuscripts presenting 48 miracles from various periods and places, all collected, collated, and published by Ludwig Deubner. The collection in this edition is based primarily on cures obtained through incubation in the church of the Cosmidion in Constantinople, probably between the fifth–sixth and thirteenth centuries. The earliest textual strata may date to the sixth–seventh centuries, but the collection was continuously enlarged until the thirteenth century.[32] Deubner organizes the miracles in their apparent chronological order and distinguishes six separate units.[33]

The London Codex (*Codex Londoniensis*, hereinafter *CL*) is an alternative version of Cosmas and Damian's miracles written in a simple Greek in an inventory-like way; the manuscript, dating from the tenth century, was found near Edfu in Egypt and now resides in the British Library. Its first owner, Robert de Rustafjaell, had already argued that the London Codex represented an earlier

[32] The most useful guidance on the maze of different versions and transmissions of these miracles is M. van Esbroeck, "La diffusion orientale de la légende des saints Cosme et Damien" in *Hagiographie, Cultures et Sociétés IV–XII. Siècles: Actes du Colloque organisé à Nanterre et à Paris (2–5 mai 1979)* (Paris, 1985), pp. 61–77.

[33] I: *Miracles* 1–10; II: *Miracles* 11–19 (*Miracles* 20 is an addition, which was originally in the fifth series); III: *Miracles* 21–6; IV: *Miracles* 27–32 (this series is supposed to be an extract from a longer collection, probably written by the author of Section III); V: *Miracles* 33–8; VI: *Miracles* 39–47, written by Maximus the Deacon (thirteenth century); *Miracle* 48 was performed in the saints' lifetimes and does not belong to any of the six series.

version of the *Miracles* (and probably an earlier phase of the cult as well), pointing to its unpretentious style and straightforward narration.[34] The editor of the text, Deubner's disciple Ernst Rupprecht, called it the "*antiquissimum quod novimus exemplum graecum*."[35] The *Vita* at the beginning of the *Miracles* introduces the nonmartyr version of the saints' life which belongs to the earliest layer of the tradition. In addition to this, the text twice unmistakably locates the origin of the saints' cult in their hometown and burial place, Pheremma near Chyrresticon in Syria. Besides the 14 miracles that figure in this collection but not in *KDM*, the uniqueness of the London Codex lies in its Egyptian coloring and in its Monophysite leanings. The hagiographer divides the corpus into 47 sections, with each miracle story being given a number and a title; there are no traces of the "units" found in the *KDM* corpus. There is a huge lacuna in the Codex, as *Miracles* 12–20 are missing.

I will compare these two related traditions—the Egyptian and the Constantinopolitan—in the next section and will examine the ways in which the presentation of the narrator changes through time and space. Here I limit myself to a general characterization of the longer and more complex corpus of *KDM*. The hagiographers of Cosmas and Damian's miracles belong to a continuous hagiographic tradition; only in the later layers do we find a personal voice and statements of authorial intentions. The hagiographer of Section III (*KDM* 21–6) places himself in the midst of his fellow pilgrims and listeners, describing himself as a healed patient who recorded the stories he heard while staying at the church. The hagiographer of Section IV (*KDM* 27–32) forsakes this sort of immediacy and instead pictures himself as a *narrator–I* in contrast to the *you* of the reader. In addition, he says this *you*—his audience and the addressee of the collection—is a certain Florentinus, a friend of his who asked or encouraged him to embark on this task of recording miracles. In Section V (*KDM* 33–8), the hagiographer depicts himself with a New Testament parable: he offers his contributions by adding new stories to the saints' known miracles, just as the poor widow once offered her two mites.[36] The thirteenth-century hagiographer who

[34] R. de Rustafjaell, *The Light of Egypt from Recently Discovered Predynastic and Early Christian Records* (London, 1909), p. 90: "The text of the manuscript ... in all probability refers back to an original of greater antiquity than those of any of the current texts."

[35] Rupprecht, *Cosmae et Damiani sanctorum medicorum vita*, p. vii.

[36] Mark 12.41–4: "And Jesus sat over against the treasury, and beheld how the people cast money into the treasury: and many that were rich cast in much. And there came a certain poor widow, and she threw in two mites, which make a farthing. And he called unto him his disciples, and saith unto them, Verily I say unto you, That this poor widow hath cast more in, than all they which have cast into the treasury: For all they did cast in of their abundance; but she of her want did cast in all that she had, even all her living"; cf. also Luke 21.1–4.

wrote Section VI of the *KDM* collection (*KDM* 39–47) is the only identified author/compiler in the corpus. Called Maximus the Deacon, he belonged as a monk to the monastery attached to the saints' church in Constantinople. This community of monks, like the monastery complex around the church of Thecla, was certainly a repository for the conservation and transmission of miracle traditions. Maximus' acknowledged goal is twofold: he ambitiously aims to express well-known miracles in a better style and he also wishes to enrich the collection with stories from his own lifetime.[37] He gives a lot of information about his own hagiographical activity, especially in the preface of *KDM* 40: he sees himself as far less insignificant and humble than the nameless hagiographers of the preceding miracle stories.

The Hagiographer of Saint Artemius

Artemius' hagiographer is similar to Thecla's in that he establishes, with the help of the miracles from his own and directly preceding generations, the credit due to the earlier miracle of his saint. In other words, he cites what he could still collect from living witnesses or from their children. It is remarkable that although this corpus is the most medical in its character, with detailed descriptions of the physical features of illness (male hernia), the overture of this collection is also the most aesthetically refined. In the first lines of the collection, the hagiographer defines his role in a long simile about the ecstasy of a man walking in a park full of gorgeous flowers, overwhelmed by the dilemma of what flowers to pick:

> Just as when someone enters a park and beholds the shapes of many delightfully beautiful trees and the variegated hues of different flowers uncloying in fragrance, and to him everything seems praiseworthy; then departing from there and coming to another place, he desires to report the spectacle of excellence to his neighbours also.[38]

The Hagiographer as Characters within the Incubation Miracle Stories

The hagiographers of our collections do not usually stop at self-introduction by comparing their writing activity to that of other professions and situations. They consciously reflect on their art of collecting, writing, and organizing

37 Cf. Festugière, *Sainte Thècle, Saints Côme et Damien*, p. 191, line 1.

38 Crisafulli and Nesbitt, *The Miracles of St. Artemios*, p. 77.

the miracles. The highest level of self-display is when the hagiographer writes himself and his enterprise into his stories—sometimes openly, at other times with subtlety and cunning—using his art of structuring and composition to hide himself as a hagiographer and to emerge as a character in the narrative.

The Miracles of Thecla

If we examine closely when and under what circumstances the hagiographer appears in the 46 miracles of the Thecla collection, we come to the following conclusion: the hagiographer comes into sight at certain intervals in the corpus which occur in a fairly regular rhythm (his appearances in the text are in bold face):

Introduction
1–4: victory over ancient pagan deities (Thecla and her immediate cult place)
5–6: saving Seleucia and Iconium (the place of the cult in a larger context)
7–12: **the priests of the sanctuary** (5)
7–8: Dexianus (contemporary, Thecla's priest already under Symposius)
9, 9b: Menodorus
10: connecting link: Symposius
11: a relative or compatriot of Symposius
12a, 12b: the hagiographer versus Basil, bishop of Seleucia
13–15: noblemen;
15–16: journey by sea and journey by land
18–21: women (4)
21–2: theft
23–5: eye complaints
26–8: Thecla as warrior
  26: Thecla appears on her feast day in the sky, upon a carriage in flames, and similarly protects the town of Dalisandrus during a siege
  27: she protects the town of Selinunte during a siege
  28: she protects her own sanctuary
28–30: **she protects her sanctuary and cult**:
29–35: punishment, protection of her people
  29: revenge, protection of her cult and feast
  30: revenge, protection of her cult
  31: the hagiographer; Thecla appears and encourages him
  32: punishment of Dexianus
  33: punishment of Orention (woman-affair)

34: punishment (woman-affair)
35: punishment, for stealing money from orphans
36–7: healing spring
38–40 (+41?): **Greek rhetoricians**
38: Greek rhetorician, converts
39: Greek rhetorician, refuses to convert
40: Greek rhetorician, suppliant of Sarpedonius, refuses to convert
41: healing of the hagiographer (classified as a converted Greek rhetorician)
42–6: women
Epilogue

After his first mention of himself at the end of the *Vita*, which is also an introduction to the Miracles and which explains his literary enterprise, the author appears in *MT* 12, 31, and 41. Each of these miracles belongs to a single thematic group.

In the first story of the double miracle in *MT* 12, the hagiographer tells us that, suffering once from anthrax, he was told by his doctors that his finger had to be amputated. Full of fear, he fell asleep: he (very strangely) saw himself sleeping in the atrium of the church, whereupon he was attacked by wasps.[39] Thecla entered and, having removed her shawl from her head, began to chase the wasps from the hagiographer's body by slapping them with her hands and trampling them with her feet (*MT* 12). Regarding the symbolic character of this dream, we should remember that Thecla's hagiographer overtly claimed (exactly because of the pagan connotations) that the saint did not work through riddles and enigmas—methods that, according to the hagiographer, belonged to the traps of Greek *daimones*. Nevertheless, when it came to interpreting his own dream, he could not avoid confronting the inherent symbolism of the dream. This is all truer for the more enigmatic dream recorded in the same miracle, which foretold the hagiographer's excommunication from the Church. Prior to receiving the actual sentence, he saw in a dream a midget—a short black boy (who was, it seems, a real figure of the town)—offering him a dirty black coin. He reluctantly took it and the next day, when news of the excommunication arrived, interpreted the repellent black boy as the bishop Basil of Seleucia and the dirty coin as a substitute for the host.[40]

---

[39] That is, he had a dream about his own incubation experience.

[40] For the Eucharist in incubation miracles and for the host taken in as medicine, see I. Csepregi, "Mysteries for the Uninitiated. The Role and Symbolism of the Eucharist in Miraculous Dream Healing," in I. Perczel, R. Forrai, and G. Geréby (eds), *The Eucharist in*

MT 12 ends the thematic unit that speaks about the bishops of Thecla's church (Dexianus, the hagiographer's contemporary and Thecla's favorite bishop; Menodorus, Bishop of Cilicia; and Symposius, an earlier bishop of the sanctuary: *MT* 7–11). The text underscores the fact that, just as the miracles of the collection are part of a longer series of miracle stories that record Thecla's deeds, this healing miracle of the hagiographer is but one of the miraculous recoveries Thecla performed on his behalf. Aside from the fact that here he does not give the patient's (that is, his own) name and other personal information as in his other stories, the miracle narrative does not differ in its illness/dream-healing story pattern from rest of the collection. The hagiographer naturally tells his story in the first person, but we get the impression that this apparently innocent healing miracle is just a prelude to telling a far more significant event shaped into a miracle. In connection with Thecla's healing power, the hagiographer puts himself in the role of a beneficiary; when talking of himself, he begins another story that is unconnected to his illness but expresses the grace Thecla has shown him. This involves the hagiographer's confrontation with the new bishop (the successor to Dexianus), who in this story is a dishonest drunkard but who became known in ecclesiastical history as Basil of Seleucia. From the transition, the reader gets the impression that the hagiographer had given us his story of recovery from illness, not only in order to insert himself into the collection but also because Thecla's healing miracle, which conforms to the nature of the other miracle narratives, will strengthen belief in the miraculous intervention into ecclesiastical politics which follows. Along with his effort to establish credibility, the hagiographer emphasizes that here he is narrating Thecla's personal help toward him in his conflict as a priest with his bishop. According to the narrative, the background of events was formed by the circumstances of Basil's episcopal election. As an omniscient narrator, he underlines especially the gravity of the way things happened by not speaking about it: "How he became a bishop, and how he got the church into his power, this man who is unworthy even to appear on stage in the theatre, I now omit."[41]

The hagiographer's next appearance in *MT* 31 is an emblematic representation of how he sees his own role as narrator and how he makes Thecla perceive it. During the redaction of the miracles, the hagiographer was oppressed by fatigue and negligence. At this moment, Thecla, in the very place where the hagiographer usually consulted his books, appeared as he was transcribing a

---

Theology and Philosophy: Issues of Doctrinal History in East and West from the Patristic Age to the Reformation (Leuven, 2006), pp. 97–130.

[41] *MT* 12.45–6: τὸ μὲν ἐπίσκοπός τε ἐγένετο καὶ τῆς ἐκκλησίας ἐκράτησε, τὸ μηδὲ σκηνῆς ἄξιον, ἀφείσθω τὰ νῦν.

draft version of a miracle on a tablet.[42] She began to read the finished part and was greatly delighted by it! After this encouraging apparition, the hagiographer redoubled his efforts to continue the collection. I would again like to suggest that the context of this miracle points to a homogeneous thematic group. From *MT* 26 onward, Thecla appears in her character as a warrior-saint and protector of her besieged city and her sanctuary. From *MT* 29 onward, the text is concerned with retaliation and punishment miracles that protect those for whom Thecla cares. It should be noted here that Thecla's attention is dedicated to those who are under her protection not only in a general sense (like the orphans of *MT* 35) but who also stand in a direct relation to her cult (such as the cult objects of her sanctuary, the woman who celebrates Thecla's feast day, or a nun who lives at the sanctuary). It is not accidental that the hagiographer writes himself into the stories where Thecla works for "her own people."

The last occurrence (indeed a spectacular appearance) of the narrator in the collection (*MT* 41) belongs to the closing miracle of a well-defined thematic group and is at the same time a precious piece of information about the image the hagiographer wished to record of himself. All the previous three miracles (*MT* 38, 39, and 40) concern Greek rhetors. These are completed by Thecla's intervention on the hagiographer's behalf, on the occasion of a rhetorical contest organized in her honor. On the eve of the event, the hagiographer's ear became inflamed, thereby jeopardizing his participation in the contest. He was helped by Thecla and of course won the first prize. Moreover, the hagiographer first tells two stories of Greek rhetors who, although they personally experienced the greatness of the Christian healer saint, refused to convert; he proceeds to tell two stories of converted rhetors where the latter figure is the narrator himself, and thus proves himself more worthy than the famous Aristarchus, one of the unconverted rhetors.

The hagiographer seems to compete consciously with the miracle tales of the local pagan cult hero, a rival to Thecla's fame, for he repeatedly uses a powerful image, that of silence, and describes how Thecla silenced or dumbfounded Sarpedonius:

> She rendered him voiceless, he who has so many voices and so many words saying oracles, by making the word of the Lord and King a stronghold against him: Keep silence and withhold yourself! In this way he was muted, left alone, and he hid himself. I think he even left his tomb and the place where he stayed. (*MT* 1, lines 16–20)

---

[42] Cf. Dagron's (*Vie et miracles de sainte Thècle*, p. 373 note 1) remarks about the technique of writing/rewriting/copying: "Les tablettes et le stylet servent à faire un brouillon, qui est ensuite recopié sur un quaternion de parchemin."

Thus, the imagery of total silence dominates—the heroes and the words concerning him are equally muted. And with an amazing twist, the hagiographer connects the physical presence of the healer with the stories circulating about him and his miracle-working. No miracle tales told, no cult.

In the same vein, the hagiographer also tries to silence his own rivals, the local rhetors.[43] The high level of the literary apparatus mobilized by the hagiographer is partly a response to the level of rhetoric that marked the work of the greatest poets and writers of antiquity. Just as his narrative technique was based on his classical reading, the first "narrative" of the miracle collection, not surprisingly, comprises a Herodotus paraphrase, the story of the Delphic oracle given to Croesus.[44] Nevertheless, the inspiration for storytelling and rendering the miraculous words of the miracle narratives originates from Thecla. The merit is hers not only in the recording of her miracles but also when, during the annual panegyric competition, the words to praise the saint themselves became the *thauma* of eloquence.[45]

Thecla's hagiographer thus constantly foregrounds himself as a beneficiary of miracles and as protagonist of four, detailed stories, two of which focus on his literary activity. Although we do not know his name, we learn far more about his personality than we do about those of the other hagiographers. At the end of the collection, he reveals a hitherto concealed, very much down-to-earth motif for embarking on his task of collecting and writing the miracles. The hagiographer, who must have had a serious row with a certain Porphyrius, calls him a dog, a pig, and a bastard. He appeals for Thecla's help against this man and to overcome his own wrath. Dagron has suggested that this Porphyrius might have been the new bishop of Seleucia (who succeeded Basil of Seleucia sometime after 468), a successor to the good bishops who lived under Thecla's guidance—hence the prominence of the stories about them.[46]

Thecla's corpus is the most consciously structured of the miracle collections, with well-elaborated thematic groups, connecting themes, and reappearing figures. This is in sharp contradiction to Johnson's statement that "the *Miracles of Thekla* are more casual in their approach to collection, arranging their material with no real structure or overarching argument."[47]

---

[43] Cf., for example, *MT* 30.

[44] In the introduction to the miracles; see note 25 above.

[45] *MT* 41.25–7: οὕτω δέ μοι τὴν χεῖρα καὶ κάριν συνεπέδωκεν ἡ μάρτυς, ὡς εἶναι τι καὶ δόξαι, καὶ εἰρηκέναι μετρίως, καὶ θαῦμα πλεῖστον ἐπὶ μηδενὶ θαυμαστῷ τῶν ἐμῶν ἀπενέγκασθαι λόγων.

[46] Dagron, *Vie et miracles de sainte Thècle*, p. 16.

[47] Johnson, *The Life and Miracles of Saint Thekla*, p. 196.

Sophronius

In his collection, Sophronius used alphabetical ordering and numerical proportions, and was methodical in composing his own intrusions as well. He places himself at the beginning and the end of the collection, in this way dividing the circumstances of his healing into two narratives. The introductory *Laudes* before the first miracle of the collection and *MCJ* 70 complement each other in order to give the entire story. It is not by chance that the tenth-century Latin compiler and translator of the corpus, Peter of Naples, combined these two stories into one. The narration of *MCJ* 70 differs at several points from the other miracles of the collection, despite the fact that Sophronius emphasizes here too his familiarity with the formal requirements of the incubation miracle structure. He is carried away partly by his own personal message and partly by his efforts to push his extensive experiences into the usual narrative elements. Accordingly, at the beginning of his story, after a longish introduction and still in the first person, he quickly makes it unmistakably clear what should follow, as per the requirements of the incubation narrative:

> I shall tell soon my name, my town, my country and my monastery, where I am coming from, where I was—by God's will—consecrated, and afterwards my eye-complaint and the divine visit of the saints, as I have done in the previous miracles. (*MCJ* 70)

When he comes to the facts, Sophronius switches to third-person narrative and continues in this way until the end, unfaithful to his promise of concise and informative narration.

The miracle differs from the others not only by its exceptional length, but because Sophronius, for greater effect, places the obligatory narrative elements in a new position. The hagiographer himself does not sing the praises of his hometown, Damascus, but gives the word instead to the apostle Thomas. As a patient he is not just a patient, his illness is not only an illness, for Sophronius immediately assimilates himself to the blind Homer and makes the saints address him accordingly. Such an approach is quite strange, as Cyrus and John, unlike Saint Thecla, were not at all sympathetic to Greek learning. Sophronius diligently explains that the two "authors," Homer and himself, are analogous *only* in their blindness. His taste for the uncommon is also manifest when the saints are described, on their appearance, as not simply in monks' clothes. Saint Cyrus reveals himself in the likeness of the hagiographer's friend John, probably John Moschus, while Saint John appears as Peter, the *praefectus praetoriorum* of Alexandria. Concerning the illness, we learn that it was *xêrophthalmia*, that

Sophronius was visited by doctors, and that a Byzantine eye specialist made the diagnosis.[48]

The Hagiographers and Rewritings of the Miracles of Saints Cosmas and Damian

The consecutive, chronological order of the *KDM* sections is at odds with the London Codex, since the latter contains miracles from all the first five series, ranging from *KDM* 1 to 33. The miracles of the London Codex also to some extent undermine the distinction that Deubner and Festugière made regarding the separate "authorship" of the different sections. The first two sections do not have much to say about their author or their narrator. The miracles follow one another without particular authorial comment or personal remarks. More interesting is Section III (*KDM* 21–6), especially when compared to the respective stories of the London Codex. I shall examine each of these miracle stories and their corresponding versions in the London Codex in order to illustrate how that hagiographer depicts telling, listening to, and recording miracles.

In *KDM* 21–6, the hagiographer describes how newly healed patients told their own stories during the *pannychis*, the all-night vigil, one after the other. The narrator-protagonist of the first miracle of the section (*KDM* 21) was a recently recovered patient, of whom we learn at the end of the story (from the hagiographer), who since the miracle happened to him became, and still was, a regular visitor to the church. The hagiographer thus establishes a continuity between the time of the narration and that of recording, trying in this way to give credit to the story and depicting the subject and source of the miracle (the narrator) and the recorder (the hagiographer) as living witnesses to the saints' deeds.

The beginning of the next miracle (*KDM* 22) remains within the framework of this communal storytelling. It starts by saying that as soon as the previous patient ends his story, another recently recovered patient takes up the thread. In the London Codex, each story begins with the words *meta tauta*. Here in the *KDM* collection, the "after these events" *incipit* is enlarged into a framed narration, as each patient leaves as the next arrives. However, this narrative situation undergoes a change in the next miracle (*KDM* 23), as we learn only from interpolated half-sentences that the sick person is the narrator himself. Moreover, in the epilogue added to the end of the miracle, it is made clear that as soon as the patient left the sanctuary, he continued to spread the saints' miraculous deeds that he had personally experienced. In the fictitious narrative framework of the next miracle, *KDM* 24, the storytellers within the sanctuary

[48] A particularly interesting feature of the dream pattern here is that Sophronius sees himself from the outside, just as Thecla's hagiographer saw himself practicing incubation.

keep telling their miracle accounts and actually interrupt each other as they are telling their story. The miracle in *KDM* 24 is noteworthy for several reasons.[49] One of the most famous miracles in the corpus, it was known to Sophronius and was paraphrased by the hagiographer of Saint Menas. The narrator was also a healed patient on this occasion, although not the recipient of the cure described in the miracle; rather, he was a witness to the miracle—a third patient lying between the two people healed by the same miracle. This storytelling technique (what may be called the "narration of the third") appears on other occasions in the corpus[50] and in Thecla's collection[51] as well.

The closing miracle of this section, *KDM* 26, takes us back to the all-night vigil: the heretic protagonist of the story learned from hearsay about the miracle-working of the saints (apparently from outside the sanctuary) and was taken with a desire to participate in the Saturday night vigil. He was not ill, but the stories he heard had piqued his curiosity. Despite the fact that he was not a patient, the saints appeared to him in a dream and proposed a remedy for the illness of the noblewoman lying next to him. In the story, it was a test of his faith whether or not he would have the courage to believe and report the dream he received. He was hindered from telling the wondrous event because of the difference in rank between the woman and himself, and even more so by the fear that if he told the story, nobody would believe it and he would be ridiculed. Thus, the telling of the miracle was both the prerequisite for the woman's recovery and a test of the man's faith. The hagiographer tells us that he had been told that although the man remained a heretic, he put down in writing the miracles of the saints when the prophecy that the saints had told him concerning his future was fulfilled. This part of the story concludes with an epilogue in which the hagiographer turns to his patron, saying "Here, at your request, I have compiled the saints' miracles for you. If you like them, I shall send more later." Werner Kelber summarizes this phenomenon: "One may thus find inscribed in the newly mediated story a rationale for its own medium and history."[52]

---

[49] The story runs that on the right side of our "narrator" lay a mute noblewoman and on his left side a paralyzed man. The saints appeared to the paralyzed man in a dream and ordered him to approach the woman; when he finally made an attempt, the mute woman cried out and the paralyzed man ran away. In order that the miracle element of the story could be made clear, it was essential within the coherence of the narrative that the paralyzed man *tell* his dream to a third person, since this legitimized his action and demonstrated the saints' intervention.

[50] E.g., *KDM* 25, 26.

[51] *MT* 46.

[52] W. Kelber, *The Oral and Written Gospel: The Hermeneutics of Speaking and Writing in the Synoptic Tradition, Mark, Paul and Q* (Philadelphia, 1983), p. 129.

The same miracles are found in the London Codex: *KDM* 21–6 are analogous to *CL* 33, 34, 26, 11, and 35, respectively. *CL* 33 starts with the customary first words *meta tauta*. The repeated cures of the patient, the timeframe of the recovery that extends over years, have placed the patient in a different relationship with the narrator of the story, since there is no hint of personal contact or direct oral transmission between them. That the ultimate source for the miracles was in general the healed patient is mentioned casually in a half-sentence: "He hurried to the saints' church and told what happened to him by the virtue of the saints." The other analogous miracles also begin with the usual catalog-like *meta tauta* formula. In none of them is there any trace of the framework of communal or personal storytelling set up by the later *KDM* hagiographer. Nevertheless, in *CL* 35, the moment of the miracle is indeed the Saturday night vigil. The stories that figured in this earlier, less elaborate, and indeed rather inventory-like collection show that the hagiographer of *KDM* created a context of oral tradition for the miracles, an age-old narrative method that was to have a long future.[53]

The "fiction" of communal listening/direct storytelling does give credit to the hagiographer's compositional creativity, but it also well reflects the actual way in which these stories were transmitted. However well it accords with the way the community preserved its miracle traditions, it is important that the hagiographer emphatically builds communal listening into the narrative—to the extent of creating the fiction of a direct, personal experience.[54] Most probably, the editors of the *KDM* miracle corpus worked from written and perhaps oral sources as well, transforming both into written descriptions of personal and oral sources. Written sources are presented as the miracles read aloud in the church, while the oral sources are presented as stories heard from the patients themselves. It can generally be said that the London Codex did not refer to its sources, although its hagiographer was familiar with the idea of the genealogy of miracles, a tradition that received new layers generation by generation, as he wrote after the first three miracles in a short prologue:

[53] M. Chabon, "The Game's Afoot," *New York Review of Books* 52(3) (24 February 2005): p. 4: "Nearly all the Holmes stories, therefore, are stories of people who tell their stories, and every so often the stories these people tell feature people telling stories (about what they heard or saw, for example, on the night in question), and if this sounds like a dubiously metafictional observation then we may have forgotten how fundamental such stories within stories have always been to popular art from Homer to Green Acres, and how lightly worn."

[54] Cf. Kelber's (*The Oral and Written Gospel*, p. 116) remarks concerning the Gospel of Mark: "The text, although a written artefact, conveys the sense of 'realism' that in its total impact exceeds that of orality. More to the point, this 'realism' is the logical outcome of the manufactured text. Written language, exempt from concerns for self-preservation, is allowed full play. It can live and create its own interior potential."

> While these miracles happened right after the consecration of the Church of Saints Cosmas and Damian, in the past, we should not ignore those succeeding miracles that happened at our place, by their intervention. One generation shall praise thy works to another ... says David the prophet for the glory of God, who urges even now for praise, showing to us, descendants, similar miracles performed by Saints Cosmas and Damian.

Although André-Jean Festugière considered the third section of the *KDM* miracles connected to Section IV of the corpus (*KDM* 27–32),[55] the different ordering of the London Codex alters this picture. Moreover, we find in Section IV the hagiographer working in a completely different way, as embedded storytelling is not evidenced in the miracles; instead, he establishes directness of transmission differently. The two actors of the oral speech-act, the narrator and the listener, hitherto assume that the patient is the narrator and the hagiographer the listener (together with the others who make up the "we"). Now, a new aspect of textual formation comes to the fore. It is emphatically the hagiographer who assumes the role of "I," while the reader/listener is the public "you." The means of achieving this immediacy, or even intimacy, is the way the hagiographer turns to his audience at the end of the narrative: "Do you see, my beloved friend, how the saints succour those whom they love?" (*KDM* 27).[56] The addressee here may still be the real or fictitious friend mentioned earlier, Florentinus, but there was also a more general audience before the hagiographer's eyes: "Do you all see what great things faith is capable of, when combined with the grace of the Saints?" (*KDM* 28).[57] This narrator's aside is expanded to such an extent that by the time *KDM* 31 was written, the miracle itself occupied only a third of the narrative—the larger part was devoted to a universal message addressed by the hagiographer to his reader-friend, an excursus packed with biblical references and at the same time personalized by a simile about the emperor's servant.

A more explicit version of this same narrative situation is apparent in the much later fifth section (*KDM* 33–8), clearly from the hands of a different hagiographer. The section is introduced in a lengthy prologue where the hagiographer describes the motivations for his work, the sources on which he has relied, and his own compositional principles. He compares himself and his collection to the poor widow with two mites. His statement that his work is a "partial narrative" (*meros exêgêseôs*) immediately informs the reader that it is

---

55 Festugière, *Sainte Thècle, Saints Côme et Damien*, p. 165, line 1.

56 Deubner, *St. Kosmas und Damian*, p. 170, lines 56–7: ὁρᾷς, ἀγαπητέ, πῶς φθάνουσιν τοὺς φιλοῦντας αὐτοὺς οἱ ἅγιοι.

57 Ibid., p. 172, line 27: ὁρᾶτε ὅσα μετὰ τῆς τῶν ἁγίων χάριτος ἡ πίστις δύναται.

an addition to already-existing miracle traditions,[58] that the hagiographer has composed his work in fulfillment of a vow and, at the same time, is motivated by a desire to record the stories, already familiar, of the miracles that he himself had just heard first hand: "as I was listening to the reading of the miracles here in the church." The first words of the prologue provide valuable witness that there was in the cult place a written record of the saints' deeds that was regularly read out and "written down in various and multiple ways." However, the stories told by newly healed patients present fresh sources for the enthusiastic recorder: "as I have heard them day by day, in every hour ... either from the mouth of those who were cured, or from those who were eyewitnesses or the servant of the healed person." In Section V of *KDM*, a recorded miracle reveals that the hagiographer learned his tale from an interesting source. The beneficiary of the miracle did not narrate what had happened to him, but instead handed it to the hagiographer in written form; the latter even admits to having incorporated the patient's own words into the narrative.[59]

Section VI of *KDM* was the work of the thirteenth-century Maximus the Deacon. We learn from him that he composed his set of miracles by using the stories that reached his ears and that he did it in view of a certain audience: "for you, my listeners," "for you, all gathered here." The style of address may be rhetorical, but it doubtless represents an attempt to reconstruct an oral performance-context for the act of narration. Mention of eyewitness testimony is made in reference to sources at the end of *KDM* 42. The majority of the stories (*KDM* 43–7) are connected to the monastery—the community that was centered on the church complex and the most natural transmitter of miraculous cures that took place in the sanctuary. The hagiographer remarks at one point that the beneficiary of the miracle was a member of this very community. Elsewhere he simply recalls a case "which happened recently and is well known to all of us." Maximus calls attention not only to the truth of the miracles but also to the well-proportioned structure of the narratives, "since ... Nature ordained for all living creatures that their limbs should be proportionate to the whole of their bodies; it is the same in my case: during the act of writing the parts of the narrative should necessarily be ordered proportionally, with nothing superfluous or useless."

The self-display of the hagiographer's *persona* in the miracles of Cosmas and Damian, and especially in Section III of the *KDM*, attests in the most exemplary way how a compiler-hagiographer can style himself into an author-hagiographer, consciously shaping the presentation of his person in the text, and

---

58 Festugière, *Sainte Thècle, Saints Côme et Damien*, p. 177.

59 ἀνήρ τις ... διηγήσατό μοι, μᾶλλον δὲ καὶ ἐγγράφως ἐξέθετο (οὕτινος αὐτὰς τὰς λέξεις τῇ προκειμένῃ ἐνέθηκα πραγματείᾳ) ...

mobilizing (as a kind of reality effect) the idea of sources and methods, especially the collection of miracles first hand from people in the church. He can present himself as a patient, healed by the saints, who makes of his text a votive offering commissioned by a named friend.

The "fiction" of communal listening to the miracles and the context of direct storytelling give credit to the hagiographer's compositional creativity, even as listening was probably the real medium for the transmission of these stories. Importantly, the hagiographer emphatically builds communal listening, which accords well with how the community preserved its miracle traditions, into the narrative, to the extent of creating the fiction of a direct, personal experience.

The Hagiographer of Saint Artemius

Regarding Artemius' hagiographer, it has been supposed that we should look behind the figure he presents—a man intimately at home with the special medical terminology and with the contemporary doctors of Constantinople—for a real physician/hagiographer or, as J. Grosdidier de Matons has written, one of the *hypourgoi* (church servants who helped around the patients),[60] a man like the protagonist of *MA* 22. But we should remember that medical knowledge and its vocabulary were rather fashionable among the literary intellectuals of Byzantium.[61] Lennart Rydén has formulated another speculative but plausible hypothesis about the hagiographer's identity. In most miracles the patients are all named, while the reappearing protagonist of *MA* 18 and 22 is, as Rydén says, "conspicuously" anonymous. In this middle-aged, experienced protagonist, an

---

60 J. Grosdidier de Matons considered this a typical case of filariasis; see his "Les Miracula Sancti Artemii: Note sur quelques questions du vocabulaire," in E. Lucchesi and H. D. Saffrey (eds), *Mémorial André-Jean Festugière: Antiquité païenne et chrétienne* (Geneva, 1984), pp. 263–6, at p. 265.

61 As John Scarborough ("Introduction to the Symposium on Byzantine Medicine," *Dumbarton Oaks Papers*, 38 [1984]: pp. ix–xvi, at pp. x–xi) aptly points out: "Literary sources further verify the typical presupposition of a sophisticated medical knowledge, widely diffused among the upper strata of the Byzantine Empire; such medicine was practiced by skilled professionals, well schooled in the theory of medicine. Illustrative are the following: Procopius' *Wars* and *Anecdota* contain numerous instances of medical knowledge, often on a rather high plane; Photios' review of important books include Dioscorides, among other medical authors, Psellus' *Chronographia* gives details of the illness and death of Romanus III that rest upon close acquaintance with technical medical theory and their approaches to treatment; Anna Comenna's *Alexiad* not only has many examples of medicine and medical learning, but also the 'death scene' of Alexios Commenos which suggests a long-standing awareness of therapeutics and medical theory; and John Tzetzes' *Letters* show a deeply embedded expertise in 'ancient' medical writings, particularly Galen."

adherent of the cult and member of the all-night vigil society, it may not be difficult to find the hagiographer himself.[62] Recently, Stephanos Efthymiadis has elaborated on Rydén's hypothesis while examining in detail the two anonymous miracles: "In writing Mir 18 ... the author's main intention was not to make an objective report of a given miracle story, but rather to record reality through the emotional experience of the bachelor-hero."[63] In Efthymiadis' view, the hagiographer wants to make the impression that some time passed between the events of *MA* 18 and *MA* 22. The first might have happened to him in old age and the second much earlier, as the protagonist claims to have been serving the saint from the age of 10. In the protagonist's devotion, Efthymiadis has discovered "the isolation and loneliness of the hero whose only friend turns out to be St. Artemios."[64] Moving forward from Rydén's hypothesis, Efthymiadis groups *MA* 15 with those miracles that seem to conceal the presence of the hagiographer in the text. The protagonist of this story is a free man voluntarily serving a man of prominence, still young and similarly a member of the all-night vigil sodality. Scholars are of one opinion, however, that our hagiographer must have been a learned man with some knowledge of and interest in medicine, a man who understood his connection to the saint and his cult to be a special one, and who also unveils a particular talent for describing the busy social life of the capital. He was familiar with its streets, its churches and church officials, its factions, and its key figures, whether actors, officials, or physicians. Efthymiadis sees in the miracles constructed around the nameless figure of the hypothetical hagiographer a marked deviation from the usual conventions of incubation narrative, in that these two miracles do not involve healing but a burglary that takes place partly in a secular environment, and instead of being solicited, Artemius appears on his own initiative. Although I think that a general typology of incubation stories shows that these miracles do not differ too conspicuously from the others (we have several cases when saint-healers appear in daytime, even outside their church, or care for the suppliants' lost and stolen property), we should, nevertheless, admit that despite their emphatic conformity to the other miracles in the corpus, the miracles with the hagiographer as a character are all in some way atypical.

62 L. Rydén, "Kyrkan som sjukhus. Om den helige Artemios' mirakler," *Religion och Bibel*, 44 (1985): 3–16, at p. 15 note 5.

63 S. Efthymiadis, "A Day and Ten Months in the Life of a Lonely Bachelor: The Other Byzantium in Miracula S. Artemii 18 and 22," *Dumbarton Oaks Papers*, 58 (2004): pp. 1–26, at p. 3.

64 Ibid., p. 12.

The Personal Stamp of the Hagiographer

It is not easy to summarize the overall impact a hagiographer wished to make on his collection. Thecla's hagiographer, a converted and learned Greek rhetor, dismissed the residuum of pagan cults but colored his narratives with similes and literary references to Homer, Herodotus, Euripides, and Plato, thereby showing by example that Greek learning might fruitfully be used to praise a Christian saint. In my opinion, the hagiographer's personal stamp can be found most especially in the urge to create a Christian *paideia*, a new narrative canon—hence his constant thematized concern with the continuous dilemma as to what to include and what to dismiss. Like his contemporary and compatriot Theodoretus of Cyrus, he wished to create, at least in writing, the Seleucia in which he desired to live—an educated city that values Greek eloquence. He places himself in it as its greatest rhetorician and makes Thecla the patroness of Greek literary learning blended with Christian faith. Just as personal is what Sophronius wanted to communicate with his *Thaumata*: like his Alexandrian friends around John the Almsgiver, he was a fighter for Chalcedonian Orthodoxy. In a Monophysite Egypt, Sophronius turned the saints into the mouthpiece of this conviction. He placed in the center of the corpus harsh punishment miracles performed on Monophysite Christians and included scenes like the heretic's dream where the saints take the Eucharist in the Orthodox way, make a public confession of the Chalcedonian creed, or order their perplexed patients to do the same as a condition of a cure. Sophronius' choice to make the saints into the defenders of Orthodoxy was conscious, and I am prone to think that this, alongside his own experience of their healing power, was his chief reason for making the whole collection. We can see further down-to-earth motivations for the hagiographic endeavor in the background of the other collections as well. Thecla's hagiographer, as he reveals in passing at the end of his corpus, had a serious row and some ecclesiastical trouble with someone, and he wished to mobilize Thecla and the whole cult and his learned commitment to it in the hope he might emerge as a winner from this conflict. If the hagiographer of Artemius lies behind the figure of the man who was robbed and who magnanimously and publicly forgave the thief, a fellow member of the all-night vigil society, we may suggest that including himself anonymously in the collection of the miracles was a very telling gesture toward the church community to which he belonged.

The hagiographers' inclusions into their own stories make quite spectacular testimony for what they thought of themselves and how they wished to be seen, but also show how much they knew their craft, and what narrative and theological role they attributed to their own writing. Less openly, the hagiographers reveal a mixture of motivations and reasons for their work, sometimes personal matters and hatreds, and elsewhere more elevated convictions. Composing hagiography made one automatically a hagiographer. But composing one's own self into the miracle stories as a character in the way the incubation collections attest betrays a greater compositional talent and creative fantasy than is usually attributed to Byzantine hagiographers.

Chapter 8

Healing Dreams in Early Byzantine Miracle Collections

Stavroula Constantinou

In her relatively overlooked essay *On Being Ill* from 1930, the famous British author Virginia Woolf wrote:

> Considering how common illness is, how tremendous the spiritual change that it brings, how astonishing, when the lights of health go down, the undiscovered countries that are then disclosed ... it becomes strange indeed that illness has not taken its place with love and battle and jealousy among the prime themes of literature.[1]

Woolf's claim that disease, despite its frequent presence in human lives, is absent from literature is not valid for a considerable number of late antique and Byzantine literary texts that focus on the ill and suffering body.[2] For late antiquity, as Patricia Cox Miller notes quoting Michel Foucault, "the production of narratives of illness" was an effect of a:

> culture that was theoretically soul-oriented. Physical symptoms and bodily dysfunctions took on the huge importance that they did because ... such bodily symptoms functioned as signs of threats to the soul, that is, threats to the integrity of one's identity[3]

[1] Virginia Woolf, *On Being Ill*, reprinted ed. with an introduction by H. Lee (Ashfield, MA, 2002), pp. 3–4.

[2] See, for example, S. Constantinou, *Female Corporeal Performances: Reading the Body in Byzantine Passions and Lives of Holy Women*, Studia Byzantina Upsaliensia, 9 (Uppsala, 2005); and J. Perkins, *The Suffering Self: Pain and Narrative Representation in the Early Christian Era* (London and New York, 1995).

[3] P. Cox Miller, *Dreams in Late Antiquity: Studies in the Imagination of a Culture* (Princeton, 1994), p. 185.

For similar reasons, I would add, bodily ailments play an important role in Byzantine literature, the product of a culture that was deeply Christian, and consequently it was very much concerned with the elevation of the spirit through the dysfunction of the body.

In particular, the miracle collection, a hagiographical text in anthology form consisting of a number of independent short stories (often framed by a prologue and an epilogue) which relate a saint's miracles and which had flourished in the early and late Byzantine periods, is the disease genre par excellence.[4] The large majority of narratives included in the Byzantine Greek miracle collections that have come down to us might be described as healing miracle stories, since they refer to the miraculous cures affected over the ill bodies of individuals who, defeated by incurable diseases, visit famous healing shrines in a desperate attempt to achieve a cure, and in so doing to escape from sure death.[5]

Quite often the hagiographers describe the illnesses and the symptoms of their protagonists in such great detail that it reveals a familiarity with medicine.[6] The illnesses from which most protagonists of healing miracles suffer are mental disorders as well as eye, skin, gastroenterological, and genital ailments. Some healing saints, such as Artemius and Photeine, specialize in particular illnesses; the former cured hernias and testicular and genital diseases, the latter eye

[4] For a catalog of Byzantine miracle collections, see S. Efthymiadis, "Greek Byzantine Collections of Miracles: A Chronological and Bibliographical Survey," *Symbolae Osloensis*, 74 (1999): pp. 195–211. S.F. Johnson, in his *The Life and Miracles of Thekla: A Literary Study*, Hellenic Studies Series, 13 (Washington, D.C., and Cambridge, MA, 2006), pp. 239–49, provides a list of the early collections.

[5] See S. Constantinou, "Grotesque Bodies in Hagiographical Tales: The Monstrous and the Uncanny in Byzantine Collections of Miracle Stories," *Dumbarton Oaks Papers*, 64 (2011): pp. 43–54 and "The Morphology of Healing Dreams: Dream and Therapy in Byzantine Collections of Miracle Stories," in C. Angelidi (ed.), *Dreaming in Byzantium and Beyond* (Aldershot, forthcoming); A.-M. Talbot, "Pilgrimage to Healing Shrines: The Evidence of Miracle Accounts," *Dumbarton Oaks Papers*, 56 (2002): pp. 153–73. It should be noted that most miracle stories included in other hagiographical genres, such as the saint's *Life* and the *enkomion*, are also devoted to miraculous healings. See also the chapter by Miller in this volume.

[6] Such hagiographers include Sophronius (seventh century), author of Cyrus and John's miracles; Nicephorus Callistus Xanthopoulus (c. 1256–1335), author of a collection of miracles performed by the Virgin at the Pege monastery; and John Lazaropoulus (fourteenth century), author of a collection of Saint Eugenius' miracles. For the use of hagiography as a source for medical history, see the two articles in *Dumbarton Oaks Papers*, 38 (1984): J. Duffy, "Byzantine Medicine in the Sixth and Seventh Centuries: Aspects of Teaching and Practice," pp. 21–7 and A. Kazhdan, "The Image of the Medical Doctor in Byzantine Literature of the Tenth to Twelfth Centuries," pp. 43–51.

problems.[7] Symptoms include mad behavior, paralysis, blindness, broken and inflamed skin, and grotesquely swollen bellies and genitals. The diseased bodies in the stories in question are presented in their full materiality; they produce excessive quantities of foul substances such as vomit, diarrhea, urine, pus, blood, and viscous liquids of putrefaction that breed worms. All these bodily products function as signs of the patients' great pain, which in many cases does not remain inexpressible, contrary to Woolf's claim: "[L]et a sufferer try to describe a pain in his head to a doctor and language at once runs dry."[8] For example, the pains of Anthony, the protagonist of *Miracle* 48 from Cyrus and John's collection, are described in the following way: "The patient was shouting from pain that his inwards were awfully eaten up, and that [he felt] as if they were consumed by worms, or that they were destroyed by other awful creeping animals" (*Cyrus and John's Miracles*, 48.2).[9]

As narratives, most healing miracle stories have a standard and simple structure with a happy ending. They start by introducing the protagonist's health problem, often followed by a detailed presentation of its bodily symptoms and by the description of the unbearable pains that it causes. The protagonist's extremely bad bodily situation leads him or her to undertake a first action, namely to consult a doctor; however, the doctor, instead of solving the acute health problem, makes it even worse. Left with no other choice, the protagonist decides to seek divine assistance; he or she goes to a healing shrine and awaits a miraculous cure, which in early Byzantine miracle collections (fifth to seventh centuries) is mostly achieved through the medium of dreams.[10] As soon as the protagonist is healed, he or she glorifies the healing saint and God, the ultimate healer who cures His people through His saints, and he or she happily returns home. At this very point, the healing miracle story ends.

---

[7] For Artemius' miracle collection (seventh century), see *Varia graeca sacra*, edited by A. Papadopoulos-Kerameus (Leipzig, 1975; first printed St. Petersburg, 1909), pp. 1–75. As for Photeine's miracles (eleventh or twelfth century), see *Hagiographica inedita decem*, Series Graeca, 21, edited by F. Halkin (Turnhout and Leuven, 1989), text XI, pp. 111–25.

[8] Woolf, *On Being Ill*, p. 7.

[9] See *Los Thaumata di Sofronio. Contribucion al estudio de la 'incubatio' cristiana*, edited and translated by N. Fernandez Marcos (Madrid, 1975), p. 355. Unless otherwise indicated, the English translations of primary sources are my own.

[10] In miracle collections of the middle and late Byzantine periods and in healing miracle stories incorporated in other contemporary hagiographical genres, such as the saint's *Life* and the *encomium*, therapies are mostly achieved through the patients' immediate contact with the saints' miraculous possessions, tombs, relics, and icons, as well as by the consumption of holy oil or water, or their application on the patients' afflicted bodily parts. See Constantinou, "The Morphology of Healing Dreams."

At the very center of an early Byzantine healing miracle story lies the ill protagonist's dream, or a series of dreams, through which he or she is cured, and as a result the narrative reaches its closure. Healing dreams, like all dreams incorporated in Byzantine literature, are independent narrative units with a beginning, middle, and end. They are mostly placed in the middle of the story and they consume the most narrative space. Dreams in the miracle collections under discussion not only have a narrative significance, as I have showed elsewhere;[11] they are also esthetic vehicles that provide spirituality and religious instruction which function as remedies for both bodily and psychic illness, as the following analysis will attempt to show.

In the extract from *On Being Ill* quoted at the very beginning of this chapter, Woolf refers to the "spiritual change that it [illness] brings." Talking about her personal experience of illness, she wrote in her diary entry "Sunday 16, February 1930": "I believe these illnesses are in my case ... partly mystical. Something happens in my mind."[12] In the framework of early Byzantine healing miracles, the spiritual experiences that, for Woolf, accompany suffering and illness find their expression in the realm of dreams. It is because they are great sufferers that the protagonists of these texts become great dreamers, and as such they acquire otherworldly experiences. In other words, illness and suffering allow our heroes and heroines to communicate with the divine through the medium of dreams.

The examined texts' contemporary and later audiences share the protagonists' spirituality too.[13] This is mostly achieved by the depiction of healing dreams as live dramas that are enacted before the audiences' eyes. As pointed out by Cox Miller, the use of theatricality as an aesthetic means for bringing the holy into people's daily lives was a common practice of early Christian authors. By providing their texts with strong theatrical elements, these authors aimed at creating visual stimulants and mental spectacles that would engage their audiences' active theological imagination and would offer them spiritual experiences.[14]

The use of dreams as a device for providing a narrative with theatricality proves to be a particularly useful and effective tool in the hands of our hagiographers, since according to the famous dream theorist Carl Jung, "a dream is a theater in

[11] See Constantinou, "The Morphology of Healing Dreams."

[12] *The Diary of Virginia Woolf*, vol. 3: *1925–30*, edited by A. Olivier Bell (3 vols, London, 1980), p. 287.

[13] For the reader's or listener's spiritual communication with the divine through hagiographical writings, see C. Rapp, "Storytelling as Spiritual Communication in Early Greek Hagiography: The Use of Diegesis," *Journal of Early Christian Studies*, 6(3) (1998): pp. 431–48.

[14] P. Cox Miller, *The Corporeal Imagination: Signifying the Holy in Late Antique Christianity* (Philadelphia, 2009), pp. 14–15 and 82–101.

which the dreamer is himself the scene, the player, the prompter, the producer, the author, the public, and the critic."[15] In the case of healing dreams, which have a divine origin, the dreamer does not undertake all the roles listed by Jung. He or she is just one of the protagonists, the public and the critic of his or her own dreams. It is the healing saint who is the most important player, the prompter, the producer, and the author of the dream-drama. The healing dream's structure includes various dramatic elements: exposition, role playing, dialogues, *peripeteia*, tragic irony, crisis, *anagnôrisis*, and *lysis*. Of course, not all of these elements are always present in a single dream, and those that are employed do not in all cases acquire the same significance. Some are extended; others diminish or have a fragmentary form. For instance, the exposition may be very short or intimated by some detail. Dialogues might be rather long or have the form of stichomythia. The crisis may take up a large part or be implied. An example in which the dramatic elements listed here may be detected either in an amplified or a reduced form is the following dream from *Miracle* 23 in Saint Artemius' collection:

> After many days the disciple [Artemius] of the Great Healer of souls and bodies appeared one night in a dream to the suffering patient [a certain priest of the church of John, the Forerunner whose name is not given] while he was lying in bed with his wife.
>
> He appeared to him in the garb of the supposed doctor, I mean the Persian, just as though he had directly entered his house and gone straight to his bed to treat him. The latter, after he had seen him and thinking that this was really the Persian, when he drew near to touch him, furiously uttered a loud cry: "Really, you will no longer lay a hand on me nor will I be treated by you any longer." Artemius said to him: "Allow me to treat you." But the sick man kept shouting all the more: "You will not lay a hand on me hereafter." Again the saint exhorted him saying: "Come, let me treat you." But the former continued shouting: "You will not treat me! I gave you a *semisis* and a *trimisis* and four carats and just as many tips, and in no way whatsoever did I benefit from you. On the contrary, however many times you did anything to me, I had a bad day and got worse. Get out of my house." And Artemius said to him: "You don't seem to be acquainted with the proverbial saying: 'The sick man goes to the doctor.' Instead of your having to come to me, I came to you and you chase me out of your house. Look, I'm leaving." And as he started to leave, he said to the sick man: "Believe, you will come near me." And saying this, he left.

15 *C.G. Jung Collected Works*, vol. 8: *The Structure and Dynamics of the Psyche including "Synchronicity: An Acausal Connecting Principle,"* edited by H. Read et al. and translated by G. Adler and R.F.C. Hull (20 vols, New York, 1960), para. 509.

> But after he woke up and came to himself, he realized the purpose of the dream and said: "Alas for my sins, it is the lord. Really, master, you have spoken the truth; to you I come." While he was saying this, his wife heard and asked him saying: "With whom are you conversing, husband? What's wrong with you?" And he related the dream to her and the manifestation of the holy martyr. And upon rising early in the morning, he went to the church to do what was customarily done by those who suffer this disease. And after he waited upon the holy martyr, he was healed.[16]

The above extract has been divided into paragraphs to separate the dream in question from its frames, and in so doing to facilitate both the dream's analysis from the perspective of its dramatic structure and the examination of its impact on the dreamer. The first paragraph functions as an introduction to the subsequent dream and calls attention to it. It also gives important information concerning the dreamer's identity and his bodily condition as well as the dream's actors, namely Saint Artemius and the suffering dreamer himself. Additionally, the time and the place in which the dream takes place are also given: during the night and in the dreamer's own bedroom while he lies on his bed with his wife. As is obvious, the second paragraph is the dream itself, which in comparison to other healing dreams of the discussed collection is rather long. The last paragraph informs the reader or the listener that the dream has finished, and presents its impact on the dreamer, who now undertakes certain actions that will solve his health problem.

Concerning the dream's theatrical elements, the narrator starts his dream narrative by introducing its main actor. Saint Artemius enters the scene and goes directly to the bed of the dreamer, who is suffering from a hernia. Playing the role of the Persian doctor who has wrongly treated the patient, Artemius seems to have the intention of curing the seriously ill man. But when the doctor is about to touch him, he starts shouting, expressing, on the one hand, his great anger for the doctor's incompetence and, on the other, his strong wish not to be treated again by such a doctor. At this point, *peripeteia* is detected, since the dreamer is transformed from a suffering and miserable patient into an angry man who attacks an uninvited and unwanted visitor. Obviously, the patient's words and his strong reaction create an effect of dramatic irony. The dialogue that follows takes the form of a stichomythia in which the tension generated by the patient's anger becomes even greater. A conflict is developed between the two men, with

[16] Translation, with slight modifications, taken from V.S. Crisafulli (translator) and J.W. Nesbitt and J.F. Haldon (commentators), *The Miracles of St. Artemios: A Collection of Miracle Stories by an Anonymous Author of Seventh-Century Byzantium* (Leiden/New York/Cologne, 1997), pp. 139, 141.

the doctor insisting on treating the patient and the patient strongly resisting. The situation reaches a climax when the patient asks the doctor to get out of his house. The tension is resolved through the doctor's decision to leave the patient's house without treating him. The *lysis* to the patient's health problem is given by the doctor's last words before his departure: the ill priest will be cured when he himself goes to the doctor. The dream drama ends with the doctor's departure from the scene.

Anagnôrisis, however, takes place when the patient wakes up. The key to the process leading to this essential theatrical element is provided by the doctor's last sentence addressed to the patient: "Believe, you will come near me," which has dual meanings—a literal and a metaphorical meaning—which are analogous to the saint's double function as a doctor of both bodies and souls. On a literal level, the doctor's prophetic words mean that the patient will go to the Church of the Forerunner, where Saint Artemius' relics are kept, to prepare a votive lamp in the name of the saint, and in so doing to achieve a cure to an illness that no human being, not even the best and wisest doctor, can heal. On a metaphorical level, the sentence suggests that the patient (and those around him) will recognize the saint's miraculous powers, and as a result he will acquire the spiritual life from which he used to refrain, despite the fact that he is a priest. As the narrator informs us earlier in the narrative:

> He was suffering in the extreme and yet no thought whatever occurred to him of the holy martyr ... Remembering nothing about the martyr not even recalling to mind what those do who suffer with this disease ... he entrusted himself to doctors and although he endured many treatments he got worse. And still, not even in such circumstances did the recollection of the saint's miracles occur to him nor to those around him.[17]

Obviously, the dream provides the dreamer with a solution to both his health and spiritual problems, which are inextricably associated. His lack of spirituality leads to bodily suffering, which in turn becomes so inhuman and extravagant that it results in the acquisition of spirituality. It is in his greatest pains that he acquires another state of consciousness, which allows him to *see* both the saint and his own sins, to recognize the divine truth and the truth about his own self: "Alas for my sins, it is the lord," he exclaims as soon as he wakes from the dream; "Really, master, you have spoken the truth; to you I come." As his subsequent words and actions reveal, the hero turns to the saint to receive both bodily and spiritual health.

---

[17] *The Miracles of St. Artemios*, p. 139.

That bodily health is strongly related to spiritual health, or that the one is the effect of the other, is a recurrent theme in healing miracle stories, and this relationship often becomes more prominent through the dramatic structure of the dreams. A case in point is the first miracle story from Saint Demetrius' collection (seventh century) written by an archbishop of Thessalonica named John. Here the protagonist, a certain Marianus, eparch of Illiricon, who suffers from paralysis, has two dreams where the saint, in the disguise of one of the hero's most respected and beloved friends, offers to cure him on condition that he will not neglect his spiritual health. He says to the dreamer: "If you assure me with truthful and honest promise that you will preserve your soul's health after your body is healed ... Christ will cure you through me."[18]

The dream dramas in Demetrius' first miracle story are also remarkable for their strong instructive character:

> He sees in his dream a certain Demetrius, one of his real friends, a known and illustrious person in the court, who says to him: "What is wrong, my precious friend and you are so sad? Tell me immediately and I might be able to give you a useful advice." The eparch answers in his dream: "... What is it that you could do, my dearest friend? What kind of advice could you give to an individual who has sunk to such a great calamity, and to a sea of diseases?" The supposedly true Demetrius replies to him: "First of all I advise you to cheer up, and not to bury yourself into soul-destroying sadness, to keep your hopes to the providence of God, who has created everything. Because you know well that each illness is sent by our Creator's provident force, and aims at the sufferer's benefit: if he is a right man the illness is given to him for not becoming proud, or rather for becoming more notable; just as the gold in a melting pit becomes more genuine through fire. If he is a sinner the illness is given to him to clear his sins ..." And the eparch replies: "You have spoken rightly provided that the patient endures his illness with pleasure, but if he loses his temper through continuous suffering, and utters ill words, the evil is double: not only does the body suffer more, but also more sins are added to the sins of his soul, that is what I see happening to me now." The supposedly beloved Demetrius says to him: "I witness, most honored friend, your humbleness, which suggests your heavenly glory. For this reason you will be soon released from your bodily illness with the power given to me by our savior Jesus Christ. Come to my house, and lie down, and there you will see God's glory that will be revealed to you through me."[19]

---

[18] See P. Lemerle, *Les plus anciens receuils des miracles du saint Démétirus*, vol. 1: *Le texte* (2 vols, Paris, 1981), §20.

[19] Ibid., §16.

In this dream drama, a dialogue is structured between the two actors who, in contrast to the actors of the dream examined earlier, behave in extremely friendly terms, and as a result there is no tension. Here the healing saint acts as a psychiatrist in the first part and promises to cure the patient's bodily illness in the second. Marianus' bodily cure is achieved in another healing dream that takes place as soon as he goes to the saint's "house," which is the Church of Saint Demetrius in Thessalonica. As a psychiatrist, the saint heals through instructive words his patient's psychological distress, which is the effect of his incurable illness. Demetrius' words offer such courage and bravery to Marianus that he eventually bears his misery and suffering with joy, a fact that causes the saint to revisit the patient in a second dream in order to cure his suffering body too. The therapeutic power of Demetrius' words lies both in their divine source and in the kind and tenderly manner in which they are expressed. Acting as a real friend, the saint shows genuine interest in and concern for his friend's bad situation.

Through Marianus' dream drama, so full of effectively acted strong emotions, the dreamer and by extension the text's readers or listeners who find themselves in a similar situation are encouraged to bear their sufferings with patience, and to consider them not as obstacles but as spiritual opportunities. They are asked not to lose courage in such tribulations, for it is God who has prepared them for their own glory. They should be aware—as Woolf repeats many centuries later, without having in mind the *Miracles* of *Demetrius* or any other religious texts expressing similar ideas—that it is through bodily affliction that they may defeat mental weakness and thereby achieve spirituality.

Chapter 9
Hospital Dreams in Byzantium

Timothy S. Miller

For historians interested in Byzantine hospitals (often called *xenônes* in medieval Greek), the rule of the twelfth-century Pantokratôr monastery in Constantinople has provided the most complete picture of how these medical institutions were supposed to function.[1] By the side of this invaluable document, however, I would place several descriptions of *xenônes* found in dream narratives. These accounts record dreams that sick men and women claimed to have experienced either while they were patients in a hospital bed or while they were sleeping in a church associated with a hospital.[2] Indeed, descriptions in dream narratives have confirmed almost all the details about medical care and administrative practices found in the *Pantokratôr Typikon* (*typikon* means a monastic rule in medieval Greek) and contain additional information about how these philanthropic medical institutions actually carried out their obligation to cure the sick. Dream narratives have proven more valuable for hospital historians than any other single category of primary source.

How is it that the dreams of sick patients have provided so much information about hospitals? Until I began research on this chapter, I had never considered the extent to which dream narratives had contributed to my work. Even critics who have questioned some of my conclusions about *xenônes*—that they were exclusively institutions to cure patients and return them to the world of the healthy, not centers to provide comfort and care—have failed to notice the

1 *Pantokratôr Typikon*, especially pp. 82–113 (for a bibliography of primary sources used in this chapter, see the Appendix below). E. Kislinger ("Der Pantokrator Xenon, ein trügerischer Ideal?," *Jahrbuch der österreichischen Byzantinistik*, 37 [1987]: pp. 173–9) has pointed out that regulations such as these hospital rules for the *Pantokratôr* are only an ideal, not the reality of daily hospital service. For this reason, the descriptions in dream narratives of how patients perceived their *xenôn* stay offer an important source to corroborate what the *Pantokratôr Typikon* mandates.

2 The dream narratives appear in the following collections of miracle tales: *Miracles of Cosmas and Damian*, *Miracles of Artemius*, and *Miracles of Sampson*. For editions and translations, see the Appendix.

influence of dream narratives.[3] Although several have attacked me for relying too heavily on the *Pantokratôr Typikon*, none so far has accused me of giving too much credence to the nocturnal fantasies of seriously ill patients, many of whom would have been suffering from high fevers.[4] How reliable could such dream narratives be? And, perhaps more importantly, why do these narratives contain such detailed descriptions of hospitals? We will return to these two questions at the end of this study.

Since 1978, I have been studying Byzantine philanthropic institutions, in particular the medical hospitals. In this I was inspired by the research of Father Demetrius Constantelos, who also used dream narratives in describing Byzantine *xenônes*. Neither he nor I ever paused to examine the dream narratives as a distinct type of primary source, nor did we examine the narratives from the perspective of the dreamer. Both of us were interested only in extracting concrete information about *xenôn* architecture, medical therapies, and staffing.[5] In this chapter, I widen the focus to include not only the places where the dreams occurred (the hospitals) but also the dreams themselves and the dreamers who experienced them.

The first dream narrative to include a hospital description is found in the collection of miracle tales recounting the healings performed through the intercession of Saints Cosmas and Damian.[6] These miraculous cures took place at their famous church of the Kosmidion, located just outside the walls of Constantinople. According to legend, Cosmas and Damian had practiced medicine, usually for free, during their lifetime (c. 300), and after their deaths, Christ had granted them the gift of healing. Because they cured their patients at no charge, Eastern Christians often called Cosmas and Damian the *anargyroi* (without silver).[7]

---

3 P. Horden, "How Medicalized Were Byzantine Hospitals?," in N. Bulst and K.-H. Spiess (eds), *Sozialgeschichte mittelalterlicher Hospitäler* (Ostfildern, 2007), pp. 213–35, especially pp. 215–16. See also M. Dols, "The Origins of the Islamic Hospital," *Bulletin of the History of Medicine*, 61 (1987): pp. 367–90, at p. 371: "Fundamentally, Miller's distinction between caring and curing is not a helpful one for understanding hospitals in the medieval period; as in the third world today, care is as important as cure."

4 Horden, "How Medicalized?," p. 226; Dols, "The Origins of the Islamic Hospital," pp. 370–71; Kislinger, "Der Pantokrator Xenon," pp. 173–9; G. Ferngern, review of T. Miller, *Birth of the Hospital*, in *Transactions and Studies of the College of Physicians of Philadelphia: Medicine and History*, 5(9) (1987): pp. 138–41.

5 D.M. Constantelos, *Byzantine Philanthropy and Social Welfare*, 2nd edn (New Rochelle, 1991), pp. 113–62, especially p. 162.

6 *Miracles of Cosmas and Damian*, pp. 173–6 (*Miracle* 30).

7 For Cosmas and Damian, see B. Kötting, *Peregrinatio religiosa: Wahlfahrten in der Antike und das Pilgerwesen in der alten Kirche,* Forschungen zur Volkskunde, 33–5 (Münster,

In the mid-fifth century, Paulinus, a close friend and advisor of Emperor Theodosius II, built the Kosmidion Church outside Constantinople and dedicated it to the two saints. By the sixth century, seriously ill people were coming to this church of the physician-saints to pray for miraculous healings; some of these suppliants slept in the church or in its porticoes, waiting for Cosmas and Damian to appear to them during the night, usually in their dreams, either to heal them immediately or to prescribe an effective therapeutic program.[8]

As is well known, Byzantine Christians adopted this practice of sleeping in churches like the Kosmidion from the ancient Greek practice of incubation, which, as we have seen in other chapters of this volume, consisted of sleeping in one of the famous temples of Asclepius, who then appeared to his suppliants in dreams and recommended some course of treatment. Often the Asclepian recommendations were in accord with the principles of human medical science, but sometimes they contradicted what physicians prescribed, as we have seen in the strange therapeutic regimes described by Aelius Aristides in his *Sacred Tales*.[9]

Of the 39 miracle tales of Cosmas and Damian, which date to the sixth century, only *Miracle* 30 describes a *xenôn*.[10] According to this tale, an aristocratic citizen of Constantinople developed a serious abscess in the hollow of his upper chest. No earthly doctors could heal it. On the advice of friends, this sick man (we never learn his name) went to the Kosmidion Church and obtained a bed inside the church proper. He lived there for some time without experiencing a vision of the physician-saints in his dreams.

One day the man left the church and went outside to pray before an icon located in the courtyard, an image of Christ together with His mother Mary and the *anargyroi* saints, Cosmas and Damian. After weeping before the icon, the man returned to his bed inside the church. That night in a dream, he saw the Virgin Mary walking between Cosmas and Damian. She came toward him and told the saints: "This is the sick one; heal him." Obeying the Virgin, Cosmas and Damian lifted up their new patient and, carrying him into the *xenôn* next

1950), pp. 213–20; and D. Krueger, "Christian Piety and Practice in the Sixth Century," in M. Maas (ed.), *The Cambridge Companion to the Age of Justinian* (Cambridge, 2005), pp. 291–315, at pp. 309–10.

[8] Kötting, *Peregrinatio religiosa*, pp. 213–18.

[9] For the connection of these Christian incubation practices with the ancient cult of Asclepius, see T. Miller, *The Birth of the Hospital in the Byzantine Empire*, paperback edn with new introduction (Baltimore, 1997), pp. 38–41 and 62–7; see also S.M. Oberhelman, *Dreambooks in Byzantium: Six Oneirocritica in Translation with Commentary and Introduction* (Aldershot and Burlington, VT, 2008), p. 53.

[10] The sixth-century miracles are found in *Miracles of Cosmas and Damian*, pp. 97–197 (*Miracles* 1–39); for *Miracle* 30, see pp. 173–6.

door, brought him to the institution's surgery. In the operating room was a cot for the patient (an operating table) and a large cabinet where the medicines were stored. The dream narrative emphasizes that this medicine locker was fitted with a latticed door. The physician-saints placed the man on the operating table.

The patient thought that Cosmas and Damian were his regular physicians who previously had tried to cut out this abscess in real life. The sick man screamed that he did not want to undergo another operation. Cosmas, however, pulled out his scalpel while Damian held the patient down and anchored the sick man's feet in the lattice grill that formed part of the medicine cabinet's elaborate gate. Cosmas cut out the abscess to its roots and thoroughly cleaned the incision. He then bound up the wound, but did not treat it with any medical salve. The patient told Cosmas and Damian that they should cover the incision with a piece of wool soaked in honey because that was the procedure he had experienced during his many previous operations. The saints responded to the man's criticism: "You are carrying out medicine according to the principles of the science [*logoi*]." In their use of the term *logoi*, the saints referred to the principles of medicine based on human reason, but Cosmas and Damian practiced medicine according to the principles of God.

This short dialogue between the two doctor-saints and their patient proves that until this point, the patient still thought that what he was experiencing was treatment in a real hospital under the care of earthly physicians. In other words, nothing that he had seen and undergone in the hospital of his dream differed from his experiences in real hospitals. In fact, most of what appears in this hospital dream is corroborated by other sources. Only the medicine cabinet with the grill-work on the door is unique to this account. Using the lattice work for anchoring a patient's feet also seems as though it would not correspond to normal operating-room procedures, but the sick man did not question this practice as unusual, only bandaging the incision with no soothing honey compress.

After this exchange, Cosmas and Damian carried their patient back to his bed in the church. When the sick man awakened, he saw the bandages, but when he attempted to touch them with his hand, he felt no bandages, only the abscess just as it had been before the dream. Of course, he was bitterly disappointed, but he decided to remain at the Kosmidion until the Saturday vigil service, an important liturgical event at the church.[11] During this service, the clergy distributed *kêrôtê* to the suppliants. *Kêrôtê* was a mixture of oil and wax made

[11] The Saturday night vigil was also important at the Church of Saint John Prodromos. See John Nesbitt's introduction to *Miracles of Artemios*, pp. 26–7. Almost the same ceremony took place at the Church of Saints Cosmas and Damian in Kosmidion (see Krueger, "Christian Piety and Practice," pp. 309–10).

from candles and lamps burning in the Kosmidion sanctuary. The suppliants applied this salve as a kind of spiritual medicine.[12]

The sick man did not attend the actual service because he was afraid he would offend the other people in the church. Apparently his ulcer was frightening to behold and may have given off an unpleasant odor, although the miracle tale never states this. Instead of going to the vigil, the man remained in his bed. This implies that the man's cot was not in the central part of the church building, but somewhere in a side aisle. Eventually, the man fell asleep, and again Cosmas and Damian approached him in a dream bringing him a cloth soaked in *kêrôtê*. They unbound his bandages and placed the cloth on the abscess. The man felt a wrenching pain as the *kêrôtê* pulled the disease from every extremity of his body. In his dream, the man removed three handfuls of fluid from the abscess. Upon awakening, however, he could see the cloth with the *kêrôtê* covering the abscess, but, just as before, when he tried to touch the cloth, he could not feel the compress. This time, however, he had been healed of the ulcer.

When the sick man had awakened from his first dream and found that he still suffered from the abscess, the author of the *Miracle Tales of Cosmas and Damian* never mentioned that the patient sought any help in interpreting what the dream had meant. Indeed, in none of the five dream narratives that describe hospitals do any of the dreamers seek assistance in understanding the meaning of their dreams. They consult neither dream interpreters nor any dreambooks.

It is possible that the author or authors who committed these 39 miracle tales to writing did not want to associate the incubation customs at the Kosmidion Church with a practice like dream interpretation (which had strong links with the pre-Christian cults of ancient Greece), especially since the tradition of incubation was already recognized as having close associations with the pre-Christian god Asclepius. Moreover, both classical and Byzantine experts on dreams emphasized that those dreams sent by the Greek deities or by the Christian God were perfectly clear and did not require interpretation.[13]

It is also possible that the sick man in this miracle tale and those patients in the other four hospital dream narratives did not consult a dream interpreter because such experts never frequented the churches of *anargyroi* saints like that of Cosmas and Damian. Dream interpreters had also been absent at the temples of Asclepius at Epidaurus and Pergamon during classical and Hellenistic Greece. Since the dreams sent by the god to his suppliants did not predict the future but rather brought healing, they required no expert to decipher what they

[12] For an excellent description of the *kêrôtê*, see Nesbitt's detailed commentary in his introduction to *Miracles of Artemios*, p. 26.

[13] Oberhelman, *Dreambooks in Byzantium*, p. 22 (theories of Artemidorus) and pp. 41–2 (theories of Synesius and Calcidius); see also Synesius, pp. 74–5 (cap. 15).

foreshadowed.[14] This observation would also apply to the Kosmidion Church of Cosmas and Damian.

Another interesting feature of *Miracle* 30 is the confusion the sick man experienced when he first awakened after each of his dreams. After the first dream, he saw bandages on his abscess, but when he touched the afflicted area of his chest with his hands, he felt no covering. When he awakened from his second dream, he saw the cloth soaked in *kêrôtê*, but again with his hand he felt no medicinal compress. In recounting these strange misperceptions, the compiler of the miracle tales includes a detail that confirms the observations of Synesius of Cyrene who, in about 400 AD, wrote the most perceptive essay on dreams to survive from classical and Byzantine times. Synesius notes that many dreams have two characteristics: first, they often present a narrative that routinely violates the laws of nature; and, second, they leave vivid impressions that remain with the dreamer after he or she has awakened.[15] The way in which the author of *Miracle* 30 describes the sick man's confused perceptions upon awakening from each dream closely follows Synesius' observations.

The second hospital dream narrative comes from the *Miracle Tales of Saint Artemius*, composed about a century later at the Church of Saint John the Baptist in Oxeia. Saint Artemius' body rested in the crypt of this Constantinopolitan church where a healing cult had developed around his relics. Seriously ill men and occasionally women came to this shrine to sleep close to the saint's tomb and to wait for a dream. Just as at the Kosmidion Church of Cosmas and Damian, the clergy celebrated a Saturday vigil in honor of Saint Artemius at which they distributed *kêrôtê*. Unlike Cosmas and Damian, however, Artemius specialized in healing diseases of the groin.[16]

According to *Miracle Tale* 22, a member of the lay confraternity attached to the Church of Saint John fell ill from water in the chest.[17] One of the man's neighbors, who happened to be the director of the Christodôtês Xenôn, noticed that this sick individual lived alone with no one to care for him. The director found him a bed in the hospital and told the *archiatroi* (chief physicians) and the professional nurses (*hypourgoi*) to care for him. The man stayed in the hospital

---

14 G. Guidorizzi, "L'interpretazione dei sogni nel mondo tardoantico: oralità e scrittura," in T. Gregory (ed.), *I sogni nel medioevo, seminario internazionale Roma, 2–4 ottobre 1983*, Lessico Intellectuale Europeo, 35 (Rome, 1985), pp. 149–70, at pp. 164–5, but see also the chapter by Downie in this volume.

15 Synesius, pp. 82–5 (cap. 19); see also Guidorizzi, "L'interpretazione dei sogni," p. 154.

16 For a description of the Artemius cult, see Nesbitt's introduction to *Miracles of Artemios*, pp. 1–30.

17 For the text of *Miracle Tale* 22, see *Miracles of Artemios*, pp. 130–37.

for 10 months, but his condition only grew worse. The disease settled in his testicles and made it difficult to walk. When he showed this new problem to the *archiatros*, the physician declared the illness incurable and prescribed only some palliative salves.

The sick man began to pray fervently to Saint John, the patron of his confraternity, and to Saint Artemius. "Show your wonderworking power in me," he exclaimed. He made this prayer on Christmas Eve. When he fell asleep, Artemius appeared in a dream but disguised as the man's friend who worked in the office of the City Prefect of Constantinople. Artemius removed the bandages, pulled out a scalpel, and merely touched the right testicle with the instrument. In the dream, the man raised his head to see that he was healed. When he awoke, however, he still had the great swelling in his testicles, but a stream of fluid was issuing from a small hole in the right testicle where the scalpel had touched it in the dream.

Because it was Christmas, none of the doctors made their evening rounds that day; they were all at home relaxing on the holiday. Only one *hypourgos* (trained physician's assistant) was on duty in the hospital. He went to sleep, leaving the *hypêretai* (nurses' assistants) to keep watch through the night. As the *hypourgos* was sleeping, he also had a dream of Saint Artemius who again disguised his identity; this time Artemius appeared as the chief physician who was in charge of the *xenôn* that month. He told the *hypourgos* to run to the hospital and treat the man with the swollen testicles.

When he awakened, the *hypourgos* ran to the *xenôn*, told the *hypêretai* to bring lanterns, and went straight to the sick man. The *hypourgos* uncovered the patient and found that a thin ribbon of viscous fluid was coming out of the small incision in the right testicle. With his fingers, the *hypourgos* pulled out of the opening more and more fluid, pus, and blood. He extracted two buckets full of discharge. Then he cleaned the wound according to the principles of medical science. Just as in the first dream narrative, the author uses the word *logos* to refer to the principles of medical science based on human knowledge. The *hypourgos* then applied topical medicines following specific instructions that Artemius had given him in the dream.

The following day, while the *archiatros* was making his rounds of the patients together with this same *hypourgos*, the physician came to the patient with the swollen testicles. When he removed the sheets and examined the man, he was amazed to see how the patient's condition was improving. In 30 years of practice, he had never seen such a radical change in a patient with a supposedly incurable condition. Later on, the *hypourgos* and the *archiatros* revealed their dreams to one another, and both realized that the healing was a miracle obtained through the intercession of Saint Artemius.

The two dreams, described in *Miracle Tale* 22, differ from the dreams in the Cosmas and Damian tale in that both dreamers—the patient and the *hypourgos* on duty—had their dreams in the hospital itself, whereas the suppliant of Cosmas and Damian experienced his dream in the Kosmidion Church, probably in the north aisle. Therefore, in the Artemius dream, much of the information about the hospital environment appears in the narrative preceding and following the dream experience, whereas in the Cosmas and Damian dream, the *xenôn*'s operating room appears only in the dream narrative proper.[18]

Miracle Tale 22 of Artemius has proven extremely valuable to scholars in reconstructing how Byzantine hospitals were organized, for it confirms many details of hospital practice found in the twelfth-century *Pantokratôr Typikon*: a three-tiered medical staff consisting of chief physicians (*archiatroi*), medical assistants (*hypourgoi*), and nurse's assistants (*hypêretai*); monthly shifts for the chief physicians; and daily rounds of the patients conducted by the *archiatroi*.[19] This Artemius story also proves that Byzantine hospitals had evolved into highly organized medical facilities by the seventh century, if not earlier in the sixth century.[20] Moreover, this structure lasted at least into the twelfth century with only minor changes.

Why would the author of *Miracle Tale* 22 add so much information about the Christodôtês Xenôn both in his description of the hospital and in the dream that the *hypourgos* experienced? Could it be that the author wished to stress the medical setting of the hospital to underscore how ineffective medical science

---

18 Cf. *Miracles of Cosmas and Damian*, pp. 173–6 (*Miracle* 30). Regarding the location of where patients slept during the night in the Church of Saint John in Oxeia, we know that most of them slept in the north aisle of the church. See Nesbitt's introduction to *Miracles of Artemius*, pp. 11–13. Since the cult of Saint Artemius at the Church of Saint John shared so many characteristics with the cult of Saints Cosmas and Damian at their church in Kosmidion—incubation, Saturday night vigils, and the distribution of *kêrôtê*— it is likely that the sleeping arrangements were also similar. For the routines at the Church of Cosmas and Damian in Kosmidion, see Krueger, "Christian Piety and Practice," pp. 309–10.

19 See *Pantokratôr Typikon*, pp. 84–7 (lines 937–84) for details about the medical staff at the Pantokratôr Xenôn.

20 There can be no doubt that the *archiatroi* of the Graeco-Roman cities were transferred to the Christian hospitals by Emperor Justinian (r. 527–565). See the evidence presented in Miller, *Birth of the Hospital*, pp. xxii–xxv and 152–5. Horden ("How Medicalized?" pp. 230–32) has claimed that such a change never occurred, but in his article, he fails to address the clear evidence that after the reign of Justinian, *archiatroi* were always associated with hospitals. See, for example, *Kletorologion*, p. 183, where *archiatroi* accompany their administrative superiors (the *xenodochoi* or "directors of hospitals") during ceremonies at the emperor's court in the ninth century.

was, even in its most advanced theater where the best physicians supervised treatment and where trained medical assistants were on duty 24 hours a day?

Three additional hospital dreams are found in a short series of tales dealing with miracles attributed to the doctor-saint Sampson. According to tradition in Constantinople, Sampson had studied medicine in ancient Rome before coming to the Eastern capital and opening a small hospital in the fourth century. Later, during the reign of Justinian(!), Sampson cured the famous emperor of a serious ailment. Out of gratitude, Justinian rebuilt Sampson's hospital on a grand scale.

In the tenth century, Symeon the Metaphrast rewrote Sampson's *vita* in more eloquent Greek as part of his project to collect and rephrase many biographies of famous Byzantine saints. In his introduction to Sampson's short biography, Symeon admits that the surviving versions of Sampson's life suffered from grave inaccuracies. Most glaring was the claim that he had lived in the fourth century and yet managed to treat the sixth-century emperor Justinian. Symeon did not have access to additional documents with which he could have corrected these inaccuracies, but he decided to append descriptions of nine miracles that had occurred in Sampson's Xenôn in Constantinople during the mid-tenth century. Three of these miracle tales describe dreams of hospital patients.[21]

The first of the Sampson hospital miracles recounts the case of Genesius,[22] who served as an assistant of some sort in the chapel attached to the hospital. The dream narrative does not call him a priest or a deacon. Was he a lay sacristan? For 30 years he had assisted the liturgies in the chapel. As the years passed, however, he grew lazy and failed to carry out his duties properly. One night, Sampson appeared to him in his sleep and, after berating Genesius for his negligence, struck the man. In describing this dream, Symeon comments that this vision was more than a dream since it had concrete effect; upon awakening the next morning, Genesius was unable to speak and had black pustules around his mouth.[23] For three days he could not talk at all. Eventually, Leo the Droungarios, a high officer of the imperial administration and the patron of the Sampson Hospital, found out what had happened to him. He rushed to the hospital and tried to interrogate Genesius, but because of the sick man's condition, he learned little. Leo made a profound prayer to Sampson to heal this poor man. Shortly thereafter, Genesius began to stutter and soon had his voice back.

---

[21] For Symeon Metaphrastes' introduction to the *Vita* of Saint Sampson, see *Miracles of Sampson*, cols. 277–80; for the short *vita* of Sampson, see cols. 279–92.

[22] For the miracle of Genesius, see *Miracles of Sampson*, cols. 299–302.

[23] Cf. Synesius, pp. 82–3 (cap. 19), where he maintains that dreams often move the emotions in such a way that feelings of love, fear, and revulsion continue after a dreamer awakens, but not that actual physical effects from dreams are seen in reality.

In this dream narrative, the role of the healing saint has been reversed. Rather than healing a suppliant, Sampson punished a negligent sacristan through a dream. In this case, however, Sampson's physical punishment led to a spiritual healing, since Genesius repented of his lazy ways and rededicated himself to Sampson's chapel. Nowhere in the dream narrative does it state specifically that Genesius had a bed in the hospital, but the whole story assumes that all the action has unfolded at the Sampson Xenôn where Genesius apparently lived.

The second Sampson miracle benefited a man named Bardas, a powerful person in tenth-century Constantinople.[24] Bardas belonged to the personal retinue of Emperor Romanus II. Moreover, he had obtained the office of *xenodochos* (chief administrator) of the Sampson Hospital, a clear sign that by the tenth century, the Sampson *xenôn* was administered by the imperial government, not by the patriarch of Constantinople or by some monastic community. Like the contemporary orphanage of Constantinople, the Sampson Hospital had been reorganized as an imperial institution.[25]

Bardas suffered from a severe case of anthrax that had infected his lungs. The physicians of the Sampson examined him and declared his case incurable. On the vigil of Saint Sampson's feast day (27 June), Bardas lay alone in the hospital since the physicians and the administrative staff (*chartoularioi*) had all left the institution to prepare for the following day's liturgy at the Church of Saint Mokios, where Sampson's tomb was located.[26] That night Bardas saw an elderly man, who appeared to be a monk, come out of the *xenôn* chapel into the main part of the building (what Symeon's text calls the *oikeia*). The older man turned to Bardas and told him to get up. This happened three times, and on the third appearance the elderly figure added the command "Go to the celebration at Sampson's tomb!" Bardas struggled to get out of bed. The man appeared a fourth time and disappeared. As Bardas rose from his bed, his pain disappeared. When he squeezed his chest, he felt air escaping from his lungs. Bardas summoned a female nursing attendant to help him remove his bandages. The woman removed the bindings around Bardas' chest to reveal that he had been completely healed. The next day Bardas was strong enough to join the rest of the *xenôn* staff at Sampson's tomb.

---

[24] For the miracle of Bardas, see *Miracles of Sampson*, cols. 301–6.

[25] For the close connection between the Sampson Xenôn and the Orphanotropheion, see T.S. Miller, "The Sampson Hospital of Constantinople," *Byzantinische Forschungen*, 15 (1990): pp. 101–35, at p. 113. For the Orphanotropheion as an imperial institution, see T.S. Miller, *The Orphans of Byzantium: Child Welfare in the Christian Empire* (Washington, D.C., 2003), pp. 184–5.

[26] For the history of Sampson and the reason why he was buried at the Church of Saint Mokios, see Miller, "The Sampson Hospital," pp. 104–13.

Although the dream narrative never states specifically that Bardas was sleeping when he saw Sampson, Sampson's emergence from the chapel three times indicates that Bardas was in fact dreaming: in dreams recorded in Byzantine sources, key events are often depicted as reoccurring three times.[27] Moreover, Bardas was lying in his hospital bed when Sampson appeared to him.

Unfortunately, for hospital historians, the dream narrative does not state clearly where Bardas had his hospital bed. Symeon states only that when Sampson came out of the chapel, the saint stood in the middle of the *oikeia* (literally, "house"). Does this refer to the central ward where all the patients were? If this were the case, this would mean that a man, who was one of the emperor's personal retainers and the director of the institution, shared a bed with the other hospital patients. Or does *oikeia* mean some sort of hallway from where Sampson could see Bardas sleeping in a private room? The dream narrative does not provide enough information to answer this question. It does prove, however, that very powerful and wealthy people were able to stay in a Byzantine hospital. In other words, these were not institutions exclusively for the poor.

In the last miracle tale from the Sampson collection, Irene, the wife of an employee on the hospital staff, fell ill with dropsy.[28] She obtained a bed in the *xenôn*, but the hospital physicians were unable to cure her. One night in a dream, she saw Saint Sampson standing close to her together with Cosmas and Damian. According to Symeon's account, Sampson often appeared in dreams together with these renowned physician-saints. Sampson asked Irene what was wrong with her. It seemed to Irene that she was able to answer him. Sampson conversed with one of the *anargyroi* (the dream narrative does not identify which of the doctor-saints Sampson spoke to) and finally said: "It is necessary to make an incision in her thigh."[29] One of the *anargyroi* obeyed and made the incision. Irene suddenly felt a pain that awakened her from her sleep. Though conscious again, she had no idea what had happened or that she had been healed.

When morning came, a female attendant (*hypêretis*) approached Irene's bed and noticed a pool of liquid on the floor. Thinking that this was urine, the attendant began to scold Irene for not calling the night attendant to assist her.

---

[27] For a discussion of how descriptions of dreams by Byzantine writers often mention that significant elements in dreams were repeated three times, see G. Dagron, "Rêver de dieu et parler de soi: Le rêve et son interprétation d'apres les sources byzantines," in Gregory (ed.), *I sogni nel medioevo*, pp. 37–55, at p. 41.

[28] For the miracle of Irene, see *Miracles of Sampson*, cols. 305–8.

[29] For the *anargyroi*, see *Oxford Dictionary of Byzantium* (3 vols, Oxford, 1991), vol. 1, p. 85, s.v., "*anargyroi*." Cosmas and Damian were always considered the principal *anargyroi* saints. It seems odd that in the miracle tale of Irene, these more famous saints are the junior physicians while Sampson is portrayed as the senior physician.

Irene denied that she had soiled her bed. She pulled off her covers to show the attendant the incision and the liquid draining from it. The hospital physician confirmed that, indeed, Irene had been healed. Irene immediately left the *xenôn* and returned to her home.

Of interest to hospital historians is the section in Irene's dream narrative which mentions that Sampson and the two physician-saints, Cosmas and Damian, often appeared together in the hospital dreams. This vision reflects the manner in which the hospital physicians made daily rounds of the patients in groups. In Irene's dream, Sampson clearly acted as the senior physician. Cosmas and Damian consulted with him, but Sampson made the final decision, and one of the *anargyroi* obeyed his order. We may usefully compare this dream narrative with a poem from the twelfth century in which a senior physician is described as being in the company of two younger doctors and making rounds with them of the patients in the Pantokratôr Xenôn. The author of this poem has yet to be identified, but in modern literature he is referred to as the Mangana Poet.[30]

In his Poem 59, the Mangana Poet describes another Irene, the sister-in-law of the reigning Emperor Manuel I (r. 1143–1180), as a patient in the Pantokratôr Xenôn.[31] Poem 59 thus offers even more striking evidence that Byzantine hospitals were not designed primarily to provide care for poor patients who needed a warm bed and nourishing food, as the emperor's sister-in-law obviously had a bed and ample food in her palace. Irene was undergoing medical treatment at the Pantakratôr hospital to regain her health at the hands of the institution's physicians. According to the poem, three physicians came to visit Irene, one senior physician and two younger doctors who were still learning the practical side of their medical science. All three physicians examined Irene and prescribed treatment. The Poet portrays the student physicians as knowing more about medical science than their pompous professor.

In the Sampson miracle tale, Irene, the wife of the hospital employee, dreamed that she too was visited by three physicians: Sampson, the senior doctor, and Cosmas and Damian, who play the role of the assistant doctors. In view of Poem 59, it is possible that *xenôn* practice normally assigned three physicians to conduct the daily rounds of the patients: one senior physician and

---

[30] For a brief biography of the Mangana Poet, see *Oxford Dictionary of Byzantium*, vol. 2, p. 1726, s.v. "Prodromos Manganeios." See also the complete list of his poems, both published and unpublished, in P. Magdalino, *The Empire of Manuel I Komnenos, 1143–1180* (Cambridge, 1993), pp. 494–500. The numbering system used by Magdalino was established by Michael and Elizabeth Jeffreys for their planned edition of 144 poems written by the Mangana Poet.

[31] For a summary of the content of Poem 59 by the Mangana Poet, see Miller, *Birth of the Hospital*, p. xxi.

two students. Such a practice would have formed part of the practical training routine of Byzantine physicians alluded to in the *Pantokratôr Typikon*.[32]

Now that we have reviewed the five dream narratives, let us return to our two questions: how reliable were dream narratives in their descriptions of hospitals and why do they contain more detailed information on *xenônes* than any other category of primary source? According to Byzantine dream theory, regular dreams could be confusing and, as Synesius emphasized, often violated the laws of nature.[33] However, dreams that came through divine intervention such as these five hospital dreams were supposed to reveal clearly what was useful for healing. With the exception of the first miracle at the Kosmidion Church, the dreamers are never confused about the meaning of their dreams because, as Symeon himself points out, these visions in sleep were confirmed the next morning in reality. Indeed, the whole tradition of incubation rested on confidence in the clarity and efficacy of the dreams experienced within the sacred area of the healing shrine.

Nevertheless, several scholars have pointed out that Byzantine writers were not consistent in supporting the accuracy of even supposedly divine dreams. In texts designed to advise monks, all dreams—even those that are of divine origin—are treated with suspicion. Dreams in general are said to cause monks confusion or directly tempt them to violate their vows of chastity, or even to leave their ascetic way of life.[34] Literature, rooted in practical knowledge, also condemned dreams as poor guides for understanding the world. In his *Taktika* (a manual on military matters), Emperor Leo VI (r. 886-912) advises generals to base their decisions on their knowledge and experience and to ignore any dreams they might have had about future battles. Leo also recommends to his generals to fabricate for their troops dreams that prophesize divine favor. Such fictitious dreams would inspire the soldiers to fight more tenaciously because these men would be convinced that their commander had received assurance of God's support in battle.[35]

---

32 *Pantokratôr Typikon* (pp. 106–7, lines 1313–23) mentions the teacher of medicine for students. The text on pp. 86–7 (lines 948–54) refers to extra (*perissoi*) physicians who worked in the outpatient clinic, and on pp. 92–3 (lines 1063–73) to a promotion system from *perissoi* doctors (interns of some sort) through the higher ranks of the institution. See also Miller, *Birth of the Hospital*, pp. 15–16.

33 Synesius, pp. 82–5 (cap. 19).

34 Dagron, "Rêver de dieu," pp. 43–5.

35 For advice about ignoring dreams and relying on one's own talent as a military commander, see *Taktika*, 20.213 (pp. 612–15); for the recommendation to make up dreams prophesying victory, see 20.179 (pp. 598–9) where the author, the Emperor Leo VI, reiterates his belief that dreams do not provide reliable information for decision-making.

In view of the Byzantines' suspicions about dreaming in general and the possibility that some dream narratives might be fictitious, hospital historians must carefully confirm the details about Byzantine *xenônes* provided in dream narratives with evidence drawn from other kinds of primary sources. Indeed, in my comments on the hospital descriptions in the dreams above, I have always referred to sources outside the literature of dream narrations to confirm the information conveyed in the dream descriptions.

Of all the details in the five dream narrations, only the account of the pharmacy cabinet in the *xenôn*'s operating room cannot be confirmed by a passage from another type of primary source. Recently, however, new evidence has come to my attention which does support the operating room description in *Miracle* 30, attributed to Cosmas and Damian; it comes from a legal text written in the late eleventh century.

Among the later scholia to the *Basilika*, the tenth-century reorganization of Justinian's *Corpus juris civilis*, appears a short definition of the word *pimentarios*, a word used in Byzantine Greek to mean "pharmacist":[36] "A *pimentarios* would be one who is entrusted with the care and the guarding [φυλακή] of the medicines in the hospitals or an artisan who sells remedies or the aromatic spices which are mixed with medicines" (60.39.3).[37] This comment, definitely dating from the late eleventh century,[38] reveals that hospitals regularly employed pharmacists and that "hospital druggist" is the first meaning of *pimentarios*.[39] Of interest to our discussion is the duty of the pharmacist to guard the medicines. The scholiast uses the same word φυλακή to describe the pharmacists' duty to guard the medicines as the author of *Miracle* 30 selected to indicate the elaborate medicine cabinet in the hospital's operating room.[40] The *Basilika* scholiast therefore offers some evidence from outside the realm of dream narratives that hospitals did indeed have large medicine cabinets for surgeons in the operating room—and no doubt for outpatient clinics as well—to keep the pharmaceuticals under lock and key.

---

36 For the *Basilika* and its scholia, see *Oxford Dictionary of Byzantium*, vol. 1, pp. 265–6, s.v., "*basilika*."

37 Scholia *in Librum LX*, 39, 3.7 and 12 (p. 3748).

38 Scholia *in Librum LX*, 39, 3.4 (p. 3747) summarizes a legal brief submitted to the Emperor Constantine X Doukas (r. 1059–1067) and 39, 3.11 (p. 3748) mentions the Emperor Alexius I Comnenus (r. 1081–1118). The references to the *pimentarioi* who guarded the hospital medicines appear with these eleventh-century commentaries.

39 For the section on pharmacists, see *Pantokratôr Typikon*, pp. 88–9 (lines 996–7) where the text describes the Pantokratôr Xenôn's pharmacists as *pementarioi*.

40 Cf. *Miracles of Cosmas and Damian*, p. 174 (lines 31–2): τὴν τῶν φαρμάκων φυλακήν.

Answering our second question—why hospital descriptions in dream narratives are so detailed—is a far more difficult task. One possibility, of course, is that the authors of these miracle tale collections simply concocted the dream stories and added a lot of information about hospitals to make their fabrications seem real. Since Emperor Leo VI actually recommended fabricating dreams to trick rank-and-file soldiers, we cannot rule out the possibility of a similar ruse on the part of members of the clergy, or of confraternities attached to healing churches, to lure the faithful to their particular sanctuary. If, on the other hand, the dreamers really saw the dreams they are said to have experienced, then we can assume that these people had previously been patients in hospitals and were familiar with these institutions and their professional staff. The dreamer who thought that Cosmas and Damian were his regular surgeons had clearly been in a *xenôn* operating room before he had his dream at the Kosmidion Church.

What is puzzling, however, is why Byzantine medical texts themselves are almost totally silent about hospitals while dream narratives provide so much more concrete information on nearly every aspect of these medical institutions. The silence on the part of the professional medical literature has strengthened the arguments of scholars who are skeptical about my thesis that *xenônes* stood at the very heart of the Byzantine medical profession. I would argue, however, that most of the surviving medical texts composed after 600 AD are *iatrosophia*, works that simply list various diseases and the medicines effective against them. These remedy lists served only as memory aids for professional physicians who received most of their training not through studying systematic medical treatises such as those of Galen or the seventh-century Byzantine doctor Paul of Aegina, but through practical training in a hospital under the supervision of a senior physician, just as Cosmas and Damian are portrayed in Irene's dream as learning medicine under the older Sampson.[41]

Unlike Byzantine medical texts, the authors of the dream narratives, as well as the dreamers themselves, stood outside the medical profession. When they wanted to portray the practice of scientific medicine, they did not care about the specific drugs being applied, but they did want to place their visions in the proper setting for the practice of medicine. Thus, they reproduced many of the

[41] Oberhelman (*Dreambooks in Byzantium*, p. 4) has compared medical *iatrosophia* to dreambooks; see also his contribution in this volume. Like *iatrosophia*, dreambooks do not have a fixed text. Each version adds new elements, alters others, and eliminates still others. Moreover, Guidorizzi ("L'interpretazione dei sogni," p. 160) classifies both *iatrosophia* and *onoirokritika* as "para letteratura," as supports for what is essentially an oral tradition. The *iatrosophia* simply note down the names of effective remedies against certain maladies. These entries rarely include information on how to administer the medicines and never any information on the context in which these remedies were administered.

details concerning the ranks of hospital employees, the routines that physicians followed in making their daily rounds, and even the furniture in the operating room.

Although most surviving Byzantine medical texts are *iatrosophia* or slightly expanded treatment lists such as the tenth-century medical encyclopedia attributed to Theophanes Nonnus, one late Byzantine physician, John Zacharias (often called the *aktouarios*), wrote several longer medical treatises during the early fourteenth century. Zacharias has never been properly studied—in fact, some of his essays remain unedited. A careful examination of his treatises might reveal more about Byzantine hospitals from the perspective of a medical expert. We know that Zacharias worked in hospitals, for in one passage of his *On Urines*, he mentions an observation he had made while serving on the staff of a Byzantine *xenôn*.[42]

Despite the need for much more study of medieval Greek medical manuscripts, we know enough about Byzantine hospitals now to acknowledge their importance both in training young doctors and in delivering medical care to patients. Although the *Pantokratôr Typikon* offers the most complete guidelines for organizing a *xenôn*, the dream narratives give us the most vivid pictures of how these facilities functioned on a daily basis. Most importantly, dream narratives provide us with a picture of the hospital staff and its labors to cure the sick from the patients' perspective.

Appendix: Ancient Sources

John Zacharias, *De urinis*. In J. Ideler (ed.), *Physici et medici graeci minores* (2 vols, Amsterdam, 1963), vol. 2, pp. 3–192.

Kletorologion of Philotheos. Greek text with French translation in N. Oikonomides (ed. and trans.), *Les listes de préséance byzantines des IXe et Xe siècles* (Paris, 1972), pp. 81–235.

Miracles of Artemius. Greek text with English translation by V.S. Crisafulli, with commentary by J.W. Nesbitt and J.F. Haldon, in *The Miracles of St. Artemios* (Leiden/New York/Cologne, 1997).

Miracles of Cosmas and Damian. Greek text and commentary in L. Deubner, *Cosmas und Damianos* (Leipzig and Berlin, 1907).

[42] For Theophanes Chrysobalantes' text, see below. Although Theophanes' correct name has now been established as Theophanes Chrysobalantes, most secondary sources and even encyclopedias still reference him as Theophanes Nonnus. For a reference to John Zacharias working in a *xenôn*, see John Zacharias, *On Urines*, pp. 95–6.

Miracles of Sampson. Greek text of *vita* and miracles of Sampson with Latin translation in *Patrologiae cursus completes, Series graeca* (161 vols, Paris, 1857–1877), vol. 115, cols. 277–308.

Pantokratôr Typikon. Greek text with French translation in P. Gautier, "Le Typikon du Christ Sauveur Pantocrator," *Révue des Études Byzantines*, 32 (1974): pp. 1–145. English translation by R. Jordan in J. Thomas and A.C. Hero (eds), *Byzantine Monastic Foundation Documents* (5 vols, Washington, D.C., 2000), vol. 2, pp. 725–81.

Scholia *in Librum LX, 17–69*. In H.J. Scheltema, D. Holwerda, and N. Van der Wal (eds), *Basilicorum libri LX: Series B (scholia)* (Groningen, 1988).

Synesius, *De insomniis*. Greek text with Italian translation in D. Susanetti, *I sogni: Sinesio di Cirene: Introduzione, traduzione e commento*, Studi e Commenti, 10 (Bari, 1992).

Taktika. In George T. Dennis (ed. and trans.), *The Taktika of Leo VI: Text, Translation and Commentary*, Dumbarton Oaks Texts, 12 (Washington, D.C., 2010).

Theophanes Nonnus. In J. St. Bernard (ed.), *Theophani Nonni Epitome de curatione morborum graece ac latine* (Gotthae and Amsterdam, 1794–1795).

Chapter 10

The Stuff of Dreams: Substances and Dreams in Greek and Latin Literature

Jovan Bilbija

Ancient Greek and Latin literature harbors a wealth of information on how certain herbs, stones, metals, fabrics, liquids, and animal parts were thought to influence the formation of dreams. Both the gamut of literary genres from which this information derives and the information itself are remarkably heterogeneous. Ancient medical texts mention various substances, especially herbs, which when consumed or applied to the body cause or counteract certain types of dreams.[1] The magico-medical text called the *Cyranides* (first or second century AD) describes the use of amulets, animal parts, herbs, and other substances for inducing revelatory or disagreeable dreams, and for preventing the latter.[2] Ancient manuals on magical stones, or lapidaries, suggest various stones for achieving the same purposes.[3] Pliny the Elder appropriated from both medical and magical literature various substances that cause dreams or can be used to prevent them.[4] In addition to these, numerous other sources

[1] The medical texts referred to in this chapter are principally those written by or attributed to the following authors (in alphabetical order): Aëtius of Amida, Alexander of Tralles, Caelius Aurelianus, Dioscorides, Galen, Hippocrates and the Hippocratics, Oribasius, Paul of Aegina, Philagrius, Rufus of Ephesus, Scribonius Largus, and Simeon Seth.

[2] The standard edition of the *Cyranides* is D.V. Kaimakis' *Die Kyraniden* (Meisenheim am Glan, 1976). The Latin translation of the *Cyranides* has been edited by L. Delatte, *Textes latins et vieux français relatifs aux Cyranides* (Liège, 1942), pp. 11–206. For the passages from the first book of the *Cyranides*, I have often consulted M. Waegeman, *Amulet and Alphabet: Magical Amulets in the First Book of Cyranides* (Amsterdam, 1987).

[3] With the exception of Michael Psellus' *On the Properties of Stones* (Περὶ λίθων δυνάμεων) (= *Minor Works* 34 Duffy), the Greek lapidaries referenced in this chapter (including the Latin translation of the *Lapidary* of Damigeron-Evax) have been edited by R. Halleux and J. Schamp, *Les lapidaires grecs* (Paris, 1985). I have benefited greatly from Halleux and Schamp's commentary on these texts.

[4] For Pliny, I have used K. Mayhoff's edition: *C. Plini Secundi naturalis historiae libri XXXVII* (5 vols, Leipzig, 1892–1909). I have frequently consulted the commentary on Pliny by R. König, *C. Plinius Secundus d.Ä. Naturkunde* (37 vols, Munich and Darmstadt, 1973–2004).

provide the odd comment about some substance or other that may influence one's dream life.

The main purpose of this chapter is to provide an exhaustive list of substances that in Greek and Latin literature are said to have the potential of inducing, causing, or preventing[5] certain types of dreams. The reason I have included references from all types of literature is that this will allow the reader to contrast effectively the dream-related purposes, substances, and applications suggested in the various corpora. Another reason is that in antiquity—perhaps in some periods and places more than in others—the palette of remedies for many dream-related problems was as multicolored as what has been presented here. This is testified to most succinctly by Plutarch's Lamprias, who asserts: "They who suffer from chronic diseases, after they have renounced common remedies and accustomed regimens, turn to purifications, amulets, and dreams."[6]

Before I present the actual list of substances (III), I begin with a few preliminary remarks (I) about the structure of the list and the types of substances I have included and omitted. After this I offer some very general observations (II) about the types of substances found in the list, as well as about their applications and the sources in which they are mentioned.

I. Preliminary Remarks

I have divided the list of substances into seven categories (A to G). In each category I have gathered the substances that have the same or a similar purpose or effect: A = inducing revelatory dreams; B = sending dreams; C = causing pleasant dreams; D = causing disagreeable dreams; E = causing nocturnal emissions; F = preventing disagreeable dreams; and G = preventing nocturnal emissions.

Within each category, the substances have been ordered alphabetically, listed under their English names whenever these are known. Information about the biological classification of plants and animals has been placed in the footnotes.[7]

---

[5] I use the term "preventing" here also for treatments that aim to put a halt to chronic diseases with the recurrence of dreams as a symptom.

[6] Plutarch, *On the Face Which Appears in the Orb of the Moon* 920B: οἱ ἐν νοσήμασι χρονίοις πρὸς τὰ κοινὰ βοηθήματα καὶ τὰς συνήθεις διαίτας ἀπειπόντες ἐπὶ καθαρμοὺς καὶ περίαπτα καὶ ὀνείρους τρέπονται.

[7] To this end, I have consulted the following works: J. André, *Les noms de plantes dans la Rome antique* (Paris, 1985); *Brill's New Pauly* (16 vols, Leiden and Boston, 2002) (hereinafter *BNP*); O. Keller, *Die antike Tierwelt* (3 vols, Leipzig, 1909–1920); H.G. Liddell and R. Scott, *A Greek Lexicon*, revised and augmented throughout by H.S. Jones, 9th edn (Oxford, 1996) (hereinafter *LSJ*); D.W. Thompson, *A Glossary of Greek Birds*

Each substance is accompanied by one or more paraphrases of the relevant passages. In paraphrasing I have tried to stay true to the original text, but it must be emphasized that they are not translations. In a number of cases I have also paraphrased some other properties attributed to a particular substance. This I have done in order to show the diversity of the properties belonging to a substance or when the properties seem to have some connection with one another.

I should also point out that I do not go into the effects on dreaming caused by eating and drinking in general, that is, the effects of overeating, indigestion, or fasting.[8] I also have not included the substances mentioned in the dream rituals of the Greek magical papyri.[9] Given the fact that these rituals almost always entail the recital of incantations and frequently the performance of other magical acts as well, we cannot confidently attribute the desired effect of these rituals to the substances that are used.[10]

In some cases, more than one substance is involved. The compound amulets described in the *Cyranides* have been listed under the names of the stones.[11]

(London, 1936) and *A Glossary of Greek Fishes* (London, 1947). The scientific names conform to the validated names found in the database of the Integrated Taxonomic Information System (ITIS).

[8] Passages mentioning the negative effect of indigestion on one's dreams include Hippocrates, *Ancient Medicine* 10 (p. 131, 8 Jouanna; vol. 1, p. 594 Littré: E. Littré [ed.], *Hippocrate, Oeuvres complètes* [10 vols, Paris 1839–1861]); Galen, *On the Preservation of Health* 4.4.20 (p. 109, 12–15 Koch; vol. 6, pp. 247–8 Kühn: C.G. K Kühn [ed.], *Claudii Galeni Opera omnia* [20 vols in 22 parts, Leipzig, 1821–1833]). See also Apuleius, *Metamorphoses* 1.18 (on which see S. Panayotakis, "On Wine and Nightmares: Apul. *Met.* 1, 18," in H. Hofmann et al. [eds], *Groningen Colloquia on the Novel*, 9 [Groningen, 1998], pp. 115–29). C.A. Behr (*Aelius Aristides and The Sacred Tales* [Amsterdam, 1968], p. 180 note 17) has collected numerous ancient sources in which the effect of food and drink on dreams is discussed.

[9] On these rituals, see now S.I. Johnston, "Sending Dreams, Restraining Dreams: *Oneiropompeia* in Theory and Practice," in E. Scioli and C. Walde (eds), *Sub Imagine Somni: Nighttime Phenomena in Greco-Roman Culture* (Pisa, 2010), pp. 63–80.

[10] I have, however, included one phylactery described in the magical papyri (F10, F21). Moreover, references to substances mentioned in the magical papyri have been included in several footnotes.

[11] Waegeman (*Amulet and Alphabet*, p. 8) explains the nature of the compound amulets described in the *Cyranides*: "The First Book of *Cyranides* contains twenty-four chapters, corresponding with the twenty-four letters of the Greek alphabet. As *materia medica* a plant, a bird, a fish and a stone are used in each chapter. Their names begin with the same letter. Sometimes they are even completely homonymous ... In each case the four elements of nature are symbolized: the bird represents the air, the plant the earth, the fish water and the stone fire. In this way the sympathetic forces of the entire universe are evoked and the link that keeps the distinct ingredients together is confirmed by the magic of the letters and names."

Compound medicines are paraphrased under the names of the main ingredient (e.g., F12) or the ingredient of which the initial comes earliest in the alphabet (e.g., G1). In addition, in a few texts, two working substances (e.g., D3) or the use of subsidiary substances like water, wine, or oil (e.g., F7) are mentioned.

Substances that cause or prevent nocturnal emissions (ὀνειρωγμοί) have also been given a place in this overview (sections E and G). While it is true that most of the relevant passages do not mention erotic dreams as being part of ὀνειρωγμοί, we know from general discussions about the topic that dreams were often seen as intrinsic to the experience.[12] And even though some ancient authors believed that nocturnal emissions are possible without having erotic dreams,[13] there is generally no way of ascertaining in which of our passages this was believed to be the case.[14] Given the emphasis on the physical aspect of the ὀνειρωγμός in our passages, I will translate this term as "nocturnal emission." The verb (ἐξ)ονειρώττειν will be translated as "emitting semen during sleep" or "having nocturnal emissions."

I should also point out that in section G I have only included those substances and treatments that are explicitly said to cause or counteract *nocturnal* emissions.[15] There are many more substances that the ancients believed had an influence on sexual desire[16] or the production of semen[17] but which we never

---

[12] See, for example, Hippocrates, *Generation* 1 (p. 45, 3–8 Joly; vol. 7, pp. 470–72 Littré) and Caelius Aurelianus, *On Chronic Diseases* 5.80 (p. 902, 6–13 Bendz). Note also that Pliny attributes lascivious dreams (*insomnia veneris, libidinum imaginationes in somno*, etc.) to several substances (G10a, G13a, G16a, G19a, G22a) to which Greek authors attribute ὀνειρωγμός. Obviously Pliny may have thought that erotic dreams are the essential constituent of the ὀνειρωγμοί mentioned in his Greek sources (though see G10a).

[13] Philagrius (fr. 199.8–14 Masullo) claims that nocturnal emission can take place both with and without the stimulation of erotic dreams.

[14] What has been stated here about ὀνειρωγμός applies, *mutatis mutandis*, to the condition called ἐφιάλτης/*incubus*, generally translated as "nightmare." Though in several Greek and Latin texts this condition is said to involve types of dream images, the affliction is also said to involve physical symptoms like pressure on the chest, paralysis, and asphyxiation (see note 18 below). Our passages that refer to those suffering from ἐφιάλτης/*incubus* (F11, F12, F19) do not specifically mention the occurrence of dreams.

[15] Still, I allow one exception to this rule, namely the remedies proposed by Philagrius fr. 199 Masullo (= Aëtius of Amida 11.34), many of which are not explicitly said to combat emission during sleep. They have been included because they are preserved in Aëtius' section "On nocturnal emissions. From Philagrius" (Περὶ ὀνειρώξεων. Φιλαγρίου).

[16] On (an)aphrodisiacs in antiquity, see H.S. Denninger, "A History of Substances Known as Aphrodisiacs," *Annals of Medical History*, 2 (1930): pp. 383–93; and A.K. Dalby, *Food in the Ancient World from A to Z* (London, 2003), p. 14.

[17] Those suffering from frequent seminal emission are advised to abstain from certain types of food that are conducive to seminal production: Galen, *On the Preservation of Health*

find explicitly connected to seminal emission during sleep. Furthermore, most of the substances and treatments explicitly connected to nocturnal emission are also attested as remedies for related or encompassing afflictions such as hypersexuality (satyriasis) and spermatorrhea.

Due to limitations of space, I have omitted from the list of substances compounds that are applied directly to the loins. These are summarized in note 157 below.

II. General Observations

A. Substances for Inducing Revelatory Dreams

We come across substances for inducing revelatory dreams in the *Lapidary* of Damigeron-Evax, in the *Cyranides*, and in passages from Pliny and Fulgentius. The substances are mainly stones, though we also encounter hoopoe's heart, leaf of bay laurel, and linen. The texts instruct wearing the substance on the body, placing it under or beside the head, or sleeping under it. The stone *gnathios/epignation* requires a specific engraving and, like the stone *ceraunius* and the fabric linen, the carrier is required to live in purity. The stone *ceraunius* needs to be implored in order to receive a dream. Many of the substances have more than one purpose; they are said to offer protection or give the carrier certain desirable qualities.

B. Substances for Sending Dreams

Pliny claims that the chameleon's left shoulder was used by some for sending dreams to others. He does not explain how it was applied. Its right foot he says was used for restraining dreams.

C. Substances That Cause Pleasant Dreams

The attested substances for bringing pleasant dreams are dried fruits (dried figs, raisins) and herbs (anise, balm). The sources are Hermippus, Pliny, and Simeon Seth. The dried fruits and balm are probably intended to be taken orally; the anise is to be scattered on the pillow in order to be scented during sleep.

6.14.4 (p. 195, 3–5 Koch; vol. 6, p. 444 Kühn) (cf. Philagrius, fr. 199.27–30 Masullo); Oribasius, *Synopsis for Eustathius* 9.38.1 (p. 300, 7–8 Raeder).

D. Substances That Cause Disagreeable Dreams

In medical literature, a number of aliments and herbs are said to cause disagreeable dreams when eaten or drunk. These include pulses (broad bean, lentil, and kidney bean), cabbage, leek, parts of various herbs, and young wine. Some of the herbs mentioned in medical and other literature we know to be toxic (henbane, thorn apple). As several ancient physicians considered nightmares (ἐφιάλτης/*incubus*)[18] to be caused by indigestion,[19] we should possibly connect the bad dreams attributed to certain aliments (e.g., beans, leek, lentils, and young wine) with the gastrointestinal problems they are also said to cause.

Outside medical literature, we have Pliny, Plutarch, and various other ancient authors attributing disagreeable dreams to certain herbs or meats (hare, octopus) when eaten. In the *Cyranides*, Isidore's *Etymologies*, and Aelian's *On the Nature of Animals*, certain parts of animals (otoliths, blood, fin) are said to cause terrible dreams when eaten or applied to the body.

E. Substances That Cause Nocturnal Emissions

Two anonymous medical texts state that the cowpea (φάσηλος) causes nocturnal emission. It is possible that this characteristic of the cowpea was connected with its intrinsic heat and moistness, qualities also often attributed to semen.[20] As we shall see below (section G), substances for preventing nocturnal emission often have cooling or desiccating qualities.

---

[18] The term ἐφιάλτης (Latin: *incubo/incubus*) denotes a creature (Nightmare) or condition (nightmare) which causes a sleeping person to experience discomforts like pressure on the chest, suffocation, paralysis, terror, etc. The classic study of the nightmare (ἐφιάλτης /*incubus*) in Graeco-Roman antiquity is W.H. Roscher, *Ephialtes: Eine pathologisch mythologische Abhandlung über die Alpträume und Alpdämonen des klassischen Altertums* (Leipzig, 1900), but see now N. Metzger, *Wolfsmenschen und nächtliche Heimsuchungen. Zur kulturhistorischen Verortung vormoderner Konzepte von Lykanthropie und Ephialtes* (Remscheid, 2011), pp. 9–124. An exhaustive bibliography on the subject can be found in the latter work.

[19] Cf., e.g., Caelius Aurelianus, *On Chronic Diseases* 1.3.54 (p. 460, 12 Bendz); Aëtius of Amida 6.12 (p. 152, 13–15 Olivieri); Paul of Aegina 3.15 (p. 159, 1–2 Heiberg); Paul of Nicea 26 (p. 86, 4–6 Ieraci Bio). For more relevant passages, see Roscher, *Ephialtes*, p. 23, note 53.

[20] According to some ancient authors, if the heat and moisture of the body increase, so does the chance of emitting semen during sleep: cf. Hippocrates, *Generation* 1 (p. 45, 3–8 Joly; vol. 7, pp. 470–72 Littré); Theophrastus, *On Fatigue* 16.123–6; Aristotle, *Problems* 3.33 (876a9–14), 5.31 (884a6–15), 33.15 (963a9–12).

F. Substances for Preventing Disagreeable Dreams

In medical literature, substances for preventing disagreeable dreams are generally medicines against ἐφιάλτης/*incubus*. As this affliction was often thought to be caused by indigestion, it is not surprising to find the use of purgatives like hellebore or hiera of colocynth among the recommended treatments. Pliny and several medical authors mention the seed of peony as an effective cure for nightmares.

Most of the substances for preventing disagreeable dreams are not herbs, nor are they attested in medical literature. Pliny, the ancient lapidaries, and the *Cyranides* mention various stones that protect the sleeper against unpleasant dreams as well as against various other malignant influences. Those stones described in the *Cyranides* are to be engraved with images of specific animals or deities, and a vegetable or animal substance must be attached to it.[21] Apart from stones, we frequently encounter animal parts (eyes, teeth, tongue, intestines, shoulder, skin) as phylacteries. The use of metal objects in the protection against bad dreams is attested in the Greek magical papyri and Pliny. In some cases the wearer of a phylactery is required to live in purity.

The cures for nightmares attested in medical literature, and occasionally those in Pliny, are to be taken orally. The phylacteries attested in the *Cyranides*, lapidaries, magical papyri, and in some passages of Pliny are to be carried, worn by the sleeper, or kept in some place of his house.

G. Substances for Preventing Nocturnal Emission

Nearly all passages in which substances are suggested as remedies for frequent nocturnal emission derive from medical literature and Pliny. The proposed substances (herbs, lead, leather, water) generally aim at cooling the loins or drying up, lessening, or thickening the semen. They are either to be taken orally (herbs, water) or to be applied directly to the loins (herbs, lead, leather). The treatments are often said to be effective against venery and spermatorrhaea as well. Ancient lapidaries show no interest in preventing nocturnal emission; the *Cyranides* mention rocket as an anaphrodisiac eaten by priests.

21 See note 11 above.

III. List of Substances

A. Substances for Inducing Revelatory Dreams[22]

A1. Ammonite Shell[23]

Pliny, *Natural History* 37.167: Ammonite shell (*hammonis cornu*), of a golden color and shaped like a ram's horn, brings prophetic dreams (*praedivina somnia*).

A2. Ceraunius[24]

Lapidary of Damigeron-Evax 12: Those who beseech (*obsecrare*) the stone *ceraunius* are given oracles (*oracula*) and good dreams (*bona somnia*). It is to be carried in purity (*cum castitate*). Those who carry it will not be hit by lightning; the carrier will prevail in all things.

A3. Eumeces[25]

Pliny, *Natural History* 37.160: When placed under the head, the stone *eumeces* produces nocturnal visions (*visa nocturna*) as an oracle.

---

[22] Worth mentioning here is the comment by Plutarch (*On Isis and Osiris* 383F–4A) that the incense *kyphi* polishes (ἀπολεαίνειν) the imaginative faculty that is susceptible to dreams (τὸ φανταστικὸν καὶ δεκτικὸν ὀνείρων μόριον). On *kyphi*, see A. Lüchtrath, "Das Kyphirezept," in D. Kurth (ed.), *Edfu: Bericht über drei Surveys; Materialien und Studien*, Die Inschriften des Tempels von Edfu, Begleitheft, 5 (Wiesbaden, 1999), pp. 97–145.

[23] Ammonite shells are the fossilized shells of ammonites, an extinct group of mollusks. They often have a characteristic spiral-shaped form. The term *hammonis cornu* used by Pliny in his *Natural History* literally means "horn of Ammon."

[24] Literally, "of thunder" (κεραύνιος). For the ancient testimonies on this stone and for suggestions about its identity, see Halleux and Schamp, *Les lapidaires grecs*, p. 338; A. Bravi, "Gli imperatori della *Historia Augusta* e il luxus nelle arti," *Xenia Antiqua*, 5 (1996): pp. 5–104, at pp. 31–2, 77.

[25] Literally, "of good length" (εὐμήκης). König, *Naturkunde*, p. 187 (ad Pliny, *Natural History* 37.160): "vielleicht ein mikrokristalliner Quarz (?)." The Greek magical papyri mention a λίθος εὐμήκης in a complex ritual for acquiring an assistant (πάρεδρος) (*Greek Magical Papyri* 1.42–195). At one point during the ritual, a falcon is said to fly into the room and drop a λίθος εὐμήκης (perhaps simply a "long stone"), which the petitioner is to engrave and wear around his neck (1.65–9).

A4. Gnathios, epignathion[26]

a. *Cyranides* 1.3.32–8 Kaimakis:[27] The stone *gnathios* (γνάθιος) is to be engraved with an owl (γλαύξ) holding the fish *glaukos* (γλαῦκος).[28] The eyes of the fish are to be enclosed and it has to be worn while abstaining from pork and all vulgarity (ῥυπαρία). If it is worn in bed, it will show you truthful visions (ὁράματα ἀληθῆ). In darkness, the wearer will seem illustrious (γενναῖος) and divinely inspired (ἔνθεος) to people; during the day, people will believe everything he says.
b. *Lapidary* of Damigeron-Evax 66: This stone is to be engraved with the bird *glaucius*, which is a hoopoe (*upupa*),[29] holding in its talons the fish *glaucium*. The right eyes of both animals are to be raised and enclosed in gold. It is to be carried in purity. Those who make use of this stone during sleep will see true phantasms (*vera fantasmata*). It is not to be used at night. It shows during the day, as if in darkness, terrible demonic apparitions. People will believe everything the wearer says.

A5. Hoopoe,[30] a Stone Found in its Nest; its Heart

Lapidary of Damigeron-Evax 67: A hoopoe's (*upupa*) nest contains three little stones.[31] Taking one of these stones and placing it under the head of a sleeping person will cause him to reveal in a dream (*per somnium*) everything he has thought or said about the placer of the stone during the day. If one places the

26 Identity unknown. The name probably derives from γνάθος (jaw). For an extensive discussion of the amulet, both as it is described in the *Cyranides* and in the *Lapidary* of Damigeron-Evax, see Waegeman, *Amulet and Alphabet*, pp. 27–34.

27 Cf. *Cyranides Latinus* p. 34, 12–19 Delatte.

28 On the identity of this fish, see Waegeman, *Amulet and Alphabet*, p. 32, note 14.

29 Waegeman, *Amulet and Alphabet*, p. 33, note 25: "The identification by Damigeron-Evax with the hoopoe may be based on the fact that the hoopoe's art of prophecy was very famous." On the hoopoe in ancient and medieval folk medicine and magic, see L. Thorndike, *A History of Magic and Experimental Science* (8 vols, New York, 1923–1958), vol. 2, pp. 421–3; cf. J.G. Kunstmann, *The Hoopoe: A Study in European Folklore* (Chicago, 1938), pp. 11–21 (dream-related: pp. 12–13); M. Schuster, *RE* 8A/2 (1958): cols 2110–12; M. Waegeman, "The Gecko, the Hoopoe ... and Lice," *L'Antiquité Classique*, 53 (1984): pp.218–25. *RE* here and in subsequent notes refers to A. Pauly, G. Wissowa, and W. Kroll (eds), *Real-Encyclopädie der classischen Altertumswissenschaft* (Stuttgart, 1894–1978).

30 *Upupa epops*. For the relevant literature, see the previous note. See also A4b and D8.

31 On this stone, see Kunstmann, *The Hoopoe*, p. 15.

hoopoe's heart on the pubic area of one's sleeping wife, if she has been unfaithful, she will reveal it in a dream (*per somnium*).[32]

A6. Laurel[33]

Fulgentius 1.14 (p. 24, 15–19 Helm) (= Antiphon, fr. 81b Pendrick): In their works on dream interpretation, Antiphon,[34] Philochorus, Artemon, and Serapion of Ascalon suggested placing laurel (*laurus*) beside the head of a sleeping person for inducing[35] true dreams (*vera somnia*).[36] For this reason, the laurel was called "beloved of Apollo" (*amica Apollinis*).

A7. Linen

Philostratus, *Life of Apollonius* 8.7.16 Jones: Apollonius claims that dreams (ὀνείρατα) bring truer messages (ἐτυμώτεραι φῆμαι) "to those who lead a life as I do" (τοῖς, ὡς ἐγώ, διαιτωμένοις) when they sleep under linen (λίνον).

---

[32] The heart of the κοκκοφάδιον, perhaps the hoopoe (cf. *LSJ*, Supplement, s.h.v.; see also Thompson, *Greek Birds*, s.v. κουκούφα), is used in a similar ritual described in *Greek Magical Papyri* 7.411–16, in order to make the wife speak during sleep.

[33] *Laurus nobilis* L. On the laurel (and its use in divination), see M.B. Ogle, "Laurel in Ancient Religion and Folk-Lore," *American Journal of Philology*, 31(3) (1910): pp. 287–311; T. Hopfner, *Griechisch-ägyptischer Offenbarungszauber* (2 vols, Leipzig, 1921–1924), vol. 1, pp. 129–31; A. Steier, *RE* 13/2 (1927): cols 1431–42.

[34] G.J. Pendrick (*Antiphon the Sophist: The Fragments* [Cambridge, 2002], p. 430) thinks "the attribution of the recipe to Antiphon (or even to Philochorus) is doubtful" and he deems it "most likely" that "Antiphon's name here is purely decorative."

[35] Laurel was also endowed with prophylactic qualities (cf. Ogle, "Laurel in Ancient Religion," pp. 290–92). John the Lydian (*On the Months* 4.4 [p. 68, 20–p. 69, 7 Wünsch]; cf. *Geoponica* 11.2.7) describes laurel as a phylactery against harmful sources such as demons and as a substance for repelling apparitions (φάσματα). These prophylactic qualities of laurel, according to John, are of value to those who desire to have divine epiphanies through dreams (δι' ὀνείρων θεῖαι ἐπιφάνειαι). These people follow a diet of dried figs, and since dried figs are often kept in the same container as laurel leaves, the figs benefit from the latter's prophylactic qualities (on figs, see also C3).

[36] Laurel is also used in more complex magical rituals for sending or receiving dreams (or other types of revelations); see, for example, *Greek Magical Papyri* 1.262–347, 2.1–182, 5.370–446, 6.1–47, 7.795–845. Not surprisingly, in many of these cases, the invoked deity is Apollo. Laurel is mentioned in a treatment for inducing sleep in Pseudo-Galen, *On Easily Obtainable Drugs* 2.27.3 (vol. 14, p. 489 Kühn). In Nonnus' *Dionysiaca* (48.258–86), the maiden Aura rests her head on leaves of laurel and has a dream.

B. Substances for Sending Dreams

B1. Chameleon,[37] its Left Shoulder
Pliny, *Natural History* 28.116: Democritus[38] suggested using the left shoulder of the chameleon (*chamaeleon*) for sending dreams (*somnia*) to others.[39]

C. Substances That Cause Pleasant Dreams[40]

C1. Anise[41]
Pliny, *Natural History* 20.186: Anise (*anisum*), when applied to the pillow so that it will be scented during sleep, will lighten (*levare*) one's dreams (*insomnia*).

C2. Balm[42]
Simeon Seth 66.14–15 Langkavel: Taken before sleep balm (μελισσόφυλλον) brings good dreams (εὐόνειρον).[43]

C3. Dried Fig
Hermippus, fr. 63 Kassel-Austin (= Athenaeus 1.27E–8A): Raisins (ἀσταφίδες) and dried figs (ἰσχάδες) from Rhodes bring pleasant dreams (ἡδυόνειροι).[44]

---

37 Genus *Chamaeleo*. On the chameleon in antiquity, see Keller, *Die antike Tierwelt*, vol. 2, pp. 281–4; and A. Hermann, "Chamaeleon," *Reallexikon für Antike und Christentum*, 2 (1954): pp. 1021–31.

38 The rituals Pliny wrongly attributes in this passage to Democritus have been traced back to Bolus of Mende (third century BC). For the difficulties surrounding the ascription to Bolus, see J.P. Hershbell, "Democritus and the Beginnings of Greek Alchemy," *Ambix*, 34(1) (1987): pp. 5–20.

39 Libanius (*Orations* 1.249–50) suspected that a magical ritual involving a chameleon had been performed against him. On this incident, see C. Bonner, "Witchcraft in the Lecture Room of Libanius," *Transactions of the American Philological Association*, 63 (1932): pp. 34–44.

40 Worth mentioning here as well are the flower of henna (τὸ τῆς κύπρου ἄνθος), saffron (κρόκος), and βάκκαρις (on the identification of βάκκαρις here, see S.-T. Teodorsson, *A Commentary on Plutarch's Table Talks* [3 vols, Gothenburg, 1989–1996], vol. 1, pp. 307–8), which, according to Plutarch (*Table Talk* 647D), bring untroubled sleep (ὕπνος ἄλυπος) to those who drink them. Isidore of Seville (*Etymologies* 17.8.11) states that *amomum* makes sleep pleasant (*somnos suavificat*). On the identification of *amomum*, see S. Kottek, "Medicinal Drugs in the Works of Flavius Josephus," in I. Jacob and W. Jacob (eds), *The Healing Past* (Leiden, 1993), pp. 95–105, at p. 101.

41 *Pimpinella anisum* L.

42 *Melissa officinalis* L.

43 The effect of balm on dreams is contrasted with that of cabbage (κράμβη) (cf. D2b).

44 Rhodian figs are also commended by Lynceus of Samos (fourth–third century BC), fr. 12 Dalby. On figs, see also note 35 above and G1.

C4. Raisin

Hermippus, fr. 63 Kassel-Austin (= Athenaeus 1.27E–8A): see C3.

D. Substances That Cause Disagreeable Dreams

D1. Bean[45]

a. Aristotle, fr. 242 Rose = 735 Gigon (= Plutarch, *Table Talk* 734E–F): The bean[46] (κύαμος) causes disagreeable dreams (δυσόνειρος) and disturbs visions seen during sleep (αἱ καθ' ὕπνον ὄψεις). Those who practice divination through dreams (ἡ διὰ τῶν ὀνείρων μαντική) abstain from beans.
b. Apollonius, *Miracles* 46:[47] The Pythagoreans forbade the consumption of beans (κύαμοι), among others, because they cause flatulence, are hard to digest, and bring about disturbed dreams (ὄνειροι τεταραγμένοι).[48]
c. Cicero, *On Divination* 1.62:[49] Plato offered the advice to engage in dreaming with bodies brought into such a state that no error or perturbation can affect the soul (*animus*).[50] It is believed that for this reason, the Pythagoreans forbade the consumption of the bean (*faba*) because it causes flatulence and opposes the tranquility of a mind (*mens*) in search of truth.
d. Pliny, *Natural History* 18.118: Beans dull the senses and cause dreams (*insomnia*). For this reason, they were condemned by the Pythagoreans.
e. Dioscorides 2.105:[51] The Greek bean (κύαμος Ἑλληνικός) brings disagreeable dreams (δυσόνειρος). It causes flatulence and is difficult to digest.
f. Tertullian, *On the Soul* 48.3: In order to reach the state of purity (*castimonia*) required for obtaining revelatory dreams, Pythagoreans reject the bean as an aliment because of its heaviness and the fact that it causes flatulence.

---

45 *Vicia faba* L.

46 The same things are said of the head of the octopus (cf. D14a).

47 Cf. Clement of Alexandria, *Miscellanies* 3.3.24.2.

48 On the Pythagorean abstinence from beans and its many explanations, see F. Olck, *RE* 3 (1899): cols 619–20; A.S. Pease, *M. Tulli Ciceronis de divinatione*, Illinois Studies in Language and Literature, 6 (Urbana, 1920), p. 365 (ad 1.62); and W. Burkert, *Lore and Science in Ancient Pythagoreanism* (Cambridge, MA, 1972), pp. 183–4.

49 Cf. Aulus Gellius 4.11.3.

50 Cf. Plato, *Republic* 571D–2B.

51 Cf. Dioscorides *Latinus* 2.88 (p. 213, 20–21 Stadler).

g. Diogenes Laertius 8.24:[52] Pythagoras ordered his disciples to abstain from beans. This makes the imaginations during sleep (αἱ καθ' ὕπνους φαντασίαι) smooth (λεῖαι) and calm (ἀτάραχοι). Abstention from beans is also better for the stomach.
h. Didymus[53] *apud Geoponica* 2.35.4, 8: According to physicians, beans dull (ἀμβλύνειν) the minds (καρδία) of those who eat it. They hinder the formation of vivid dreams (εὐθυονειρίαι) because they cause flatulence (πνευματώδεις). Amphiaraus was the first to abstain from beans for the sake of divination through dreams (ἡ διὰ τῶν ὀνείρων μαντική).
i. Simeon Seth p. 114, 24–5 Langkavel: Beans are reputed to cause troublesome and untruthful dreams (ὄνειροι ταραχώδεις καὶ οὐκ ἀληθεῖς). For such reasons, the Pythagoreans kept away from them.

D2. Cabbage[54]

a. Simeon Seth p. 51, 1–2 Langkavel: Cabbage (κράμβη) disturbs sleep through unpleasant dreams (ἐναντίοις ὀνείροις καθ' ὕπνους θορυβεῖ).[55] It is hot and dry and it stimulates the production of atrabilious juices.
b. Simeon Seth p. 66, 15–16 Langkavel: Cabbage brings bad dreams (δυσόνειρος).

D3. Dorycnion[56]

Dioscorides 4.143:[57] Drinking the fruit (καρπός) of great bindweed (μῖλαξ λεία) with *dorycnion* (δορύκνιον), one Attic *triobolon* of each, is known to cause many disturbing dreams (ἐνύπνια ταραχώδη).

---

52 Cf. Suda π 3124.

53 Possibly Didymus of Alexandria (fourth–fifth century AD); cf. E. Oder, "Beiträge zur Geschichte der Landwirtschaft II, " *Rheinisches Museum*, 45 (1890): pp. 212–22 ; and M. Wellmann, *RE* 9 (1903): col. 445 no. 7.

54 *Brassica oleracea* L. or the wild variant *Brassica cretica* Lam. On the various types of cabbage in antiquity, see André, *Les noms de plantes*, s.v. "brassica"; König, *Naturkunde*, pp. 217–18 (ad Pliny, *Natural History* 20.78–9).

55 See also F3 where cabbage is said to prevent dreams.

56 On the identification and etymology of δορύκνιον, see J.-M. Jacques, *Nicandre, Oeuvres; Tome III: Les Alexipharmaques; Lieux parallèles du Livre XIII des Iatrica d'Aétius* (Paris 2007), pp. 170–72. In our passage (Dioscorides 4.143), δορύκνιον should perhaps be identified with στρύχνον μανικόν, which is thorn apple (*Datura stramonium* L.) (cf. D16).

57 Cf. Dioscorides *Latinus* 4.139 (p. 63, 10–11 Stadler).

D4. Gnaphêsios,[58] its Otoliths
Cyranides 4.12.3–5 Kaimakis: The stones (λίθοι)[59] found in the head of the fish *gnaphêsios* (γναφήσιος), when eaten, cause troublesome dreams (ἐνύπνια χαλεπά). When worn, the stones cause sleeplessness.

D5. Great Bindweed,[60] its Fruit
Dioscorides 4.143: see D3.

D6. Hare[61]
Plutarch, *Life of Cato the Elder* 23.6: According to Cato the Elder, hare (λαγώς) is light and it benefits those who are weak, except that those who eat it dream (ἐνυπνιάζειν) a lot.[62]

---

58 Identity unknown. It should probably be identified with the fish γναφεύς (fuller), mentioned in Athenaeus 7.297C. In this passage, a certain Dorion (possibly first century BC; cf. M. Wellmann, "Dorion," *Hermes*, 23 [1888]: pp. 179–93, at p. 193) is said to have claimed that the liquid from the boiling of γναφεύς can be used for removing stains. Thompson (*Greek Fishes*, s.v. γναφεύς) believes this "looks like a popular interpretation of an obscure and alien word." Regardless of whether Thompson is right, the *Cyranides* (4.12), like Dorion, seems to allude to the use of the fish for making a detergent. We read that the broth of the γναφήσιος mixed with κονία στακή, which is an alkaline fluid, brightens (λαμπρύνειν) old eyes (ὀμμάτια παλαιά) and relieves them from tiredness. The verb λαμπρύνειν (brightening) already evokes associations with a cleaning process, but it is the κονία στακή that is of particular interest here, for what is alluded to in this passage of the *Cyranides*, and possibly also by Dorion, may very well be the process of saponification, that is, the conversion of triglycerides (here, the fat from the fish) into soap by treating them with a strong base (here, κονία στακή). If the γναφεύς/γναφήσιος was indeed ever used for making soap, it seems probable that it was deemed suitable on account of its high fat content.

59 These stones are probably the so-called otoliths, small particles in the inner ear that are important for movement, balance, and hearing. Fish otoliths are referred to by Aristotle (*History of Animals* 7.19 [601b.29–32]) and Pliny (on which, see König, *Naturkunde*, pp. 164–5 [ad Pliny, *Natural History* 9.57]).

60 *Calystegia sepium* (L.) R. Br.

61 *Lepus europaeus*; cf. C. Hünemörder, *BNP*, s.v. "Hare."

62 A quotation from Cato the Elder by the Latin grammarian Diomedes (1.362.22–3 Keil) shows that the former attributed not dreams but sleep (*somnus*) to those who eat hare: *lepus multum somni adfert qui illum edit* (cf. Pliny, *Natural History* 28.260). The Latin *somnus* (sleep) may have been confused with *somnium* (dream); cf. H. von Staden, "Liminal Perils: Early Roman Receptions of Greek Medicine," in F. Jamil Ragep et al. (eds), *Tradition, Transmission, Transformation* (Leiden, 1996), pp. 369–418, at p. 382, note 33.

D7. Henbane[63]

Isidore, *Etymologies* 17.9.41: The plant henbane (*hyoscyamos*; *calicularis*) is called *insana*; when drunk or eaten, it will cause insanity or a disturbed image during sleep (*somni imaginem turbidam*).[64]

D8. Hoopoe,[65] its Blood

Isidore, *Etymologies* 12.7.66:[66] If one anoints oneself (*inungere*) with the blood[67] of the hoopoe (*upupa*) before going to sleep, one will see oneself being strangled by demons.[68]

D9. Hyena Fish,[69] its Right-Hand Fin

Aelian, *On the Nature of Animals* 13.27: The right-hand fin (πτέρυξ) of the hyena fish (ὕαινα ἰχθύς), if placed under a sleeping person, will cause him to see all sorts of disagreeable and unwelcome apparitions and dreams (ἐνύπνια ἕτερα οὐδαμῶς εὐμενῆ καὶ φίλα).[70]

D10. Kidney Bean[71]

Dioscorides 2.146:[72] The kidney bean (σμῖλαξ κηπαία) causes bad dreams (δυσόνειρος). It is diuretic.

---

63 Genus *Hyoscyamus* L. Pliny (*Natural History* 25.35–6) distinguishes between four types of *hyoscyamus*. The one he designates as "common" (*vulgare*) is probably black henbane (*Hyoscyamus niger* L.). Henbane contains the toxins hyoscyamine and hyoscine (scopolamine).

64 Pliny (*Natural History* 25.35) remarks that all types of *hyoscyamus* cause insanity (*insania*) and vertigo (*capitis vertigines*).

65 *Upupa epops*. See also A4b and A5.

66 Cf. *Lapidary* of Damigeron-Evax 67.5. Halleux and Schamp (*Les Lapidaires grecs*, p. 342, note 2) believe the passage from the *Lapidary* of Damigeron-Evax was taken from Isidore.

67 On magical use of the hoopoe's blood in medieval folklore, see Kunstmann, *The Hoopoe*, pp. 12–13.

68 See Kunstmann, *The Hoopoe*, p. 12, note 7 for parallels from medieval bestiaries.

69 In Athenaeus 7.326E–7A (cf. Archestratus, fr. 22 Brandt = 23 Olson-Sens; Epicharmus, fr. 65 Kaibel; *Supplementum Hellenisticum* 580), the fish called ὗς (pig) is identified with the fish ὕαινα. The ὕαινα ἰχθύς is probably the sharpsnout seabream (*Diplodus puntazzo*), a striped fish common in the Mediterranean (cf. Thompson, *Greek Fishes*, s.v. ὕαινα; S. Douglas Olson and A. Sens, *Archestratos of Gela* [Oxford, 2000], p. 101). In Greece, the fish is still referred to as οὔαινα, οὔαινα, etc. (cf. Thompson, *Greek Fishes*, s.v. ὕαινα), in Bulgaria as *морска хиена*, and in Romania as *hiena mării*.

70 The fish ὕαινα probably obtained these properties because of its association with the hyena, whose body parts in antiquity were sometimes endowed with magical powers (cf. F14).

71 *Phaseolus vulgaris* L.

72 Cf. Dioscorides *Latinus* 2.132 (p. 228, 10–11 Stadler).

D11. Leek[73]

a. Dioscorides 2.149:[74] Leek (πράσον κεφαλωτόν) causes ill dreams (δυσόνειρον). It causes flatulence and dim-sightedness; it is diuretic, unwholesome, and eases the bowel.
b. Simeon Seth p. 88, 2 Langkavel: Leek (πράσον) causes ill dreams (δυσόνειρον). It is hot and dry, diuretic, unwholesome, and bad for the stomach.

D12. Lentil[75]

a. Dioscorides 2.107:[76] The lentil (φακός) causes bad dreams (δυσόνειρος). It causes dim-sightedness and is difficult to digest and bad for the stomach.
b. Simeon Seth p. 116, 19–20 Langkavel: Lentils (φακοί) cause bad dreams (δυσόνειροι) because of the atrabilious vapors that issue from it. They are cold and dry and have thick juices (παχύχυμοι).

D13. Leontopodion,[77] its Seed

Pliny, *Natural History* 26.52: The seed (*semen*) of *leontopodion*, when drunk, produces frantic dreams (*lymphatica somnia*).

D14. Octopus,[78] its Head

a. Aristotle, fr. 242 Rose = 735 Gigon (= Plutarch, *Table Talk* 734E–F): The head of the octopus (πολύπους) causes bad dreams (δυσόνειρος) and disturbs visions seen during sleep (αἱ καθ' ὕπνον ὄψεις).[79] Those who practice divination through dreams (ἡ διὰ τῶν ὀνείρων μαντική) abstain from it.
b. Plutarch, *How the Young Man Should Study Poetry* 15B: The head of the octopus (πολύπους), though pleasant to eat, causes sleep filled with bad dreams (ὕπνος δυσόνειρος) and it welcomes confused and strange imaginations (φαντασίαι ταραχώδεις καὶ ἀλλόκοτοι).

---

[73] *Allium porrum* L.

[74] Cf. Dioscorides *Latinus* 2.135 (p. 228, 24–5 Stadler); Paul of Aegina 7.3 (p. 254, 14–15 Heiberg).

[75] *Lens culinaris* Medik.

[76] Cf. Dioscorides *Latinus* 2.90 (p. 214, 31–p. 215, 1 Stadler).

[77] Possibly the lion's leaf (*Leontice leontopetalum* L.); cf. André, *Les noms de plantes*, s.v. "leontopodium"; König, *Naturkunde*, p. 240 (ad Pliny, *Natural History* 26.52).

[78] *Octopus vulgaris*; cf. Thompson, *Greek Fishes*, s.v. πολύπους; C. Hünemörder, "Cuttlefish II.2," *BNP*.

[79] The same things are said of beans (cf. D1a).

D15. Pycnocomon,[80] its Seed/Fruit

a. Pliny, *Natural History* 26.57: The seed of *pycnocomon*, when a drachma of it is drunk with wine, causes tumultuous dreams (*somnia tumultuosa*).
b. Dioscorides 4.174:[81] The fruit (καρπός) of *pycnocomon* (πυκνόκομον), when the amount of one drachma is drunk, causes many disturbed dreams (ταραχώδη καὶ πολλὰ ἐνύπνια).

D16. Thorn Apple,[82] its Root

Dioscorides *Latinus* 4.69 (p. 40, 1–3 Stadler): The root of thorn apple (*strigno manicon*), one drachma drunk with wine, will bring about bad dreams and imaginations (*insomnia non bona et fantasmata*). Two drachmas drunk for three or four days will cause insanity (*mania*). Drinking four drachmas is lethal.[83]

D17. Young Wine

Dioscorides 5.6:[84] Young wine (οἶνος νέος) causes bad dreams (δυσόνειρος). It causes flatulence, is difficult to digest, and is diuretic. Middle-aged and old wines do not have these side-effects.

---

80 The identity of this plant is uncertain. Suggestions include *Leonurus cardiaca* L., *Chaiturus marrubiastrum* (L.) Erhr. ex Rchb. (= *L. marrubiastrum* L.), and *Valeriana tuberosa* L. See André, *Les noms de plantes*, s.v. "pycnocomon"; König, *Naturkunde*, pp. 243–4 (ad Pliny, *Natural History* 26.57).

81 Cf. Dioscorides *Latinus* 4.169 (p. 85, 8–9 Stadler).

82 *Datura stramonium* L. It contains the toxins hyoscyamine, atropine, and hyoscine (scopolamine).

83 Cf. Dioscorides 4.73.2, where one drachma of στρύχνον μανικόν drunk with wine is said to bring a multitude of "not unpleasant imaginations" (φαντασίαι οὐκ ἀηδεῖς). Note that the Latin version speaks of dreams that are "not good" (*non bona*), while the Greek states that they will be "not unpleasant" (οὐκ ἀηδεῖς).

84 Cf. Dioscorides *Latinus* 5.9 (p. 170, 9–10 Stadler).

E. Substances That Cause Nocturnal Emissions[85]

E1. Cowpea[86]

a. Anonymus Medicus, *On the Properties of Foods* p. 469, 28–30 Delatte: The cowpea (φασίουλος) increases nocturnal emissions (ὀνειρωγμοί). It is hot and moist, causes flatulence, and is diuretic.
b. Anonymus Medicus, *On Foods* 2 (p. 231, 19–22 Ermerins): The cowpea (φάσηλος) causes nocturnal emission (ἐνυπνιασμὸς κακός). It is hot and moist, causes flatulence, and is diuretic.

F. Substances for Preventing Disagreeable Dreams

F1. Adamas[87]

Lapidary of Damigeron-Evax 3: The stone *adamas* repels all visions of dubious dreams (*visiones incertorum somniorum*), specters, poisons, and lawsuits.[88]

F2. Aloes[89]

Paul of Aegina 7.4.3 (p. 276, 1–3 Heiberg): Aloes (ἀλόη) can be administered as a purgative to those who see fantasies during sleep (οἱ ἐν τοῖς ὕνοις φαντασιώδεις) but have no fever.

---

[85] It is worthwhile to draw attention here to Pliny's (*Natural History* 23.48–9) warning never to give wine to a person who suffers from hypersexuality (*libido*) or from seminal emission during sleep (*si per somnos genitura effundetur*). I should also mention here the myrtle (μύρτος), the plant sacred to Aphrodite-Venus and connected with libidinous dreams in a passage of Nonnus' *Dionysiaca* (48.258–300). After Aura wakes up from her erotic dream, which she saw while sleeping under a laurel bush (δάφνη), she reproaches Daphne and her plant for allowing her to see such a lewd dream. The proximity of the laurel is supposed to prevent seeing erotic dreams, but οὐ νέμεσις παρὰ μύρτον ὀνείρατα ταῦτα νοῆσαι (It is no cause for anger having such dreams near a myrtle, 48.291).

[86] *Vigna unguiculata* (L) Walp.

[87] The term *adamas*, like the Greek ἀδάμας, was used for a variety of very hard substances, including the diamond. See Pliny, *Natural History* 37.55–61 with J.F. Healy, *Pliny the Elder on Science and Technology* (Oxford, 1999), pp. 190–92. Halleux and Schamp (*Les lapidaires grecs*, pp. 238–9) think the *adamas* in *Lapidary* of Damigeron-Evax 3 is the diamond.

[88] For other sources mentioning the prophylactic qualities of *adamas*, see Halleux and Schamp, *Les lapidaires grecs*, p. 239, note 1.

[89] Aloes is the bitter juice of aloe (genus *Aloe*) which was used for various medical purposes, notably for healing wounds and for purgation (cf. Dioscorides 3.22; Oribasius, *Medical Collections* 11.α.32; Aëtius of Amida 3.24; Paul of Aegina 7.4.3).

F3. Cabbage[90]

Pliny, *Natural History* 20.82:[91] According to Cato the Elder, cabbage (*brassica*), when it is boiled and eaten with oil and salt, removes (*tollere*) *insomnia* (sleeplessness or dreams)[92] and lying awake (*vigiliae*).[93]

F4. Chameleon,[94] its Right Foot

Pliny, *Natural History* 28.116: Democritus[95] suggested using the right foot of the chameleon (*chamaeleon*) for dispelling dreams (*somnia*) that have been sent with use of the chameleon's left shoulder.[96]

F5. Coral[97]

a. *Cyranides* 4.67.2–7 Kaimakis:[98] Placing seal skin (φώκης τὸ δέρμα) with a coral (κοράλλιον) attached to it inside the house will repudiate various harmful influences such as demons and nocturnal visitations (νυκτερινὰ συναντήματα).
b. *Orphica, Lithica Kerygmata* 20: Through its counteracting influence (ἰδίᾳ ἀντιπαθείᾳ), coral (κοράλιος) drives away dreams (ὄνειροι) and apparitions (φαντάσματα) (20.15). Placed inside the house, coral protects against demons, apparitions, and thunderbolts (20.19).
c. *Lapidary* of Damigeron-Evax 7: Through its remedial powers (*suo remedio*), coral (*corallius*) repels the mockeries of dreams (*somniorum*

90 See note 54 above.

91 Cf. Gargilius Martialis, *Medicines from Vegetables and Fruits* 30 (p. 167, 8–9 Rose).

92 An interpretation of *insomnia* here as "sleeplessness" agrees with what Cato says in *On Agriculture* (157.8), namely that cabbage benefits those who are sleepless (*insomnis*) or languid (*seniosus*). *Thesaurus Linguae Latinae* 7.1, 1938.31–3, however, interprets *insomnia* in *Natural History* 20.82 as "dreams," possibly because the *Geoponica* (12.17.15) speaks of cabbage (κράμβη) preventing φαντασίαι (~ *insomnia*, "dreams") and ἀγρυπνία (~ *vigiliae*, "sleeplessness"); cf. R.J. Getty, "Insomnia in the Lexica," *American Journal of Philology*, 54 (1933): pp. 1–28, at p. 22. Still, it is not impossible that the φαντασίαι from the *Geoponica* ultimately go back to the *insomnia* of Pliny (on a connection between Pliny and the *Geoponica* through Apuleius, see E. Oder, "Beiträge zur Geschichte der Landwirtschaft bei den Griechen I," *Rheinisches Museum*, 45 [1890]: pp. 58–99, at pp. 79–81).

93 See D2, where cabbage is said to cause bad dreams.

94 See note 37 above.

95 On this attribution, see note 38 above.

96 See B1.

97 On the magical properties of coral, see Pliny, *Natural History* 32.23, 37.164 (*gorgonia*); Halleux and Schamp, *Les lapidaires grecs*, pp. 160–62, 242, 326–7.

98 Cf. *Cyranides Latinus* p. 202, 5–9 Delatte.

ludibria) (7.2). Placed inside the house, coral protects against all harm, shades of demons, empty dreams (*vana somnia*), and thunderbolts (7.9).

F6. Donkey,[99] its Hide

Cyranides 2.31.21–2 Kaimakis:[100] He who sleeps on a donkey's hide (δορὰ ὄνου)[101] will not be frightened by demons, Gello,[102] or nocturnal apparitions (νυκτερινὰ συναντήματα).

F7. Draco,[103] its Tongue, Eyes, Gall, and Intestines

Pliny, *Natural History* 30.84: Rubbing oneself morning and evening with the tongue, eyes, gall, and intestines of a *draco*, a mixture that has been boiled in wine and oil and left to cool outside during the night, will free one from maltreatment by gods of the night (*nocturni dii*) and Fauni.[104]

F8. Eagle Stone[105]

Lapidary of Damigeron-Evax 1.15: The eagle stone (*lapis aetites*) prevents the occurrence of dreams (*visa somnientur*). It protects pregnant women against miscarriages and speeds up the delivery; it will increase one's property and give

---

99 *Equus asinus*.

100 Cf. *Cyranides Latinus* p. 123, 3–5 Delatte.

101 In *Greek Magical Papyri* 36.361–71, the donkey's hide (δέρμα ὄνου) serves as a writing surface for a spell of attraction.

102 On the child-killing demon Gello, see S.I. Johnston, "Defining the Dreadful: Remarks on the Greek Child-Killing Demon," in M.W. Meyer and P.A. Mirecki (eds), *Ancient Magic and Ritual Power* (Leiden, 1995), pp. 361–87; and K. Hartnup, *"On the Beliefs of the Greeks": Leo Allatios and Popular Orthodoxy* (Leiden, 2004), pp. 85–172.

103 The term *draco*, like the Greek δράκων, can denote various types of serpents, including mythical creatures (cf. C. Wick, *M. Annaeus Lucanus, Bellum civile, liber IX* [2 vols, Munich, 2004], vol. 2, pp. 306–7). In our passage (Pliny, *Natural History* 30.84), *draco* possibly denotes the Indian rock python (*Python molurus*) (cf. C. Hünemörder, *BNP*, s.v. "Snake B3").

104 Elsewhere, Pliny explicitly associates Fauni with nightmares (*Natural History* 25.29; cf. 27.86). On Faunus/Fauni and nightmares, see E.C.H. Smits, *Faunus* (Leiden, 1946), pp. 58–61; and P.F. Dorcey, *The Cult of Silvanus: A Study in Roman Folk Religion* (Leiden, 1992), p. 38, note 20.

105 The eagle stone, or Aetite (ἀετίτης, *aetites*), is a stone that according to ancient sources is found in the nests of eagles. As it contains another stone and is thus "pregnant," it was thought to protect pregnant women (cf., e.g., Pliny, *Natural History* 36.149; Dioscorides 5.160; *Cyranides* 1.1 Kaimakis). The ancient sources and theories are discussed in Halleux and Schamp, *Les lapidaires grecs*, pp. 336–7. The eagle stone is probably a hollow geode containing loose concretions.

a good name; it protects children; it is effective against abominable terrors (*terrores nefandi*).

F9. Emerald[106]

Cyranides 1.6.20–22 Kaimakis:[107] The emerald (σμάραγδος),[108] engraved with an ἅρπη[109] having a moray (σμύραινα)[110] under its feet, and with a root of the great bindweed (σμῖλαξ)[111] enclosed under the stone can be worn against disturbing dreams (ταραχώδη ἐνύπνια). It is also a remedy for colic.

F10. Gold

Greek Magical Papyri 10.24–35: Inscribe a golden (χρυσῇ) or silver (ἀργυρᾷ) plate (λᾶμνα) with magical symbols and words,[112] consecrate it, and wear it in purity (καθαρίως). It is a restrainer of anger (θυμοκάτοχον) which protects the wearer against dream-apparitions (φαντασμοὶ ὀνείρων). It protects against enemies, accusers, robbers, and terror.[113]

---

106 On the amulet in *Cyranides* 1.6.19–24 Kaimakis, see Waegeman, *Amulet and Alphabet*, pp. 47–54.

107 Cf. *Cyranides Latinus* p. 43, 1–5 Delatte.

108 Spelled as ζμάραγδος. Like all four elements of this entry of the *Cyranides*, the initial is (conformed to) a zeta (cf. Waegeman, *Amulet and Alphabet*, p. 48). In *Greek Magical Papyri* 5.239–43, instructions are given for engraving an emerald (σμάραγδος) with a scarab (κάνθαρος) and with Isis.

109 The ἅρπη is the ζῷκος πτηνόν mentioned in the title of *Cyranides* 1.6. Waegeman (*Amulet and Alphabet*, p. 48) thinks that the ἅρπη could be the Egyptian vulture (*Neophron percnopterus*), but deems it more likely that it is some kind of hybrid creature.

110 Spelled as ζμύραινα. This is the Mediterranean moray (*Muraena helena*); cf. Waegeman, *Amulet and Alphabet*, p. 48.

111 Spelled as ζμῖλαξ. This is the *Calystegia sepium* (L.) R. Br. As Waegeman (*Amulet and Alphabet*, p. 49) points out, Dioscorides (cf. D3) claims the great bindweed (μῖλαξ λεία) *causes* disturbing dreams (ἐνύπνια ταραχώδη). "This contradiction," Waegeman explains, "is not surprising when we bear in mind the rule of homoeopathy: *similia similibus curantur*."

112 The symbols and words are provided on lines 29–35.

113 The spell for restraining anger described in *Greek Magical Papyri* 7.579–90 can also be inscribed on a plate of tin. It protects against demons, apparitions, illnesses, and suffering.

F11. Hellebore[114]

a. Rufus of Ephesus *apud* Oribasius, *Medical Questions* 7.26.177: Hellebore (ἐλλέβορος) can be administered as a purgative (καθαρτήριον)[115] to those who are throttled at night by a nightmare (ἐφιάλτης).[116]
b. Oribasius, *Synopsis for Eustathius* 8.2 (p. 245, 10–12 Raeder):[117] Hellebore is especially useful to those who suffer from nightmares (ἐφιαλτικοί). They should be given one drachma of black hellebore (μέλας ἐλλέβορος) mixed with three obols of scammony (σκαμμωνία)[118] and some aromatics like anise, wild carrot, or parsley.

F12. Hiera of Colocynth[119]

a. Scribonius Largus 100:[120] The hiera called *picra* or *diacolocynthidos*[121] offers relief to those who suffer from shortness of breath, asphyxiation, and nightmare *(incubo)*. To those who suffer from nightmare, the medicine should be administered the day after they have been afflicted, once they have taken sufficient walks. The amount to be given is one denarius or one and a half denarii depending on the patient, mixed with four or five *cyathi* of water in which hyssop (*hysopum*) or horehound (*marrubium*) has been boiled. After three or four hours, the patient should be given cream of barley (*cremor ptisanae*).

---

114 In our passages, it is the purgative black hellebore (*Helleborus cyclophyllus* Boiss.); cf. C. Hünemörder, *BNP*, s.v. "Hellebore." The term ἐλλέβορος was also used for *Veratrum album* L.

115 Elsewhere, Oribasius (*Medical Questions* 7.26.15 [p. 228, 31–p. 229, 3 Raeder]) mentions purgation as a remedy for frightening and disturbing dreams (ἐνύπνια φοβερὰ καὶ ταραχώδη).

116 On ἐφιάλτης, see note 18 above.

117 Cf. Aëtius of Amida 6.12 (p. 152, 28–30 Olivieri) and Paul of Aegina 3.15 (p. 159, 12–14 Heiberg).

118 From the root of scammony (*Convolvulus scammonia* L.), a purgative was made.

119 Hiera (ἱερά, *hiera*) of colocynth (κολοκύνθη, σικυωνία, *colocynthida*, *cucurbita silvestris*, all of which here denote the *Citrullus colocynthis* [L.] Schrad.) is a name that can be given to various compound purgatives with colocynth as one of the main ingredients and/or which were called hiera of colocynth (e.g., *hiera diacolocynthidos*; ἡ διὰ τῆς σικυωνίας ἱερά) in antiquity. For more on the hiera of colocynth in ancient medical practice, see Metzger, *Wolfsmenschen und nächtliche Heimsuchungen*, pp. 39–40.

120 Cf. Marcellus Empiricus 20.4.

121 The hiera described in this source is attributed to the Greek physician Paccius Antiochus (cf. Scribonius Largus 97). Scribonius provides the recipe, which has 16 ingredients, in caput 106. Marcellus' version of the recipe (20.13) has 15 ingredients; it lacks the ingredient horehound (*marrubium*). Another difference is that it includes myrrh (*myrrha*) among the ingredients, which have to be ground in a mortar with honey. Scribonius' recipe includes myrrh, but it does not prescribe its grinding.

b. Oribasius, *Synopsis for Eustathius* 8.2 (p. 245, 12–13 Raeder):[122] The hiera of colocynth[123] (ἡ διὰ τῆς σικυωνίας ἱερά) is very serviceable to those who suffer from nightmares (ἐφιαλτικοί). Patients should keep their diet light and avoid flatulent food.

c. Aëtius of Amida 6.12 (p. 152, 27–8 Olivieri): When a person suffers from nightmares because of an unhealthy state of the humors (κακοχυμία), one may purge him with the hiera of Archigenes (ἡ ἱερὰ Ἀρχιγένους).[124]

F13. Hephaestites[125]

Cyranides 1.7.17–21 Kaimakis:[126] The stone *hephaestites* (ἡφαιστίτης), engraved with a flamingo (φοινικόπτερος) with a scorpion (σκορπίος) at its feet, and with a root of the plant eryngo (ἤρυγγος)[127] placed under the stone, will keep the wearer safe from nocturnal apparitions (ἰνδαλμοὶ νυκτερινοί). Other properties: it is also a phylactery against venomous animals and all malice (βασκανία).

F14. Hyena,[128] its Eyes; its Tooth

a. *Cyranides* 2.40.35–8 Kaimakis:[129] If you remove the eyes[130] of a living hyena (ὕαινα) and carry them around your arm in a purple rag, you will

[122] Cf. Paul of Aegina 3.15 (p. 159, 14–15 Heiberg), where it is said to be the hiera of Rufus.

[123] Oribasius provides a recipe of hiera of colocynth, the one attributed to Rufus, in his *Synopsis for Eustathius* 3.210 and *Medical Questions* 8.47. For variants of the hiera of Rufus, see the commentary of Daremberg-Ruelle at Rufus of Ephesus, fr. 46 (*Oeuvres de Rufus d'Ephèse* [Paris, 1879]).

[124] Aëtius provides a recipe of this hiera of colocynth at 3.115 (p. 304, 9–16 Olivieri).

[125] Identity unknown. The stone is said to be also known as πυρίτης (*Cyranides* 1.7.17 Kaimakis), a name given to a variety of stones. On the possibility of it being our pyrite, see Waegeman, *Amulet and Alphabet*, p. 59. On the amulet in general, see Waegeman, *Amulet and Alphabet*, pp. 47–54.

[126] Cf. *Cyranides Latinus* p. 44, 12–17 Delatte.

[127] Spelled as ἠρύγγιος. Probably the *Eryngium creticum* Lam.

[128] The species of hyena known in antiquity were the striped hyena (*Hyaena hyaena*) and the spotted hyena (*Crocuta crocuta*) (cf. C. Hünemörder, *BNP*, s.v. "Hyena"). On the magical properties of body parts of the hyena, see Pliny, *Natural History* 8.106, 28.92–106, 37.168; *Greek Magical Papyri* 7.204–8 (cf. bYoma 84a); *Cyranides* 2.40 Kaimakis. See further the references in Hünemörder, "Hyena."

[129] Cf. *Cyranides Latinus* p. 132, 4–8 Delatte.

[130] Pliny (*Natural History* 37.168) mentions a stone called *hyaenia* found in the eyes of the hyena. If placed under the tongue, this stone allows one to predict the future (cf. Isidore, *Etymologies* 16.15.25). The Orphic *Lithica kerygmata* (53) mention the magical stone ὑαινίτης, which is found in the heart of the hyena. It offers many powers, including sharp-sightedness (ὀξυδορκία).

chase away every terror of the night (φόβος νυκτερινός). It also puts to flight the child-killing Gello and every demon.

b. Pliny, *Natural History* 28.98: It is said that wearing a large tooth[131] of a hyena (*hyaena*) on a linen thread (*linum*) will help those who suffer from nightly terrors (*nocturni pavores*) and dread of ghosts (*umbrarum terror*).

F15. Nail

Pliny, *Natural History* 34.151: Nails (*clavi*) pulled out from a tomb and then driven into one's threshold will prevent nocturnal frenzies (*nocturnae lymphationes*).

F16. Nemesis Stone[132]

Cyranides 1.13.23–5 Kaimakis:[133] The Nemesis stone (νεμεσίτης) is engraved with the goddess Nemesis, standing with her foot on a wheel and holding a cubit-rule and wand in her hands. Under the stone is enclosed the tip of a duck's wing (ἀκρόπτερον νήσσης) and a small piece of the plant mullein (νεκύα).[134] It averts demonic imaginations during dreams (φαντασίαι δαιμόνων ἐπὶ τῶν ἐνυπνίων), the frightfulness of children, and nocturnal visitations (νυκτερινὰ συναντήματα). It will make a demon leave a possessed person and it cures the moonstruck. The person who wears it must desist from all wicked things.

F17. Obsidian[135]

Lapidary of Damigeron-Evax 25.2: Obsidian (*obsianus*) is excellent against dubious dreams (*somnia incerta*). It aids those who wish to inflict harm; he who inscribes it with the sun and moon and carries it consecrated will lead a good life.

---

131 Cf. F22.

132 This stone is said to be "removed from an altar of Nemesis." Concerning the identity of this stone, Waegeman (*Amulet and Alphabet*, p. 105) suggests that "the Nemesis stone is not a specific mineralogical variety, but ... any kind of stone 'removed from a Nemesis altar' or any kind of stone showing the picture of Nemesis." On the amulet described in *Cyranides* 1.13.16–29 Kaimakis, see Waegeman, *Amulet and Alphabet*, pp. 103–9.

133 Cf. *Cyranides Latinus* p. 68, 4–6 Delatte.

134 The plant νεκύα is said to be the φλόμος (*Cyranides* 1.13.3 Kaimakis), which is mullein (genus *Verbascum* L.). On the magical properties attributed to mullein, see Waegeman, *Amulet and Alphabet*, pp. 105–7.

135 On the identification of *obsianus* as obsidian, see Halleux and Schamp, *Les lapidaires grecs*, p. 307, note 8.

F18. Onyx
Michael Psellus, *On the Properties of Stones*, lines 73–4 (*Minor Works* 34, Duffy): Onyx (ὄνυξ) dispels nocturnal fantasies (φαντασίαι νυκτεριναί).

F19. Peony,[136] its Seed

a. Pliny, *Natural History* 25.29: The peony (*paeonia*; *pentorobos*; *glycyside*) is a remedy for the mockeries of Fauni during sleep (*Faunorum in quiete ludibria*).[137]
b. Pliny, *Natural History* 27.86: The black grains (*grana*) of peony (*paeonia*; *pentorobos*; *glycyside*) help against nocturnal oppression (*suppressiones nocturnae*). Fifteen seeds should be taken, drunk with wine. It helps against stomach pains and for dispersing suppurations.
c. Dioscorides 3.140:[138] Drinking 15 black grains (κόκκοι) of peony (γλυκισίδη) with hydromel or wine will help those who are throttled (οἱ πνιγόμενοι) by nightmares (ἐφιάλται).[139] It also helps those with stomach problems and it relieves women with a suffocating or painful womb.
d. Dioscorides, *On Simple Medicines* 1.28: Those who are often suffocated by nightmares (οἱ ὑπὸ τῶν ἐφιαλτῶν πνιγόμενοι) are healed by frequent drinks of a mixture of 15 black grains of peony (γλυκισίδη) with water.
e. Oribasius, *Synopsis for Eustathius* 8.2 (p. 245, 13–15 Raeder):[140] Those who suffer from nightmares (ἐφιαλτικοί) will benefit from frequently drinking 15 pounded grains of peony (παιωνία) with water.

F20. Seal,[141] its Skin
Cyranides 4.67.2–7 Kaimakis: see F5a.

F21. Silver
Greek Magical Papyri 10.24–35: see F10.

---

136 In our passages, either the European peony (*Paeonia officinalis* L.) or the wild peony (*Paeonia mascula* [L.] Mill.).

137 On peony as a remedy for nightmares, see Roscher, *Ephialtes*, pp. 26–7; and Metzger, *Wolfsmenschen und nächtliche Heimsuchungen*, pp. 43–4, 96–8.

138 Cf. Dioscorides *Latinus* 3.152 (p. 439, 16–17 Stadler).

139 Peony is called ἐφιαλτία in Aëtius of Amida 1.84 (p. 50, 1–2 Olivieri) and ἐφιάλτειον (see *testimonia* in Roscher, *Ephialtes*, p. 27, note 62).

140 Cf. Aëtius of Amida 6.12 (p. 152, 30–p. 153, 1 Olivieri) and Paul of Aegina 3.15 (p. 159, 16–18 Heiberg).

141 Genus *Phoca*.

F22. Wolf,[142] its Tooth

Cyranides 2.23.10–12 Kaimakis:[143] Wearing a tooth (κυνόδους)[144] of a wolf (λύκος) will preserve those who see dreadful dreams (ὄνειρα πονηρά). It will also help those who are moonstruck or terrified.

G. Substances for Preventing Sexual Dreams and Nocturnal Emission

G1. Ajowan,[145] its Seed

Philagrius, fr. 199.47–9 Masullo:[146] Patients (suffering from nocturnal emission) are given a compound consisting of six grains of ajowan (ἄμι), six grains of fennel (μάραθρον), and 30 leaves of rue (πήγανον). The compound is to be administered at least once a month, with three dried figs (ἰσχάδες).

G2. Calamint[147]

a. Galen *apud* Aëtius of Amida 11.33 (p. 122, 9–12 Daremberg-Ruelle): An effective compound against spermatorrhea and nocturnal emissions (ὀνειρωγμοί) is that consisting of seven drachmas of the fruit of willow (ἰτέας καρπός), six drachmas of calamint (καλαμίνθη), five drachmas of the seed of the chaste tree (ἄγνος), four drachmas of rue (πήγανον), and two drachmas of the seed of hemlock (κώνειον). It is to be mixed with water and administered with hazelnut (κάρυον ποντικόν) and three *kyathoi* of sour wine mixed with water (ὀξύκρατον).
b. Philagrius, fr. 199.39–40 Masullo: The continuous intake of calamint (καλαμίνθη) is said to make a person sterile (ἄγονος).
c. Philagrius, fr. 199.77–82 Masullo: In order to cool the loins of those who emit semen during sleep (ὀνειρώττων), scatter dried herbs under the bedclothes mixed with leaves of the chaste tree (ἄγνος), rue (πήγανον), calamint, and roses (ῥόδα).

G3. Chaste Tree,[148] its Seed; Leaves and Flowers

a. Dioscorides, *On Simple Medicines* 2.104: see note 157.

---

142 *Canis lupus*. On the wolf in magic and medicine, see C. Hünemörder, *BNP*, s.v. "Wolf IV."

143 Cf. *Cyranides Latinus* p. 116, 17–p. 117, 1 Delatte.

144 See F14b.

145 *Trachyspermum copticum* (L.) Link.

146 Philagrius, fr. 199 Masullo (= Aëtius of Amida 11.34).

147 Genus *Calamintha* Mill.

148 *Vitex agnus-castus* L.

b. Galen, *On the Preservation of Health* 6.14.11 (p. 195, 33–p. 196, 1 Koch; vol. 6, pp. 446–7 Kühn): To prevent nocturnal emissions (ὀνειρώττειν), one can scatter the tender twigs (κλῶνες) of the chaste tree (ἄγνος) and rue (πήγανον) under the bedclothes. Also effective is frequently eating the seed (σπέρμα) of these plants.
c. Galen *apud* Aëtius of Amida 11.33 (p. 122.9–12 Daremberg-Ruelle): see G2a.
d. Philagrius, fr. 199.30–31 Masullo: Roasted seed of the chaste tree can be given to those who emit semen during sleep (ἐξονειρώττοντες). The leaves and flowers of this plant, when eaten, drunk, or scattered under the bedclothes, are said to have the same effect.
e. Philagrius, fr. 199.77–82 Masullo: see G2c.
f. Paul of Aegina 1.38 (p. 26, 15–17 Heiberg): Scattering the tops (ἄκροι) of the chaste tree under the bedclothes will prevent nocturnal emissions (ὀνειρωγμοί). It has a cooling effect.

G4. Dill,[149] its Seed
Oribasius, *Books for Eunapius* 4.107 (p. 485, 7 Raeder): The seed of dill (ἄνηθον), drunk with wine, will stop nocturnal emissions (ὀνειρωγμοί).[150]

G5. Fennel,[151] its Seed
Philagrius, fr. 199.47–9 Masullo: see G1.

G6. Flax,[152] its Seed
a. Philagrius, fr. 199.53–74 Masullo: see note 157.
b. Paul of Aegina 1.38 (p. 26, 17 Heiberg): Eating linseed (σπέρμα τοῦ λίνου) will prevent nocturnal emissions (ὀνειρωγμοί).

G7. Hemlock,[153] its Seed
a. Dioscorides, *On Simple Medicines* 2.104: see note 157.
b. Galen *apud* Aëtius of Amida 11.33 (p. 122, 9–12 Daremberg-Ruelle): see G2a.
c. Oribasius, *Synopsis for Eustathius* 9.38.2 (p. 300, 9–12 Raeder):[154] see note 157.

---

149 *Anethum graveolens* L.
150 Cf. Dioscorides, *On Simple Medicines* 2.103.
151 *Foeniculum vulgare* Mill.
152 *Linum usitatissimum* L.
153 *Conium maculatum* L.
154 Cf. Paul of Aegina 3.55 (p. 267, 24–6 Heiberg).

G8. Honeysuckle,[155] its Fruit

Rufus of Ephesus, *On Satyriasis and Gonorrhea* 29 (p. 75, 13–p. 76, 1 Daremberg-Ruelle): Drinking the fruit (καρπός) of honeysuckle (περικλύμενον) will help against nocturnal emissions (ὀνειρωγμοί) and venery.

G9. Ivy,[156] its Clusters

Philagrius, fr. 199.41 Masullo: Drinking three clusters (κόρυμβοι) of the ivy (κισσός) can make a person sterile (ἄγονος).

G10. Lead

a. Pliny, *Natural History* 34.166: When applied to the loins (*lumbi*),[157] a plate (*lamina*) of lead (*plumbum*) will inhibit venereal dreams that are accompanied by spontaneous emissions (*visa in quiete veneria sponte naturae erumpentia*).

---

155 In our passage, it is the Etruscan honeysuckle (*Lonicera etrusca* Santi).

156 *Hedera helix* L.

157 Medical texts mention numerous cooling herbs that, when applied to the loins, are said to prevent nocturnal emission. Due to limitations of space, I will mention these herbs here rather than in the running text. Dioscorides, *On Simple Medicines* 2.104: the following plasters (καταπλαττόμενα) can be applied to the private parts: plaster of seed of hemlock (κώνειον) or of root of water lily (νυμφαία), or anoint with juice of *korion* (cf. André, *Les noms de plantes*, s.v. "corion") and of *strychnon* (cf. note 173 below), or of sodium carbonate (νίτρον) with juice of *rhamnos* (cf. André, *Les noms de plantes*, s.v. "rhamnus") and pulp of purslane (ἀνδράχνη). Apply with barley (ἄλφιτον), or with the leaves of the chaste tree (ἄγνος) with barley, or cumin (κύμινον) mixed with Cimolian earth (Κιμωλία). Philagrius, fr. 199.53–74 Masullo (cf. Galen, *On the Preservation of Health* 6.14.6–10 [p. 195, 10–27 Koch; vol. 6, pp. 445–6 Kühn]): The following unguents with a moderately cooling effect can be applied after bathing: oil from unripe olives (ἔλαιον ὀμφάκινον), of rose (ῥόδινον), and of apples (μήλινον). A thicker unguent: mix one part wax with four parts oil and add refreshing juices like that of houseleek (ἀείζωον), *strychnon*, navelwort (κοτυληδών), fleawort (ψυλλίον), *polygonon* (cf. André, *Les noms de plantes*, s.v. "polygonos"), thistle (τρίβολος; cf. André, s.v. "tribolus"), *perdikion* (cf. André, s.v. "perdicium"), water lily, and purslane. Add some more juice, especially that of unripe grape (ὄμφαξ) and of roses, but suitable is also that of lettuce (θριδακίνη), endive (σέρις), water lettuce (στρατιώτης), and lentils (φακοί). Linseed (λινόσπερμον) boiled in water offers a moderately refreshing juice. The juice of the leaves of *rhamnos* is effective as well. Oribasius, *Synopsis for Eustathius* 9.38.2 (p. 300, 9–12 Raeder) (cf. Paul of Aegina 3.55): the loins can be anointed with cooling herbs like coriander (κορίαννον), parsley (σέλινον), hemlock, white lead (ψιμύθιον), and purslane. They are more effective with vinegar. Caelius Aurelianus, *On Chronic Diseases* 5.84 (p. 904, 23–6 Bendz): one of the following cooling substances can be applied to the affected part: flower of wild pomegranate (*balaustium*), acacia (*acacia*), cytinus (*hypoquistida*), fleawort (*psyllium*), each used on their own or with dates (*palmulae*).

b. Galen, *On the Preservation of Health* 6.14.11 (p. 195, 27–9 Koch; vol. 6, p. 446 Kühn): In order to prevent nocturnal emissions (ὀνειρώττειν), some athletes place a plate of lead (μολυβδίνη λεπίς) under their loins (ψόαι).[158]
c. Galen, *On the Powers of Simple Remedies* 9.23 (vol. 12, p. 232 Kühn): Whenever they emit semen during sleep (ὀνειρώττειν), athletes place a plate of lead under the loins to keep them cool.
d. Philagrius, fr. 199.74–6 Masullo: It is very good to place a plate of lead under the loins of him who emits semen during sleep (ὀνειρώττειν). It has a cooling effect.
e. Oribasius, *Books for Eunapius* 1.13.9 (p. 330, 12–13 Raeder):[159] Placing a plate of lead under the loins will prevent seminal emissions during sleep (ὀνειρωγμοί).
f. Oribasius, *Books for Eunapius* 4.107 (p. 485, 4–5 Raeder): A plate (πλάτυσμα) of lead placed under the loins will benefit those who experience nocturnal emissions (ὀνειρώττοντες).
g. Caelius Aurelianus, *On Chronic Diseases* 5.84 (p. 904, 21–2 Bendz): Place a plate of lead (*lamina plumbea*) under the buttocks of the patient for cooling purposes.
h. Alexander of Tralles 2.497.20–21 Puschmann: Lead, placed on the loins, will benefit those who emit semen during sleep (ὀνειρώττοντες).
i. Paul of Aegina 7.3 (p. 243, 3–4 Heiberg): A plate (ἔλασμα) of lead carried on the loins will stop nocturnal emissions (ὀνειρωγμοί).

G11. Leather

Philagrius, fr. 199.83–4 Masullo: Those who emit semen during sleep (ὀνειρώττοντες) should sleep on a leather bed (στρωμνὴ δερματίνη) and not on a soft material.

G12. Lentil[160]

a. Philagrius, fr. 199.34–5 Masullo: A decoction (ἀφέψημα) made of lentils (φακοί) puts an end to (genital) tensions (ἐντάσεις).
b. Philagrius, fr. 199.53–74 Masullo: see note 157.

---

[158] According to Philostratus (*On Gymnastics* 49, 52), emitting semen, both in waking and in sleep, was thought to weaken athletes.

[159] Cf. Paul of Aegina 1.38 (p. 26, 14–15 Heiberg).

[160] *Lens culinaris* Medik.

G13. Lettuce,[161] its Seed; Juice

a. Pliny, *Natural History* 20.68: The seed of cultivated lettuce (*lactuca sativa*), pounded and taken in wine, represses all libidinous imaginations during sleep (*libidinum imaginationes in somno*).
b. Dioscorides 2.136:[162] The seed of cultivated lettuce (θρίδαξ ἥμερος), when drunk, helps those who frequently emit semen during sleep (ὀνειρώττοντες), and it deters sexual intercourse. The seed and juice of wild lettuce (ἀγρία θρίδαξ) can accomplish the same, but the juice is less effective.
c. Dioscorides, *On Simple Medicines* 2.105: Nocturnal emissions (ὀνειρωγμοί) can be stopped by drinking the seed of lettuce and purslane (ἀνδράχνη) with water.
d. Galen, *On Powers of Simple Medicines* 6.8.6 (vol. 11, p. 887 Kühn):[163] The seed of lettuce stops spermatorrhea (γονόρροια) and is given as a drink to those who suffer from nocturnal emission (ὀνειρώττοντες). It is both moist and cold.
e. Philagrius, fr. 199.35–7 Masullo: The seed of lettuce, when drunk, quenches the semen (γονή) by cooling it.
f. Philagrius, fr. 199.53–74 Masullo: see note 157.
g. Paul of Aegina 7.3 (p. 216, 11–12 Heiberg): When it is drunk, lettuce stops spermatorrhea and the emission of semen during sleep (ὀνειρωγμοί). It is both moist and cold.

G14. Maidenhair[164]

Galen *apud* Aëtius of Amida 11.33 (p. 122, 25–30 Daremberg-Ruelle): Maidenhair (ἀδίαντος), beaten and ground, mixed with vinegar (ὄξος), or the juice of parsley (σέλινον), or endive (σέρις), or fleawort (ψυλλίον), can be used against spermatorrhea and nocturnal emissions (ὀνειρωγμοί). One must guard against lascivious thoughts.

G15. Mint[165]

Pliny, *Natural History* 20.146: Wild mint (*mentastrum*) inhibits lascivious dreams (*somnia veneris*).

---

161 *Lactuca sativa* L.

162 Cf. Dioscorides *Latinus* 2.121 (p. 226, 4 Stadler).

163 Cf. Oribasius, *Books for Eunapius* 2.1.θ.14 (p. 361, 27–30 Raeder), 4.107 (p. 485, 2–3 Raeder); Aëtius of Amida 1.165 (p. 76, 13–14 Olivieri); Alexander of Tralles 2.497.16–17 Puschmann; *Geoponica* 12.13.14.

164 *Adiantum capillus-veneris* L.

165 Genus *Mentha* L. In our passage (Pliny, *Natural History* 20.146), it is probably wild mint (*Mentha arvensis* L.).

G16. Purslane,[166] its Leaves; Seed

a. Pliny, *Natural History* 20.214: Purslane (*porcilaca*) inhibits venery and lascivious dreams (*veneris somnia*).
b. Dioscorides, *On Simple Medicines* 2.104: see note 157.
c. Dioscorides, *On Simple Medicines* 2.105: see G13c.
d. Philagrius, fr. 199.35–7 Masullo: Purslane (ἀνδράχνη), when eaten, quenches the semen (γονή) by cooling it.
e. Philagrius, fr. 199.53–74 Masullo: see note 157.
f. Oribasius, *Synopsis for Eustathius* 9.38.2 (p. 300, 9–12 Raeder):[167] see note 157.

G17. Rocket[168]

a. *Cyranides* 1.5.12–13 Kaimakis:[169] Fresh rocket (εὔζωμον) inhibits (ψύχειν) sexual intercourse, frequent erections, and nocturnal emissions (ὀνειριάζειν). It is for this reason that priests (ἱερεῖς) and those in temple precincts (οἱ ἐν τοῖς ἱεροῖς διατρίβοντες) eat it continuously.[170]

G18. Rose,[171] its Petals; Extract

a. Philagrius, fr. 199.53–74 Masullo: see note 157.
b. Philagrius, fr. 199.77–82 Masullo: see G2c.

G19. Rue,[172] its Leaves; Seed

a. Pliny, *Natural History* 20.143: Rue (*ruta*) is given as an aliment to those who often have lascivious dreams (*venerem crebro per somnia imaginantes*).
b. Galen, *On the Preservation of Health* 6.14.11 (p. 195, 33–p. 196, 1 Koch; vol. 6, pp. 446–7 Kühn): see G3b.
c. Galen *apud* Aëtius of Amida 11.33 (p. 122, 9–12 Daremberg-Ruelle): see G2a.
d. Philagrius, fr. 199.38–9 Masullo: When eaten, rue (πήγανον), with its heat, will destroy (διαφθείρειν) and coagulate (πηγνύναι) the semen (γονή).
e. Philagrius, fr. 199.47–9 Masullo: see G1.

---

166 *Portulaca oleracea* L.

167 Cf. Paul of Aegina 3.55 (p. 267, 24–6 Heiberg).

168 *Eruca vesicaria* ssp. *sativa* (Mill.) Thellung.

169 Cf. *Cyranides Latinus* p. 40, 4–6 Delatte.

170 Cf. Pseudo-Galen, *On Easily Obtainable Drugs* 3 (vol. 14, p. 543 Kühn).

171 Genus *Rosa* L. For the various species known in antiquity, see André, *Les noms de plantes*, s.v. "rosa."

172 *Ruta graveolens* L.

f. Philagrius, fr. 199.77–82 Masullo: see G2c.
g. Alexander of Tralles 2.499.7–10 Puschmann: Rue, being hot, thickens (παχύνειν) the semen (γονή). For this reason, it helps to prevent having frequent nocturnal emissions (ὀνειρώττειν) and seminal discharge.
h. Paul of Aegina 1.38 (p. 26, 15–17 Heiberg): Scattering rue under the bedclothes or eating its seeds will prevent nocturnal emissions (ὀνειρωγμοί).

G20. Strychnon[173]

a. Hippocrates, *Regimen* 2.54 (p. 174, 31–p. 176, 1 Joly and Byl; vol. 6, p. 558 Littré): *Strychnon* has a cooling effect (ψύχειν) and it prevents emitting semen during sleep (ἐξονειρώσσειν).
b. Dioscorides, *On Simple Medicines* 2.104: see note 157.
c. Philagrius, fr. 199.53–74 Masullo: see note 157.

G21. Water

a. Rufus of Ephesus *apud* Aëtius of Amida 3.165 (p. 339, 18–19 Olivieri): Drinking water (ὕδωρ) is suitable for those who suffer from frequent nocturnal emissions (ὀνειρώττοντες) and spermatorrhea.
b. Philagrius, fr. 199.42–3 Masullo: Drinking the water in which iron has been extinguished reduces the amount of semen (γονή).

G22. Water Lily,[174] its Root; Seeds

a. Pliny, *Natural History* 26.94: The white water lily (*nymphaea heracleia*) removes venery and lascivious dreams (*insomnia veneris*). Applying the root of water lily to the generative organs will prevent both venery and spermatorrhaea.
b. Dioscorides 3.132:[175] The root or seed of water lily (νυμφαία) is drunk against nocturnal emissions (ὀνειρωγμοί).
c. Dioscorides, *On Simple Medicines* 2.104: see note 157.
d. Dioscorides, *On Simple Medicines* 2.105: Those who suffer from nocturnal emissions (ὀνειρώττοντες) are helped by drinking a decoction

---

173 The term στρύχνον can denote various plants (cf. André, *Les noms de plantes*, s.v. "strychnon"). In our passages, it may be στρύχνον ὑπνωτικόν or sleepy nightshade (*Withania somnifera* [L.] Dunal), the root of which is still used today in Ayurvedic medicine for treating spermatorrhea (cf. M.H. Mirjalili et al., "Steroidal Lactones from *Withania somnifera*, an Ancient Plant for Novel Medicine," *Molecules*, 14(7) [2009]: pp. 2373–93, at p. 2374).

174 In our passages, the term *nymphaea*/νυμφαία probably denotes the white water lily (*Nymphaea alba* L.). The term is also used for the yellow water lily (*Nuphar luteum* [L.] Sm.).

175 Cf. Dioscorides *Latinus* 3.143 (p. 435, 15–16 Stadler).

(ἀπόζεμα) of the root of water lily (νυμφαία ῥίζα) instead of food, or by mixing the food with dried root and seeds of water lily, and drinking a decoction of mint.

e. Rufus of Ephesus, *On Satyriasis and Gonorrhea* 29 (p. 75, 13–p. 76, 1 Daremberg-Ruelle): Drinking the root of water lily will help against nocturnal emissions (ὀνειρωγμοί) and venery.
f. Galen, *On the Powers of Simple Medicines* 8.13.9 (vol. 12, p. 86 Kühn):[176] Both the root and the seed of water lily cause to dry up. They therefore prevent various types of discharges, including that of semen during nocturnal emissions (ὀνειρωγμοί).
g. Philagrius, fr. 199.36–7 Masullo: Both the root and seed of water lily, when eaten, quench the semen (γονή) by cooling it.
h. Philagrius, fr. 199.53–74: see note 157.
i. Alexander of Tralles 2.497.21–2 Puschmann: Both the root and seed of water lily work well against nocturnal emissions (ὀνειρωγμοί).

G23. White Violet,[177] its Seed
Philagrius, fr. 199.40–41 Masullo: Drinking the seed of white violet (λευκόϊον) can make a person sterile (ἄγονος).

G24. Willow,[178] its Fruit
Galen *apud* Aëtius of Amida 11.33 (p. 122, 9–12 Daremberg-Ruelle): see G2a.

176 Oribasius, *Books for Eunapius* 2.1.v.5 (p. 374, 16–18 Raeder), 4.107 (p. 485, 5–7 Raeder); Aëtius of Amida 1.295 (p. 114, 12–13 Olivieri).

177 On the identity of this plant, see André, *Les noms de plantes*, s.v. "leucoïon."

178 Genus *Salix* L.

Chapter 11

Magic, Infidelity, and Secret Annotations in a Cypriot Manuscript of the Early Fourteenth Century (Wellcome MSL 14)

Barbara Zipser

MSL 14 is an unusual little book.[1] It consists of two very different parts written within a couple of decades of each other. The first part contains in a neat thematic sequence a variety of medical treatises, which include, among others, a high-quality version of an innovative medical text.[2] This work is one of the rare witnesses of the Greek vernacular, the language spoken at the time. The second part contains an idiosyncratic, if not chaotic compilation of mainly medical content. It is a collection of excerpts, most of which only consist of one sentence.

Both parts of the book lack a number of pages and are generally in a poor state of preservation. Clearly, the volume was handled a lot. Overall, it appears to be a common, pocket-sized handbook someone used for general reference.[3]

---

[1] The manuscript was first pointed out to me by Vivian Nutton (UCL). One of the texts contained in the book subsequently became the topic of a postdoctoral fellowship funded by the Wellcome Trust. Nikolai Serikoff (Wellcome Library) and Lara Artemis (now British Library) examined binding, cover, and watermarks found in the book. Agamemnon Tselikas identified the handwriting as an unusual Cypriot hand. This chapter was written while I held a Wellcome Trust University Award for studies on Theophanes Nonnus and Simon Ianuensis.

[2] An analysis of the thematic structure of the first part of the manuscript and basic data on the second can be found in B. Zipser and V. Nutton, "MSL 14—a Wellcome Manuscript of a Medical Practitioner," in V. Boudon-Millot, A. Garzya, J. Jouanna, and A. Roselli (eds), *Histoire de la tradition et édition des médecins grecs: Actes du VIe colloque international (Paris, Université de Paris Sorbonne—Académie des Inscriptions et Belles Lettres, 10–12 avril 2008)* (Napoli, 2010), pp. 259–70. The manuscript was first catalogued by W.R. Dawson, *Manuscripta medica: A Descriptive Catalogue of the Manuscripts in the Library of the Medical Society of London* (London, 1934), p. 24.

[3] The volume measures only 14.4 x 10.0 cm. It has been rebound at least once. In this process, some pages were cut off and pasted back together; it was subsequently bound too tightly, so that it cannot be opened fully.

When looking at the tome, one is left wondering whether the book's owners would have expected it to be at some point the center of a scholarly analysis. For us, its decidedly unacademic nature is what makes it interesting. Not many of these books survived to our times.

The focus of this chapter is on the second, slightly older part of the book.[4] Most likely, it was written by a certain Theodoulos Philagres, a Cypriot scribe of the early fourteenth century.[5] The handwriting and the general layout of the page can only be described as very odd. The characters are large, broad, and bulky, and the lower and outer page margins are unusually wide, so that each page contains on average only 30 words. Such a script would make any conventional, coherent text very difficult to follow. An aphoristic collection such as the one contained in this manuscript can, however, be read easily.

In the following, various layers of text in the manuscript will be examined: first the main text body written by the scribe, then annotations made by owners and users of the book, and finally scholia written in invisible ink.

The main text body is the oldest layer of text in the manuscript: when the book was produced, the scribe did not use any ruling, which led to an uneven spacing and script size. In effect, the lower margins do not always have the same width. The text written in invisible ink at the bottom of the page and the annotations added in the outer margins were then wrapped around the main text.[6]

---

[4] On a few pages, traces of watermarks can be found (280, 288, 312, 314, and 316). They are, however, very fragmentary, with most parts of the watermark being cut off. Some (280, 288) could be identical with watermarks found in the first part of the manuscript. These resemble entries 6913f. and 1900–1906 in V. Mosin, *Vodeni znakovi XIII i XIV vijeka* (Zagreb, 1957), where they are dated to 1358 and 1352–1366; all are described as being of Italian origin. The paper of both parts of the manuscript has laid lines 1 mm apart, and no chain lines (I owe the analysis of the paper to Lara Artemis). The paper of the second part is, however, much thicker and stronger than the first, and looks distinctively different.

[5] A sample of his writing dating from 1319 can be found on plate 44 (ms. 30) in C. Constantinides and R. Browning, *Dated Manuscripts from Cyprus to the Year 1570*, Dumbarton Oaks Studies 30, Texts and Studies of the History of Cyprus, Cyprus Research Center 18 (Washington, D.C., 1993). It also bears some similarity to a hand listed in A. Jakovljevic, *Catalogue of Greek Manuscripts in the Library of the Monastery of St. Neophytos (Cyprus)* (Nicosia, 2002), ms. 10, p. 86. Agamemnon Tselikas has dated the handwriting of our text to the third decade of fourteenth-century Cyprus. With his guidance, I was able to identify the scribe.

[6] As the boundaries of the invisible text are not indicated in the manuscript, and since the invisible text and the main text body do not overlap, this part of the book could only have been written down after the main text body was finished. The annotations in the outer margins (written in conventional ink) were clearly scribbled down on whatever space was left blank.

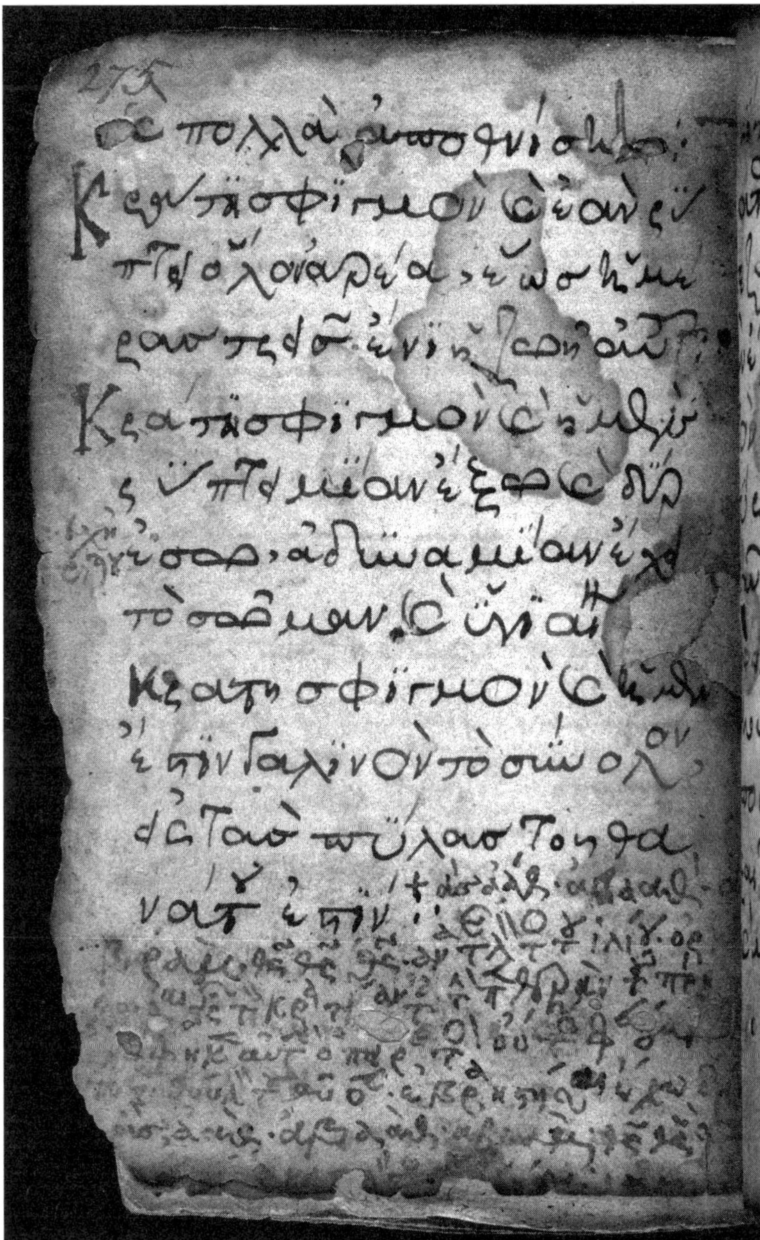

Figure 11.1 Wellcome Library, MSL 14, p. 275: The second folio of the fragment. The page is partly torn and glued together with paper strips. It contains instructions on pulse diagnosis and a magical scholion written on the lower margins by a later hand.

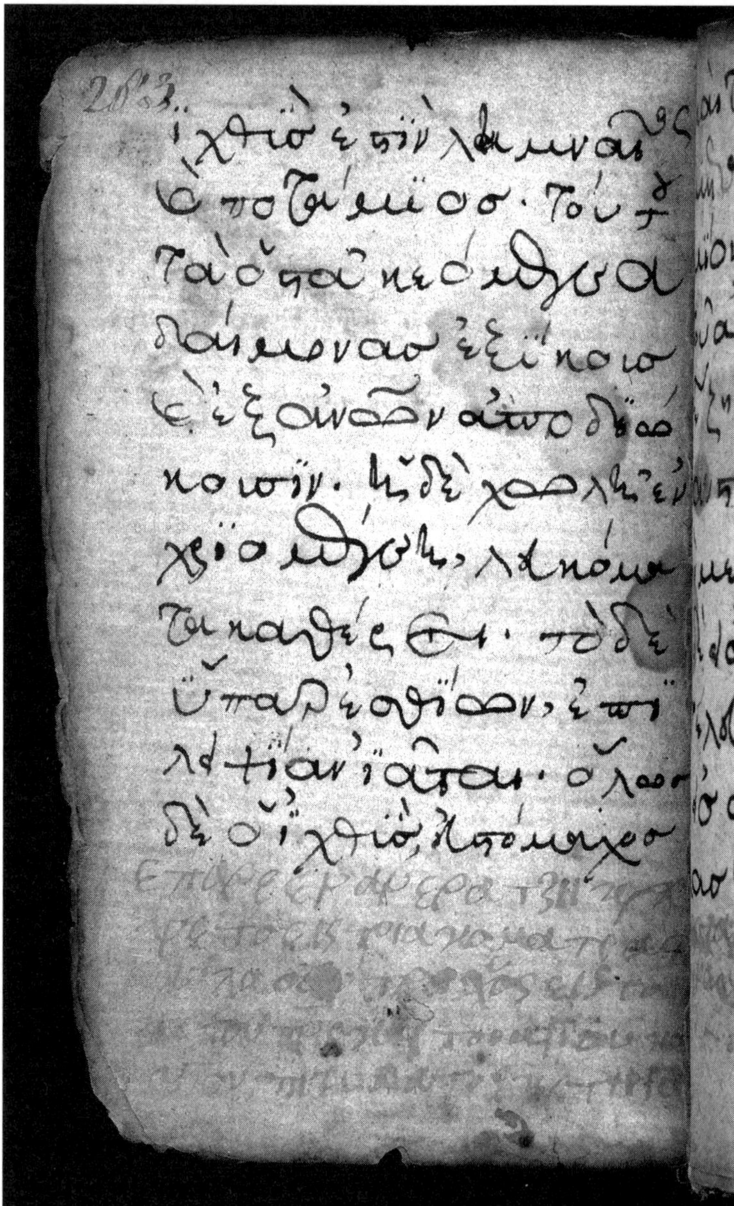

Figure 11.2 Wellcome Library, MSL 14, p. 283: The main text discusses a type of fish. On the lower margins, a borderline magical text was written in invisible ink. The photograph is digitally enhanced. To the naked eye, only a few characters are visible. The general area of the scholion has a somewhat darker appearance.

Describing the content of the main text is not an easy task. It is obviously fragmentary, with several pages missing, but the miscellaneous nature of the compilation makes it difficult for us to estimate its original length or to reconstruct the correct sequence of pages. A total of 23 folios survive—which implies that at least one more is missing, as the book would then have consisted of an even number of folios. The situation is further complicated by the fact that the pages were cut off, glued back together, and trimmed to size by a curator,[7] which eliminated any evidence on the total number of quires it once contained.[8]

The following summary presents the text roughly in the sequence it has today, with two pages being reversed. I indicate a new sheet of paper by || [9] and a gap in the text by [gap]. What we have is a compilation with at least one page missing at the beginning and at least three gaps in the text. As the end of a paragraph often coincides with the end of a folio, there may be more gaps or other reversed pages that remain undetected. Thus, we are unable to prove whether the form of the current is the original.[10] However, a number of factors do suggest that this is how the manuscript presented to a medieval reader and user; the annotations in invisible ink can only be found on pages 276–9 and 280–85, which makes it likely that these pages were at least roughly in the same section of the volume when the text was annotated. Moreover, pages 272–3 look worn out, which indicates that these were the first pages of the volume:[11]

---

7 According to data provided by Lara Artemis, this most likely happened during the nineteenth century, when the volume was rebacked.

8 The manuscript does not contain any first-hand quire marks. Greek numerals that can be found in various locations on the outer and lower margins are of a much later date. It is unclear whether they represent a quire, page or paragraph numbering, cross-references to other works, or a combination of these; in the form the manuscript presents today, the evidence can only be described as inconclusive.

9 The first two blocks of text on urine and pulse diagnosis are most likely complete and in the correct sequence of pages; thus, page breaks are not indicated in the list given above. An analysis of the texts and their sources can be found in B. Zipser, "Die uneinheitliche Überlieferung eines Fragmentes über den Puls und ein Iatrosophion," *Galenos*, 2 (2008), pp. 129–34.

10 This reconstruction was motivated by three unrelated pieces of circumstantial evidence. First, this is the way the manuscript would most likely have looked like to a medieval reader. Second, this way of reorganizing pages requires the least interventions. Third, the first part of the manuscript shows a very similar pattern of damage: most pages are roughly in the correct position, some are reversed, and a few are missing. See Zipser and Nutton, "MSL 14," pp. 265–7 for details.

11 It is often the case that the first pages of a manuscript are damaged or in fact missing. Here, page 272^r is damaged, and the preceding page is missing. Thus, page 272^r most likely was the first or second page at the time when the codex was in use.

272–9: Two larger blocks of text on urine and pulse diagnosis; longer passage on fevers; children wetting the bed; phlebotomy [gap].
282–3, 280–81: Ears (end of a paragraph); lichen; fluid building up in the chest; type of fish (|| end of paragraph), another type of fish; importance of calendar [gap].
284–9, 292–3, 290–91: Prognosis of life or death (end of paragraph, magical); teeth; fractured bones, animals and humans (|| within paragraph); wounds; unclear, perhaps heartburn; unclear, perhaps intestinal cramps (|| within paragraph, magical); spleen; belly; belly; wound (|| within paragraph); menorrhagia; predicting sex of a fetus (magical); sore throat; birth (|| within paragraph magical); induce lactation; paradontosis (|| end of paragraph).
294–7: Unclear, perhaps belly cramps; dysuria; flux from the eyes (|| end of sentence).
298–305: Unclear, on pain (end of paragraph); pain of the eye; women who do not covet (magical); paradontosis (|| within paragraph); ear; make a patient sleep; prognosis of life or death (magical); pain of the eye (|| within paragraph); flux from the eye and tears; hemorrhoids; dropsy (|| within paragraph, magical); clear eyesight; deafness; pituriasis; unclear, perhaps bedsores; cough (|| after heading) [gap].
306–17: Tongue (end of paragraph); clyster; clyster (|| within a paragraph); plague; dysuria; belly; swollen intestines; head cold (|| within paragraph); head cold; hair loss (|| within paragraph); getting rid of fleas in the house; how not to get sore feet while traveling; how not to get thirsty while traveling; pain of the eye; flux from the eyes (|| within paragraph); dropsy; unclear.

The text is written in a simplified form of learned Byzantine Greek, with some interspersed vernacular vocabulary. It consists mainly of short sentences that are easy to follow. The two fragments on prognosis have a slightly more polished style:

> Κράτη σφιγμὸν καὶ ἠμέν ἐστι γαλινὸν τὸ σύνολον εἰς τὰς πύλας τοῦ θανάτου ἐστίν.
>
> Take the pulse, and if it is generally calm, he is at the verge of death.

Most of the paragraphs in this section have a similar, clearly defined structure. They begin with "Take the pulse ..." or "If the urine is ..." followed by a description of the findings and then the prognosis.[12] Some paragraphs also contain instructions on how to treat the respective diseases.

The rest of the compilation has a different form, consisting of a number of paragraphs without any obvious thematic connection or sequence, with no more than two subsequent entries covering a similar topic.[13] The majority of the text concerns therapeutics, with a focus on diseases that are easy to recognize, such as a cough or hair loss, and notably omits rare diseases.[14] For instance, the only eye diseases mentioned are flux and pain of the eye, along with instructions on how to maintain good vision. Overall, the content contained in this collection presents remedies for diseases that may not necessarily require diagnosis by a physician.

The therapeutic measures and recipes described are equally simple: patients should eat or drink a specific medication, or the medication should be applied to the affected part. This medication would be prepared by grinding, mixing, and sometimes cooking ingredients:

> Εἰς τὴν κυλίαν. Ἔπαρον ἐρεβίνθιν καὶ ἄλεσον αὐτῶ καὶ τιγάνισον μετὰ μελ καὶ δῶς αὐτῶ καὶ ἄς τὸ φᾶ.
>
> For the belly. Take chick peas and make it smooth and fry them with honey and give him and let him eat.
>
> Περὶ τὰ οὔλοι τρογώμενα. Συνάπεως σπόρον καὶ ἀγριοσταφίδαν κοπάνισον καὶ θὲς εἰς τὰ οὔλοι.
>
> For corroded gums. Grind mustard seed and wild grapes and put it on the gums.

Generally speaking, these recipes mention fewer ingredients than one would expect to find in one of the classical and late antique manuals. Moreover, the ingredients would be available without any further difficulty.

When looking at the collection, two types of content catch the eye of a classically trained scholar. First, some of the entries concern fish.[15] It is not unusual

---

12 Structure and sources of one these texts are discussed in Zipser, "Die uneinheitliche Überlieferung."

13 Most therapeutic texts follow the so-called *a capite ad calcem* sequence, that is, diseases are arranged in a head-to-foot order, depending on their main place of manifestation.

14 These would have been included in the major therapeutic collections, such as Paul of Aegina 3.22.

15 Page 283: περὶ γλάνεον, which according to LSJ means "sheat-fish"; this corresponds with *Cyranides* 4.13 Kaimakes. Page 280: χελιδῶν θαλάσσιον ἰχθύδιον μικρόν, "flying fish," for which, see *Cyranides* 4.73. Both entries also contain some borderline magical content.

for foodstuffs to be discussed in a medical text, as nutrition was perceived to have an impact on health, and a change of diet was also used in medical treatment; for instance, the monumental works of Aëtius of Amida and Paul of Aegina contain information on nutrition.[16] However, such content would normally be found in dedicated sections of the work, rather than together with therapeutic instructions, as is the case here.

Second, the collection contains a number of passages of magical nature, which are rarely found in the established medical writers. Two of these entries are preserved in their entirety: instructions how to detect potential infidelity of one's wife and an entry on inducing birth. The latter reads (see Figure 11.3):

> περὶ τῆς γέννας τῆς γυναικὸς γράφε γυνὴ ἐκεῖ ἐδιέβην καὶ ὁ ἀρχάγγελος Γαβριὴλ εἶπεν ἔξελθε παιδίον κράζει σε ὁ χς καὶ ὑπεραγία θκς μνήσθητι κύριε τῶν ὑιῶν Ἐδώμ ἐκκενοῦται ἐκκενοῦται ἐκκενοῦται.
>
> On the birth of a child: Write "a woman went there and the archangel Gabriel said, come out child. Christ and the most holy Mother of God are calling you. Remember, lord, the sons of Edom, it shall leave, it shall leave, it shall leave."

The charm described here consists of religious incantations, with the last words quoting the Septuagint (Psalm 136:7). In all likelihood, this specific passage was chosen because it contained the word ἐκκενοῦτε, "they shall empty out (i.e. destroy or desolate)," a homophone of ἐκκενοῦται, "he/she/it shall empty itself out (i.e. leave)."[17] Some memorable words of the original quote were then added, ultimately resulting in a nonsensical text.[18]

This amulet is as such unremarkable. What is of more interest is how this short piece of text found its way into this collection. Even though we cannot identify the source for most of the medical content, it is safe to assume that the vast majority comes from a written tradition, most likely a collection such

---

[16] This would be Book 1 of Aëtius of Amida's *Libri medicinales* and Book 7 of Paul of Aegina.

[17] The original biblical quotation reads: μνήσθητι, κύριε, τῶν υἱῶν Εδωμ τὴν ἡμέραν Ιερουσαλημ τῶν λεγόντων Ἐκκενοῦτε ἐκκενοῦτε, ἕως ὁ θεμέλιος ἐν αὐτῇ (Lord, remember the day of Jerusalem when the sons of Edom say "Destroy, destroy, down to her foundations"). The wording ἐν αὐτῇ is a direct translation of the Hebrew text (בה); the classical Greek equivalent would be αὐτῆς.

[18] Intriguingly, as Figure 11.3 shows, a later hand, to judge from the ink, perhaps of the eighteenth century, added two of the missing words, again in a wrong spelling, and a redundant ἐκκενοῦται.

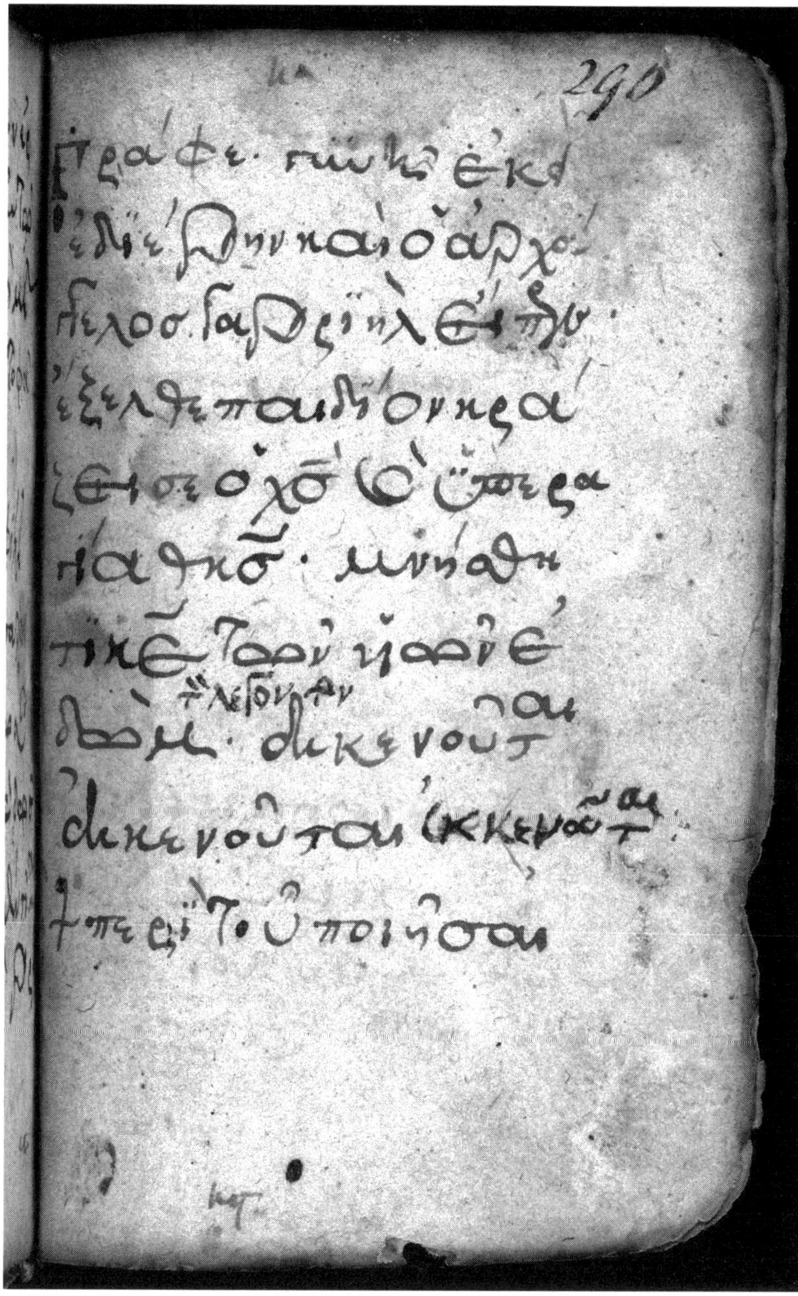

Figure 11.3 Wellcome Library, MSL 14, p. 290: Instructions on how to make an amulet to induce childbirth. A later hand corrected the Psalm quotation in blue ink and added one more word.

as the ℵ version of Ioannes archiatrus[19] or some of the Xenôn texts.[20] Even though these excerpts were simple, they do still make sense and are generally speaking in accordance with sophisticated medical writings. The amulet is of an entirely different nature. It contains factual and grammatical errors, and perhaps was never even meant to convey an intelligible text. Thus, it would have hardly have been included in one of these medical compendia, no matter how basic they were.

Surprisingly, though, parts of the text are also transmitted in an anonymous *iatrosophion*, partly written in vernacular Greek.[21] There, it can be found among medical content that is arranged in a neat thematic sequence, in a chapter on difficult birth, which also contains religious incantations and a procedure that is borderline magical. The main difference to our passage is that the Psalm text is quoted in its entirety[22] and without any addition obscuring the meaning, as in MSL 14. It is the only nonmedical content in the compilation. Since there are no further similarities between this *iatrosophion* and the text of MSL 14, a direct link between both texts, other than through an oral tradition, is unlikely.[23]

The second passage to be discussed is longer and more elaborate. It contains instructions on how to recognize the infidelity of one's wife. It reads:

---

19 Edited in B. Zipser, *John the Physician's Therapeutics: A Medical Handbook in Vernacular Greek*, Studies in Ancient Medicine (Leiden, 2009).

20 See, for instance, the texts edited in Appendices I–III (pp. 331–439) in D.C. Bennett, "Xenonika: Medical Texts Associated with Xenones in the Late Byzantine Period" (Ph.D. dissertation, University of London, 2003).

21 It is transmitted in manuscript Weimar Q 733. The *iatrosophion* covers the nature of the *kosmos*, embryology, gynecology, and general therapy. It is a carefully arranged compilation of high-quality excerpts. I am most grateful to Claudia Sode (Cologne) for pointing out the text to me.

22 The passage reads: μνίσκητι κύριε τῶν ὑιῶν ἐδῶμ τὴν ἡμέραν ἱερουσαλυμ τῶν λεγόντων ἐκκενοῦται, ἐκκενοῦται ἕως τῶν θεμελίων αὐτῖς θυγάτερ βαβυλόνος ἡ ταλαίπορος. καὶ ἐξύλθεν ὁ λάζαρος ἐκ τοῦ μνυμίου καὶ ἴωνας ἐκ τοῦ κύτους. οὕτος ἔξελθε καὶ σοὶ παιδίον ἐκ κοιλίας μητρός σου. Thus, it presents a longer excerpt from the Bible (the Psalm passage) and two shorter references to Lazarus and Jonah. These three passages were selected, apparently, because they each contain references to "leaving," one being, as outlined above, a misunderstanding.

23 The text transmitted in Q 733 remains to be described in detail. Parts of the text appear to be an excerpt from Meletius, while others come from a high-quality therapeutic work written in the vernacular. As no other witnesses for this text are known at this moment, we cannot determine whether the mention of the sons of Edom may have been an interpolation. Apart from this passage, the compilation does not contain any magical content.

περὶ γυναικὸς ἐὰν μὴ χα^τ. ὀρνιθίου στέον τὸ ἔμπροσθεν τοῦ στήθους αὐτοῦ ὅ ἐστιν εἰς τὸ δεξιὸν μέρος τὸ διχαλὸν κοιμωμένης τῆς γυναικὸς θὲς ἀπενάντι τῆς καρδίας αὐτῆς. καὶ ἂς βλέπει ἢ διχάλης τοῦ ὀστέου πρὸς τὴν κεφαλὴν αὐτῆς. πότισον δὲ αὐτὴν καὶ ὀγκάτει λίθον καὶ ὁμολογίσει ἐν τῷ ὕπνῳ ὅσα ἔπραξεν.

Concerning a woman when she does not covet. Put the bone of a bird from the front of its chest, the right part of the fork, on top of the heart of a woman while she is lying down. And let the part of the fork face towards her head. Let her drink and [unclear][24] and she will confess in her sleep to what she has done.

At first sight, one might assume that this passage describes a dream interpretation. However, there are pronounced differences between oneirocritic practices and our text.[25] Not only do these instructions describe a magical procedure—placing the right part of a wishbone on the woman's chest—it is also carried out against the woman's will.[26] Moreover, it does not involve a dream that is to be interpreted later; rather, the woman speaks while she is asleep.[27] Instead, the procedure has parallels in a Greek magical papyrus. In one spell, one places materials on a woman's genital area and during her sleep she will be forced to divulge information to anything asked of her:

Spell for causing talk while asleep: Take the heart of a hoopee and place it in myrrh. And write on a strip of hieratic papyrus the names and characters and

[24] The phrase ὀγκάτει λίθον could, with some creativity, be interpreted as a misspelled ὀγκᾶται ἤλιθον (he/she/it makes silly animal noises). With even more creativity, one could see ὀγκᾶται as a *futurum atticum*, which would better fit the context. Alternatively, the phrase could refer to letting her drink a liquid with a specific type of stone that is unknown to us. However, either of these options appears too farfetched to lead to an emendation of the text.

[25] Dream interpretation was commonly practiced and accepted in the Byzantine era. Typically, a dream would be told to an interpreter, who would then predict future events, or would be deciphered using a dream-key manual. For more information, see Oberhelman's chapter in this volume.

[26] Had it been her free will to tell what had happened, it would not have been necessary to perform the procedure.

[27] The word ὕπνος sometimes means "dream" in oneirologic texts. Thus, the last words of the sentence could also be translated as "and she will confess in a dream what she has done." However, had this been the intended meaning, the text would likely have specified to whom she would confess ("she will confess to you ..."). Moreover, since the woman is already lying down during the procedure, it would make more sense that it is in fact she who falls asleep.

> roll up the heart in the strip of papyrus and place it on her pudenda and ask your questions. And she will confess everything to you: "DARYGKO IAU IAU [there follow 21 *characters magicae*]" (add the usual, as much as you want).[28]

Spells for causing sleep and curing insomnia, for divination through dreams, and for dream revelations were part of ancient magic (Egyptian, Near Eastern, and Greek), and they worked their way into many iatrosophic texts of the Byzantine and post-Byzantine periods.[29]

Next, in the text, we have annotations by later hands. These can be divided into two categories: the attempt to systematize the collection, and the attempt to add personalized, and mainly religious or magical, content.

Annotations of the first kind cannot be easily described. Throughout the manuscript, a total of 41 Greek numerals, ranging from α′ to ξθ′, were added in the outer and lower margins.[30] As the color of the ink reveals, many of these clearly postdate the production of the manuscript by a considerable time. Most likely, these numerals were added at a stage when the manuscript had already disintegrated but still comprised more pages than are extant today. These numerals appear to have been added in an effort to systematize the collection, which in turn indicates that this manuscript was passed on to later generations, who did not keep it for purely antiquarian purposes. On the contrary, several people tried to make sense of the collection, and, as the different types of ink reveal, these editorial efforts continued over several centuries.[31]

The second set of annotations consists of mainly magical content. About one-third of these are written in conventional ink and contain the πι πι transcription of the tetragrammaton (p. 274); a longer text containing gibberish, religious incantations; instructions to perform a certain procedure at sunrise; references to the Bible (see Figure 11.1); obscure lists of symbols; and, apparently, Greek numerals, along with the letters "ni n" in Latin script—most likely another attempt to transcribe the tetragrammaton—and other texts too fragmentary to

---

28 Translation taken from H.D. Betz, *The Greek Magical Papyri in Translation, Including the Demotic Spells*, 2nd edn with an updated bibliography (Chicago and London, 1992), p. 129.

29 See in general S. Eitrem, "Dreams and Divination in Magical Ritual," in C.A. Faraone and D. Obbink (eds), *Magika Hiera: Ancient Greek Magic and Religion* (New York and Oxford, 1991), pp. 175–87; and Oberhelman's chapter in this volume.

30 For instance, in Figure 11.3, two Greek numerals in faint black ink can be seen: an 11 at the top of the page and a 16 at the bottom. It is unclear whether these numbers refer to the two chapters transmitted on the page.

31 The numbers could refer to an index, which was added later on, or to a table of contents. Alternatively, this could be cross-references to another text.

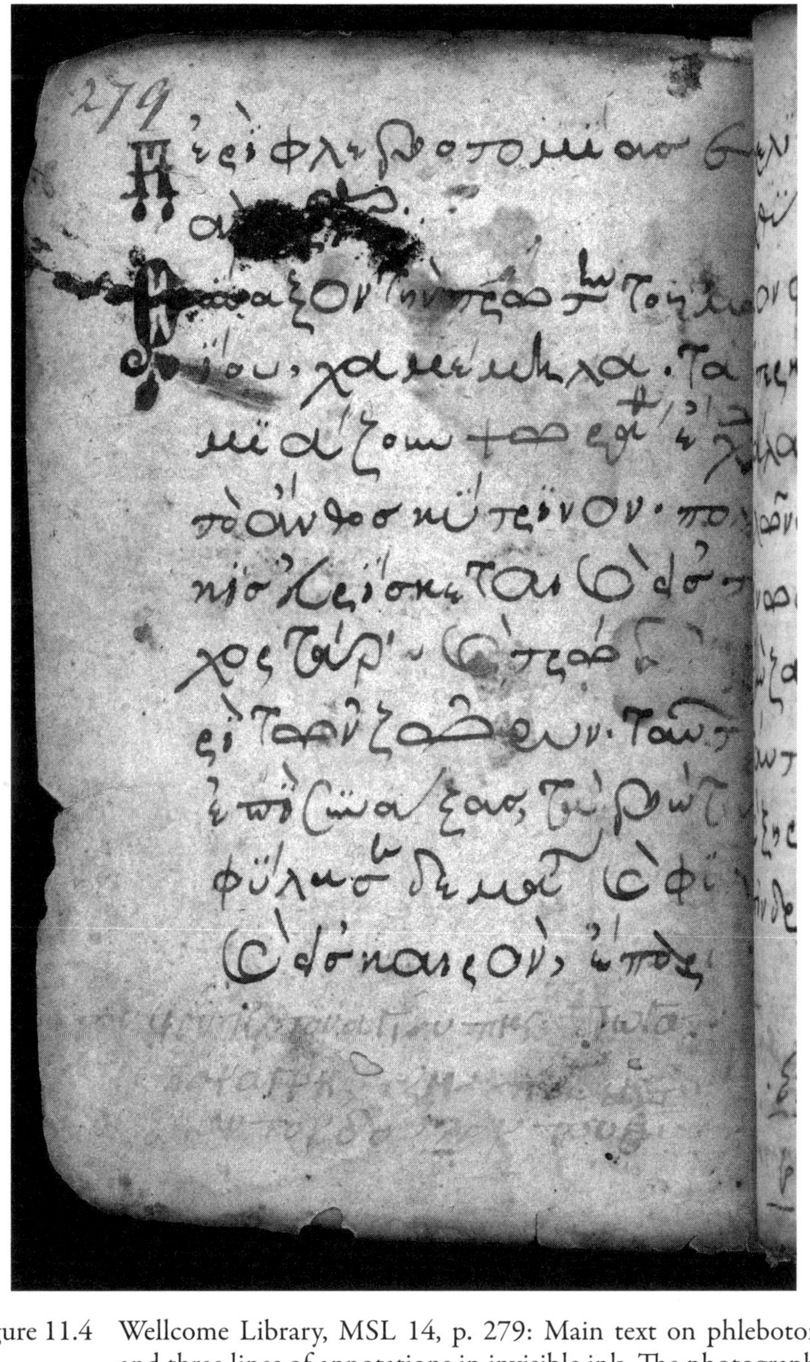

Figure 11.4 Wellcome Library, MSL 14, p. 279: Main text on phlebotomy and three lines of annotations in invisible ink. The photograph is digitally enhanced.

be analyzed here. These annotations are written in a blackish ink, which indicates that they were written at a much later date than the main text. The handwriting itself is very irregular and cannot be dated with certainty.

The other annotations are most unusual in that they are written in an invisible ink. To the naked eye, hardly a trace of the text is visible: the general area appears somewhat darker than the rest of the page, and a few stains and lines are visible (see Figures 11.2 and 11.4, which are digitally enhanced). Under ultraviolet light, three to five lines of text per page can be read.[32] They are written in a rather clumsy handwriting—after all, the scribe could not see what he had written, making it more difficult to keep the handwriting proportional.[33]

Here are a few excerpts:

> ... εἰς τὸ ὡνομαν τοῦ πρς κ ... (p. 278, last line)
>
> τοῦ φοῦ καὶ τοῦ ἁγίου πνς ... (p. 279, first line, see Figure 11.4)
>
> In the name of the Father and the Son and of the Holy Spirit.
>
> ἔπαρε ἕνα νεράζη κο
>
> ψετο εἰς τρία κομάτια
>
> κόλασε τρ.χας εἰς τα
>
> μετοῦ πρς καὶ τοῦ ἁγίου
>
> ἁγίου πνεύματος καὶ τη (p. 282, full text; see Figure 11.2)[34]
>
> Take an orange and cut it into three slices [unclear],[35] in the name of the Father and the most Holy Spirit and ...
>
> ... εἰς τὸν πόνον τῆς καρδίας ... (p. 282, last line)
>
> ... for heartburn ...

---

[32] These can be found on pages 277–9, 281–5.

[33] Under ultraviolet, the ink appeared black. However, some parts of the text were not legible, because the ink was smudged. Various pages also show water damage.

[34] I am very grateful to Agamemnon Tselikas, who deciphered the word τρία.

[35] Most likely, these words mean "join them together threefold." However, τρίχα can also mean "hair" in the vernacular.

Also found in these scholia are references to someone being in pain, quotes from the liturgy, and instructions to compress, leave, apply, or stretch items. The text also mentions ground cumin, followed by some more religious invocations and prayers.

The fragmentary nature of these annotations and the general problem of reconstructing the sequence of pages make it difficult to describe the texts in more detail. It is safe to say, however, that they contain religious incantations, magical elements (the orange being sliced into three parts), and references to medical conditions.

The most important point about the scholia is that they are not legible to the naked eye. This practice of adding secret annotations is highly unusual for Greek medical manuscripts. In the field we do encounter palimpsests, which are essentially recycled parchment books, and the odd correction, for which an existing text has been erased, but, overall, the intention of writing a text was that the text was read. Here, however, the main goal appears to have been to add a magical value to the book itself.

Overall, we encountered a number of different layers of text in the manuscript. First is the main text, a compilation of therapeutic content of unknown provenance, on various common diseases—ranging from treatment for minor issues such as children wetting the bed or sore feet to chronic conditions such as deafness, and more serious disorders such as dysuria or dropsy. In literary form, content, and vocabulary, these paragraphs very much resemble the ℵ version of Ioannes archiatrus or the Xenôn texts. Most likely, they originate from a similar written source. They are complemented by two blocks of text on prognosis. Mingled with these paragraphs are two passages on fish and instructions for various magical procedures—to induce lactation, predict the sex of a fetus, make a woman confess potential infidelity, predict death, and more. Of these, the procedures to detect infidelity are particularly striking. They are not, as one might assume, a dream interpretation.[36] Another layer of text contains magical charms in clear text. Finally, there is another layer containing instructions on magical procedures in invisible form.

---

[36] There is a definite manuscript link between therapy and dream interpretation; at some point, probably during or shortly after the eleventh century, the traditions of Alexander of Tralles and Artemidorus, two authorities in these fields, were fused when a canon of their works was formed (this canon survives in the Vat. Ott. 89 and Gonville and Caius 77). The vast majority of MSL 14 contains therapeutic writings in a simplified form. However, the instructions on how to detect infidelity are not compatible with traditional dream interpretation, so that it cannot be seen as a parallel to the developments that led to the formation of the Alexander-Artemidorus canon.

If one takes two steps back and looks at the book again, it appears to be a personalized medical handbook for practical use. The diseases covered reflect very much what one would realistically expect to encounter in real life. Magical content not commonly found in medical texts either in the scholarly field or in practical medical works[37] but very frequently encountered in the Byzantine world[38] has been incorporated into the medicine. Intriguingly, most of the later annotations are of a magical nature.

In conclusion, we may say that the book reflects the world in which it was perused, adapted, and developed. Despite its basic content and the inconvenient format, it was in continued use over centuries. More magic was added, and even the book itself was turned into a magical object, most likely while it was still being used for medical purposes.

---

37 Sometimes, magical content can only be found in one part of the transmission, an indication of an interpolation. See, for instance, Ioannes archiatrus, chapter ω 201 on infertility.

38 For an introduction to the world in which the book was used, see H. Maguire, *Byzantine Magic* (Washington, D.C., 1995). In this volume, J. Russell ("The Archeological Context of Magic in the Early Byzantine Period," pp. 35–50) presents a number of amulets.

PART THREE
The Post-Byzantine Period to the Current Day

Chapter 12

Dreams, Dreambooks, and Post-Byzantine Practical Healing Manuals (*Iatrosophia*)

Steven M. Oberhelman

For nearly four millennia, people have resorted to dream-key manuals to discover information about the present and the future.[1] A dream-key manual may be defined as a compendium of dreams or dream symbols that are interpreted for the purpose of providing a guide to present or future matters like health and illness, wealth and poverty, life and death, success and failure, and marriage and divorce. The barest (and most typical) schematic form of such manuals is the arrangement, usually alphabetically or by thematic grouping, of dream symbols that are assigned a predictive value stated either as a simple equivalence ("Eating roasted rabbit signifies disease but also wealth from a woman" or "Drinking olive oil: illness") or in a protasis-apodosis construction ("If someone dreams of eating hot pita bread, he will be afflicted with the disease of tuberculosis").[2] Theoretical

[1] The bibliography is extensive. Two recent discussions in English with relevant scholarship are Jovan Bilbija, "Ancient Dream-Books as Mirrors of Worlds," in E. Cingano and L. Milano (eds), *Papers on Ancient Literatures: Greece, Rome and the Near East: Proceedings of the "Advanced Seminar in the Humanities," Venice International University 2004–2005* (Venice, 2008), pp. 75–104; and S.M. Oberhelman, "Prolegomena to the Reconstruction of the Archetype of the Greek *Somniale Danielis*," *Quaderni di Studi Indo-Mediterranei*, 2 (2009): pp. 107–24. All translations in this chapter are my own, unless otherwise noted.

[2] As Mark Geller remarks, the same dream omens probably circulated throughout antiquity in collections that were variously translated in different cultures. Indeed, texts surviving from the earliest times of ancient Egypt, Assyria, and Babylon contain in the protases dream symbols similar to those in the dream-key manuals of Greece and Rome. It is in the apodoses, which contain the symbols' interpretations, where differences according to locality, culture, and time occur; see Geller's "West Meets East: Early Greek and Babylonian Diagnosis," in H.F.J. Horstmanshoff and M. Stol (eds), *Magic and Rationality in Ancient Near Eastern and Graeco-Roman Medicine* (Leiden, 2004), pp. 11–51, at p. 53; cf. Oberhelman, "Prolegomena," pp. 113–14, 117–19. The protasis-apodosis format extended to many genres in Assyrian and Babylonian scientific texts, for example, calendar texts, astrological omina, lunar eclipse tablets, physiognomic omina, and especially the *Diagnostic Handbook*, a medical text from the mid-eleventh century BC; for the latter, see R. Labat, *Traité Akkadien de diagnostics et prognostics médicaux* (Leiden, 1951); and N.P. Heeßel, *Babylonisch-Assyrische Diagnostik* (Münster, 2000).

discussions are rarely offered; only a few writers of dream-key manuals discuss the psychology of dreaming, attempt an analysis of dreamers, or divulge their methods of interpreting dreams.[3] Typically, dreams are drawn up in repetitive and often banal lists and are whittled down to a simple verbal action or a noun qualified by an adjective or two, with the entries often alphabetized for easy reference by the reader. Each symbol is then assigned an associative meaning, along the pattern of "if x then y" or "x = y." It is an open question whether any of the dreams preserved in these texts are historical, that is, whether people did in fact have the dreams that are recorded—although many ancient writers claimed this was the case.[4] Even if the dreams did come from real dreamers, they have been stripped of their individual specificity and recast in universal terms. Thus, a dream of eating lion meat means one thing and one thing only: a lawsuit with one's enemy. Whether the dreamer is a man or a woman, a king or a slave does not affect the predicted outcome (a lawsuit); nor are any details about the lawsuit given—what the suit may involve, the adversary's identity, the result, etc. The dreamer simply has been informed by the text he reads that a lawsuit will occur and that his opponent will be some personal enemy.[5]

Dreams and outcomes preserved and recorded in dream-key manuals reflect to a certain degree the concerns and anxieties of the culture in which

[3] The classic discussion is S.R.F. Price, "The Future of Dreams: From Freud to Artemidorus," in D. Halperin, J. Winkler, and F. Zeitlin (eds), *Before Sexuality: The Construction of Erotic Experience in the Ancient Greek World* (Princeton, 1990), pp. 365–87; cf. S.M. Oberhelman, *Dreambooks in Byzantium: Six Oneirocritica in Translation, with Commentary and Introduction* (London, 2008), Chapter 2.

[4] Artemidorus (for whom see below; Walde's chapter in this volume; and J. Bilbija, "The Dream in Antiquity: Aspects and Analyses" [Ph.D. dissertation, Vrije Universiteit, 2012], pp. 258–63) claims in his introductions to Books 1 and 5 of his treatise on dreams that during his extensive travels in Turkey, Greece, and Italy, he collected and analyzed over 3,000 dreams; he also reports that he interviewed diviners at festal assemblies and religious gatherings, and bought every book written on dreams. Anthropological research into dreams is a different matter when it comes to questions of veracity, as Stewart's chapter in this volume demonstrates, although we cannot always say whether all details in a dream recounted by a dreamer to an investigator are true or redacted or elaborated.

[5] A particular exception to this type of "one interpretation fits all" is the dreambook of Artemidorus, where symbols are assigned different meanings on the basis of the dreamer's individual circumstances and on the basis of factors like time, place, culture, law, and habits. The medieval Arabic dreambooks and the Byzantine dream-key manual ascribed to Achmet ibn Sereim (a treatise itself based on Arabic sources) also follow Artemidorus' text in offering interpretations for different dreamers (rich, poor, unmarried and married women, soldiers, etc.), but their format is an imitation of Artemidorus' dreambook which was translated into Arabic in the late ninth century; see M. Mavroudi, *A Byzantine Book on Dream Interpretation: The Oneirocriticon of Achmet and Its Arabic Sources* (Leiden/Boston/Cologne, 2002), pp. 128–67.

they were produced. The sixteenth-century version of the Greek dreambook assigned to Daniel the Prophet may serve as an example.[6] If we examine the 486 dreams and interpretations in the dreambook, we discover a pervasive fear of plots and treachery launched by enemies because of envy or hatred. A total of 20 dreams focus on dangers posed by personal enemies and 15 deal with broken alliances and friendships. We see no anxiety over external dangers like invasion or wars; rather, the enemy one should be concerned about lives next door, is a business partner, or sleeps in one's bed. Many dreams involve the making of profit or suffering loss: 30 dreams foretell the loss of property or money, while 60 predict acquisition of profit. Eleven dreams deal specifically with risky business ventures and another 12 with hindrance and impediments to one's way of life. Nineteen other dreams focus on gaining honors and ranks of office or on the opposite fate, namely losing one's status, imprisonment, or execution at the hands of the authorities. And in a world where fatality through illness and pestilence was an all-too-frequent occurrence and where people were accordingly obsessed with staying healthy, 21 dreams predict impending disease or an outbreak of plague. Jovan Bilbija provides similar statistics on dreams in Assyrian, thirteenth-century BC Egyptian, Talmudic, Hellenistic Greek, and medieval Arabic dreambooks. For example, a seventh of the dreams in the Egyptian and Assyrian dreambooks he studied focus on gain or loss, but the Assyrian texts have three times the number of dreams that deal with health.[7] Was disease more rampant in Old Babylon? Or was medical treatment more effective in the Nineteenth Dynasty? It may be a stretch to draw definitive conclusions about health care or epidemiology in any given culture on the basis of dream texts, but not too farfetched to say that if records show a high number of dreams fixated on disease and physical ailments, they may very well reflect contemporary anxieties over illness and wellbeing.

All dream-key manuals contain dreams that predict the onset of a disease or the course of an illness the dreamer has. The latter type is discussed frequently by Artemidorus and medieval Arabic writers, although a few occur in texts from ancient Assyria, Babylon, pharaonic Egypt, and Byzantium.[8] A few examples here will suffice:

[6] Much of this paragraph is taken from Oberhelman, "Prolegomena." The sixteenth-century version of the Daniel dreambook is an expanded adaptation of the original early Byzantine dreambook (fourth or fifth century AD). See the discussion, with bibliography, in Oberhelman, "Prolegomena," especially pp. 114–17.

[7] Bilbija, "Ancient Dream-Books," pp. 87–91.

[8] See Bilbija, "The Dream in Antiquity" for excellent summaries of dreams in Mesopotamia (pp. 13–43) and pp. 44–67 (Egypt); see also pp. 68–135 (Judaism).

If [a man dreams that] he eats the meat of a fox, he will be affected by a prickling sensation of the skin; for someone who is [already] ill, this is a good sign. (Assyrian Dreambook, K. 6663 + 8300)[9]

A wreath made of parsley kills both those who are ill and for the most part those who are afflicted with dropsy on account of the fact that parsley is cold and full of water [by nature] and because this sort of wreath is suitable for an athletic event held at funerals. (Artemidorus 1.77)[10]

To dream that one is sleeping in a temple foretells good health [for the dreamer] if he is ill, but disease or great worries if he is healthy; for the former will have a respite from his illness because people who are asleep have nothing to do with sufferings, but the latter will approach the gods for healing. To be sleeping amidst monuments and tombs or on a road prophesizes death for those who are ill and a lack of success for those who are healthy; [the reason is that] such activities and locales are ineffectual. (Artemidorus 1.81)

If someone dreams that he ate some [colocynths], if he happens to be ill, he will have good health; if he is not sick, he will continue to remain healthy. (Achmet 201)[11]

If someone dreams that by the order of his local ruler he was violently and forcibly hung by the neck, he will be lifted up in honor in proportion to how high he was raised when he was hung; and if the dreamer is sick or distressed, he will lose

---

9 Taken from P.J. van der Eijk, "Divination, Prognosis and Prophylaxis: The Hippocratic Work 'On Dreams' (*De Victu* 4) and Its Near Eastern Background," in Horstmanshoff and Stol (eds), *Magic and Rationality*, pp. 187–218, at p. 210.

10 I base my translations of Artemidorus' dreambook on the Greek edition of R. Pack, *Artemidori Daldiani Onirocriticon Libri V* (Leipzig, 1963). Parsley as a harbinger of death was a *topos* in antiquity; see the *testimonia* given in Pack at p. 84.

11 The *oneirocriticon* of Achmet dates to the ninth or early tenth century and was produced by a Christian living on the eastern borders of the Byzantine Empire. The author used a variety of Arabic dreambooks, although his final product was a nonliteral, Christianized translation of those materials. The work was commissioned by an imperial patron, perhaps the emperor himself, or by a dream interpreter who worked at the court, and reflects a time when Arabic works on science were being translated into Greek. See, in detail, Mavroudi, *A Byzantine Book*, especially Chapter 10. Translations of Achmet are taken from S.M. Oberhelman, *The Oneirocriticon of Achmet: A Medieval Greek and Arabic Treatise on the Interpretation of Dreams* (Lubbock, TX, 1991) and are based on the Greek edition of F. Drexl, *Achmetis Oneirocriticon* (Leipzig, 1925).

his condition, though not without violence, and he will finally become happy. (Achmet 89)

If someone dreamt that he was beheaded and his head was separated from his body and his head was separated from his body, if he is rich his wealth will diminish, and if he is poor he will become rich, and if he is a slave he will be freed, if he is in debt God will settle his debt, if he is grieved or troubled God will relieve him of it, if he is sick God will heal him, and if he is sick and there is no medical treatment to be found for his illness, this signifies his death. (Ibn Shāhīn no. 1343; translation from Mavroudi, *Byzantine Book*, p. 197)

As for salt, it is interpreted as money. Al–Kirmani says, "Whoever sees that he bought salt, or that salt was given to him, it is interpreted as dirhams. And if he is sick, God Almighty will restore him to health, since it is reported that [salt] is the cure for seventy-two diseases." (Ibn Shāhīn no. 6541; translation from Mavroudi, *Byzantine Book*, p. 440)

As these passages show, some dreams have multivalent meanings in accordance with the circumstances of the dreamer. For example, for ill people, a dream may predict recovery of health, continuation of their sick condition, even death, but for the healthy, other outcomes, unrelated to disease, await them.

Most dreams in dream-key manuals, however, have a single interpretation, universally applicable regardless of the dreamer's physical, mental, and spiritual condition. Thus, if a dream is interpreted as a harbinger of disease, that fate, and that fate alone, will befall the dreamer. Examples are as follows:

If [someone dreams that] he bathes in his own urine and that he wipes himself clean, he will be affected by [a disease called] "Hand of Istar." (Assyrian Dreambook: copy found in the great library of Assurbanipal in the series Ziqīqu)[12]

If a man sees himself in a dream stirring up his house: BAD; [it means] his falling ill. (British Museum 10683, 7.23)[13]

---

[12] Taken from van der Eijk, "Divination, Prognosis and Prophylaxis," p. 211; van der Eijk takes the phrase "Hand of Istar" to mean a disease of the genital organs.

[13] This dream text dates from the early reign of Ramesses II in the thirteenth century BC; translation in A.H. Gardiner, *Hieratic Papyri in the British Museum: Third Series, Chester Beatty Gift* (2 vols, London, 1935), vol. 1, pp. 11–19 (from which the above is taken). The Egyptian demotic dream-key manuals are much later, between the second century BC and the second century AD; for texts and commentary, see A. Volten, *Demotische Traumdeutung (Pap. Carlsberg XIII und XIV Verso)* (Copenhagen, 1942).

> Whatever festering wound or disease that someone should deem in a dream to have around his neck or in the area of his beard foretells disease for everyone equally. [The reason is that] the whole body hangs on the head and the neck, in a manner of speaking, and so when these [body parts] are healthy, the body is healthy, but when they are suffering from disease, then the body is sickly and suffers harm. (Artemidorus 1.34)

> Collecting stones signifies illness. (Daniel Dreambook 331; Oberhelman, *Dreambooks*, p. 98)[14]

> Eating cuttlefish results in a long illness. (Nicephorus Dreambook 104; Oberhelman, *Dreambooks*, p. 128)[15]

> If someone dreams that he was fighting with a cat and was wounded by its claws, he will suffer a very severe illness and be grieved. (Achmet 278)

> If someone dreams that he was wearing a broad-brimmed conical hat—especially if he normally does not wear one in everyday life—and was also holding a staff and merrily walking up and down in the royal palace, you should know that he will succumb to a harsh and terrible illness and be at the point of death. However, he will return to health because of the staff's appearance [in the dream]. (Manuel Dreambook 8; Oberhelman, *Dreambooks*, p. 197)[16]

---

[14] The interpretation is based, perhaps, on the fact that λίθος (stone) also described a renal calculus or vesical calculus.

[15] A. Dalby (*Flavours of Byzantium* [Totnes, 2003], pp. 146, 155, 156) quotes several texts that discuss how the Byzantines believed that cuttlefish, which were eaten as appetizers or side dishes or even as the main course, could cause raw or thick humors in the body. If such adverse effects on the body were common knowledge, then this would explain the interpretation above. The Byzantine Nicephorus dream-key manual is nearly contemporaneous with the Achmet dreambook, that is, it dates to the late ninth century or early tenth century, after the end of iconoclasm in the capital city of Constantinople; see Oberhelman, *Dreambooks*, pp. 8–9 for discussion.

[16] This Byzantine dreambook was written either for or by Emperor Manuel II Palaeologus (r. 1391–1425); the book was intended for the imperial court and for use by the aristocracy of Constantinople. See M. Mavroudi, "Ta'bīr al–ru'yā and ahkām al–nujūm References to Women in Dream Interpretation and Astrology Transferred from Graeco-Roman Antiquity and Medieval Islam to Byzantium: Some Problems and Considerations," in B. Gruendler and M. Cooperson (eds), *Classical Arabic Humanities in Their Own Terms: Festschrift für Wolfhart Heinrichs on His 65. Birthday from His Students and Colleagues* (Leiden, 2007), pp. 47–67, with a review of the evidence at pp. 53–5. The reason for the recovery of health in the dream above is that the staff is an oneirocritic symbol of masculinity and power.

One may wonder how many people panicked when consulting dream-key manuals like the above. After all, someone has a seemingly innocuous dream about eating hot pitta bread, but then he discovers that he will be stricken with tuberculosis (Manuel Dreambook 9; Oberhelman, *Dreambooks*, p. 198). And even when a dream may have several outcomes predicted, the situation hardly improves. For example, Artemidorus takes the dream symbol "mud" and outlines for the dreamer two unpleasant fates:

> Mud signifies disease and sexual lewdness: disease because it is neither pure water nor pure earth, but rather is a mixture of both elements and so it is neither—this being so, [mud as a dream symbol] reasonably indicates an evil blend of the body's [humors], that is to say, disease; sexual lewdness because mud leaves a stain—and yet more, the dreamer will be a male whose anus is penetrated by other males because mud [by nature] is soft and not stiff. (Artemidorus 3.29)

There are, then, two possible outcomes for a person who dreams of mud: being afflicted with disease or becoming a passive partner in homosexual anal intercourse. Neither outcome would have been a welcome prospect for a Greek, for males in that culture highly prized physical wellbeing and the prerogative of penetrating others, and highly denigrated those who were penetrated.[17]

Compounding a dreamer's confusion or fear would have been dreambook writers' disagreements among themselves and their tendency to postulate vastly different outcomes for the same dream. Now, someone may not have been too troubled over the discrepancy in the late Byzantine (c. 1400) Anonymous Dreambook in how to interpret a dream of being beheaded: "To dream that you have had your head cut off indicates being rid of great trouble; other interpreters say that you will lose your master."[18] But what of those many other times when the disagreements could portend either goodness or a horrible disaster? Which interpreter does one believe? Which interpreter is the more trustworthy? Artemidorus, for example, often claimed that his own observations were superior

---

[17] In the eyes of ancient Greek and Hellenistic Greek culture, a male was expected to penetrate, not to be penetrated. If a male was penetrated, he was considered a nonperson and assimilated into the ranks of slaves, women, and children for having received a man's penis. For dreams and gender, see J.J. Winkler, *The Constraints of Desire* (New York and London, 1990), Chapter 1; S. MacAlister, "Gender as Sign and Symbolism in Artemidoros' *Oneirokritika*: Social Aspirations and Anxieties," *Helios*, 19 (1992): pp. 140–60; S.M. Oberhelman, "Hierarchies of Gender, Ideology, and Power in Ancient and Medieval Greece and Medieval Islam," in J.W. Wright and E. Rowson (eds), *Homoeroticism in Medieval Islam* (New York, 1997), pp. 55–93.

[18] Oberhelman, *Dreambooks*, p. 167.

to those postulated by others, since it was obvious (to him) that they were incompetent or flawed in their methods. An example is his discussion (2.18) of the outcome of a dream of giving birth to a fish: "If a woman who is pregnant supposes that she gives birth to a fish, ancient dream authorities state that she will give birth to a mute child. But I have seen from experience that the child will live for only a short time; many women have also given birth to stillborns." Artemidorus' words would have offered little help to a mother-to-be already concerned about the course (and success) of her pregnancy;[19] after all, she has consulted a dream-key manual to seek answers to a bizarre dream, but in the end she has no clue whether she will deliver a mute child, a child who will be short-lived, or a dead fetus. My point is that frustration, fear, and perplexity must have been common for readers of dream-key manuals, who craved a modicum of certainty in a world of uncertainty but ended up encountering ambiguity, contradiction, and multivalency of meaning.

The greatest weakness of dream-key manuals is the absence of advice on what steps a dreamer may take to avoid his predicted fate. With the simple "if x then y" and "x signifies y" formulations, a dreamer is faced with a single destiny, and apparently nothing can prevent its actualization. What can one do to avoid the horrific death that is prophesized by a dream of being surrounded by sparrows[20] or to escape the illness that holding an elephant's tusk in a dream symbolizes?[21] Even with the more complex formulation of the interpretations in Artemidorus and medieval Arabic texts, where symbols may be multivalent and thus have differing implications for different dreamers, for example:

> The monastic cell: dreaming of a monastic cell signifies seclusion, excellence of demeanor, retirement, separation, deprivation of pleasures, divorce from one's spouse and forsaking one's brethren. Possibly this dream signifies sickness and abandonment of the desire to eat and drink. If the dreamer is sick he will die or will be protected against attacks, especially if a king dreamt of a hermitage when he was about to meet his enemy. Possibly this dream signifies [that the king] will vanquish and conquer [his enemy]. (Al-Nābulusi, vol. 2, p. 48; Mavroudi, *A Byzantine Book*, p. 307)

The dreamer here is no better off in knowing how to prepare for the future or how to take preventative steps to change or avoid it. And when illness is foretold in a dream, what course of action should the dreamer undertake? Await the

[19] For high infant mortality rates in the ancient Mediterranean, see the essays in V. Dasen (ed.), *Naissance et petite enfance dans l'Antiquité, Actes du colloque de Fribourg, 28 novembre–1er décembre 2001*, Orbis Biblicus et Orientalis, 203 (Fribourg, 2004).

[20] Manuel Dreambook 10; Oberhelman, *Oneirocritica*, p. 200.

[21] Germanus Dreambook 59; Oberhelman, *Oneirocritica*, p. 156.

fate passively and with resignation, or take proactive measures like consulting a doctor or a village woman specializing in roots and herbs or, as often happened, visiting a healing sanctuary? What does one do when a dream forecasts a horrible medical crisis, or tells a pregnant woman that she could lose her child:

> Should a woman take a reptile and hide it in her bosom and should she also derive great pleasure from it, she will commit adultery with someone who is in the great majority of cases an enemy of her husband; but if the woman is frightened or distressed, she will fall ill; moreover, if the woman is pregnant [at the time she has this dream], the embryo will perish and not be preserved. (Artemidorus 2.13)

Does a woman who has the above dream ask a dream interpreter for medical advice? From our primary sources, it seems that some dreamers did ask interpreters for advice. Artemidorus (4.22), for example, angrily heaps scorn on certain oneirocritic writers who, he claims, fabricated medical prescriptions and cures like those at Asclepian sanctuaries. Other writers

> having carelessly made extractions from the books of Aristotle on animals and from [the books of] Archelaus and Xenocrates of Aphrodisia—by what each animal is healed, what each of them is afraid of, and in what each most takes pleasure—have reinvented them into kinds of remedies and medical treatments. A certain person, who is a contemporary, does this very sort of reinvention; he has excessively utilized this very method in the third book of his treatise.

Artemidorus' polemic here is framed in the context of god-sent dreams, specifically Asclepian dream cures. Artemidorus stresses that the gods, when they offer through dreams medical relief in the form of ointments, poultices, foods, and drinks, use simple, everyday language; moreover, even if some ambiguity over the course of treatment should exist, the cure is recoverable through basic interpretive methods like analogic reasoning or wordplay. For example:

> A man who had an ailment of the stomach pleaded with Asclepius for a medical prescription. He dreamt that he went into the god's temple; the god stretched out his right hand and offered him to eat his fingers [δάκτυλοι]. Later the man ate five dates and was cured; for the fruits of the date palm, when excellent in condition, are called "fingers" [δάκτυλοι]. (5.89)

Not mentioned by Artemidorus is who may have interpreted this dream. Did Artemidorus decipher it? Did the man consult another interpreter and then Artemidorus heard of it on one of his many fact-finding trips? Or did the man do a bit of self-interpretation by resorting to a dream-key manual? We know that professional interpreters like Artemidorus did dabble in interpreting medically prescriptive dreams, as the writer of the Hippocratic *Regimen* 4 lamented.[22] Artemidorus even admitted as such when he advised his son to become acquainted with medical theory and praxis:

> Whatever medical treatment you should run across—whether you yourself interpreted it or you learned the dream's fulfillment after someone else interpreted it—you will discover once you do some investigative work that the treatment is very sound medically and does not stand outside the medical practice ... Hence let it be for you, as I have frequently exhorted you, an object of care to gain possession of medical theories to the greatest extent you can. (4.22)

How effectively dream interpreters deciphered medically prescriptive dreams is unknown. Artemidorus did try to practice his skill with professionalism, and he developed his taxonomies, methods, and theories through empirical science. But he may very well have been unique; in our ancient sources, no other interpreter approaches him in the quest for a scientific study of dreams.[23] The lack of professionalism displayed by peers and predecessors alike may explain Artemidorus' hostile attitude to his fellow practitioners, and may also account for the generally negative opinion in antiquity of oneirocriticism.[24] Physicians claimed superiority for their own methods of interpreting medical dreams, and so denigrated dream interpreters' skills in the area of prognosis and therapeutics. On those occasions when an interpreter successfully handled a medical dream,

---

[22] See van der Eijk, "Divination, Prognosis and Prophylaxis," pp. 193–8; cf. Aristotle, *On Divination through Dreams* 462b12–17. Galen's remarks on prophetic dreams appear in his *On Diagnosis from Dreams*; the best modern edition of this text is G. Guidorzzi, "L'opuscolo di Galeno 'De dignitione ex insomniis,'" *Bollettino del Comitato per la Preparazione dell'Edizione Nazionale dei Classici Greci e Latini*, 21 (1973): pp. 81–105 (Greek text on pp. 103–5). See also Hulskamp's excellent discussion of this treatise in her chapter in this volume.

[23] D. Del Corno (*Graecorum de re onirocritica scriptorum reliquiae* [Milan, 1969]) offers a comprehensive discussion of extant ancient Greek and Roman writers on dreams. Cf. G. Weber, *Kaiser, Träume und Visionen in Prinzipat und Spätantike* (Stuttgart, 2000); C. Walde, *Antike Traumdeutung und moderne Traumforschung* (Düsseldorf, 2001); and B. Näf, *Traum und Traumdeutung im Altertum* (Darmstadt, 2004).

[24] W. Harris, in his *Dreams and Experience in Classical Antiquity* (Cambridge, MA, 2009), following up on his "Roman Opinions about the Truthfulness of Dreams," *Journal of Roman Studies*, 93 (2003): pp. 18–34, offers a corrective to modern views that all ancient Greeks and Romans had favorable attitudes toward dreams and dream interpretation.

physicians attributed it to guesswork and blind luck, although one may wonder about their own success rate.[25]

Not all readers of dream-key manuals took their dream to a doctor or another medical practitioner, of whom many types were available, for consultation.[26] Some, beset with anxiety over the countless predictions of disease, trauma, and death enumerated in texts like Artemidorus', probably departed immediately for healing sanctuaries to seek divine intervention in a sort of pre-emptive strike. A few may have chosen to ignore the prognostication, or at least were skeptical about its accuracy and may have done nothing. Certainly, most readers would have considered their dream-key manual as lacking in any concrete advice on how to ward off the predicted disease or how to treat it; the manuals only warned of the onset of illness or, if the dreamer was already ill, the ailment's outcome.

There is in fact a dreambook that offers medical prophylactic and therapeutic advice to dreamers. The advice is based on an understanding of Hippocratic humoral theory and on the medical regimens typical of practical healing manuals called *iatrosophia*, which were used by doctors and healers during the Byzantine and Ottoman periods of Greece. The dreambook itself is contained in Codex 1350 of the National Library of Greece, folia 86–103, which dates to the eighteenth century.[27] The text is not complete, as it is missing several folia. Two different scribes wrote the text: one, folia 86^r–89^v and 93^r–104^v; the other,

25 Physicians and philosophers were more honest about the difficulties in using dreams in a medical context. Galen once commented that an interpretation of a dream caught him by surprise: "But since we concede that there are also prophetic dreams, it is not easy to say how these might be distinguished from the ones arising from the body. At all events, a man dreamed that one of his legs had turned to stone, and many of those clever about such matters judged that the dream pertained to his slaves, but the man was paralyzed in that leg, although none of us expected that" (*On Diagnosis from Dreams*, p. 104, 23–6 Guidorizzi); see S.M. Oberhelman, "Dreams in Graeco-Roman Medicine," in W. Haase and H. Temporini (eds), *Aufstieg und Niedergang der römischen Welt* (Berlin, 1993), part II, vol. 37.1, pp. 121–56, at p. 143 with notes and, better and more recently, Hulskamp's chapter in this volume.

26 To cite just several sources on the variety of healers in antiquity and the postclassical world: G.E.R. Lloyd, *Magic, Reason, and Experience* (Cambridge, 1979), especially pp. 38–41; D. Gentilcore, *Healers and Healing in Early Modern Italy* (Manchester and New York, 1998), especially Chapters 1, 4, and 6; V. Nutton, *Ancient Medicine* (London and New York, 2004), pp. 263–71; T.D. Walker, *Doctors, Folk Medicine and the Inquisition: The Repression of Magical Healing in Portugal During the Enlightenment* (Leiden and Boston, 2005), especially pp. 36–87 and 180–208; and J. Scarborough, *Pharmacy and Drug Lore in Antiquity: Greece, Rome, Byzantium* (Aldershot, 2010).

27 A specific date for the text itself (as opposed to the codex's date) cannot be recovered, although internal evidence (e.g., Italian florins, in use through 1523, and Turkish coins like paras, piasters, and medjidies) indicates a date after the beginning of the Tourkokratia (1453 AD).

folia 90^{r}–92^{v}. The only information we have on the author is his faith (Greek Orthodox Christianity) and his name (Blasius of Athens, a name otherwise unknown). Blasius tells us that he wrote his dream-key manual to advise the reader on how to keep his body and soul free from spiritual and physical harm.

Blasius arranges his text in paragraph format: a dream symbol, stated in the paragraph's header, is decoded and its meaning is then exemplified by a series of dreams and their interpretations.[28] This format is unusual for the dreambooks of the Tourkokratia, which follow the "if x then y" and "x signifies y" schemes, such as we see in the anonymous dreambook in Codex 1275 of the National Library of Athens, which dates to around the same time as Blasius'. Here dream symbols are listed alphabetically and are then given an "if this then that" interpretation. Medically significant dreams include the following:

> 100. If you dream that you were soiled with filth and also stained your clothes, be afraid of the great disease.
>
> 165. Withered trees that are blown to the ground by a wind: this means a worldwide deadly plague.
>
> 300. If you dream of having a red bandage on your head, you will suffer a head cold.
>
> 321. If you dream of having a scratchy throat, you will have boils.
>
> 366. A dream of vomiting is bad: fear for the health of your intestines.[29]

As Blasius states in his introductory and concluding paragraphs, a primary motivation for his writing the dreambook is to provide dreamers with the means necessary to safeguard body and soul from harm:

---

28 This is the format used by Artemidorus, Achmet, and the medieval Arabic oneirocriticsts; Blasius may well have been imitating them.

29 Each of these "medical dreams" is interpreted according to analogy or metonymy. For example, in dream #165, trees, which in the oneirocritic tradition symbolize men, are hurled to the ground by a natural force and so become a metaphor for humans dying from a plague. In dream #321, a scratchy throat is analogous to boils, which often involve scratching, while in dream #100, there is an analogy to bedridden patients who may defecate in their bed and so soil their clothes and sheets. The red bandage in dream #300 evokes the image of fumigation for head colds; contemporary medical texts recommend wrapping the sufferer's head with a cloth or towel and having him inhale vapors (see below). The interpretation for dream #366 is clear enough.

> [fol. 86ʳ] Now I beg you, as children of God, take from me but a single interpretation and you will be protected to a great extent from the artifices of the devil, and you will then congratulate me many times over for what I have written here for your benefit. [I have done this] so that you may be far from evil, enjoy goodness, and live for many years without your body suffering any harm—provided that you take into account whatever I tell you and interpret. So, please, give an attentive ear to my words ...[fol. 101ᵛ] And so this very day, I beg you, show deep regard for everything that I say and do not neglect it, [fol. 102ʳ] so that you may live for very many years to come and may not endure any evil or harm befalling your body or soul ...[fol. 103ᵛ] If you keep all [of my instructions], I tell you that you will never incur a debilitating illness, wicked people will not be able to harm you, and you will never find yourself in an evil situation.

For Blasius, a dream does not involve an unavoidable fate; although an evil outcome may be indicated by what the dreamer sees in his sleep, that evil can be overcome if Blasius' advice is followed in the waking world. The future is therefore fluid, variable according to the pre-emptive or remedial steps that the dreamer takes, thanks to Blasius, and according to God's will. A dream, in other words, offers a person a glimpse of the path that lies ahead, but that path can be changed: the person's body will not suffer disease, his enemies will not inflict harm, he and his family will remain safe, his business will flourish—provided that he follows the measures that Blasius advises (e.g., dietetics, *materia magica*, prayers, and lifestyle changes). Since most of these measures have been drawn from practical healing manuals called *iatrosophia*, it is to these texts that we now turn.

The *iatrosophion* was a literary genre of medical therapeutic text which arose during the Byzantine Empire.[30] The *iatrosophion* may be defined as a compendium of medical recipes and treatments based on the *materia medica* of ancient, Byzantine, and post-Byzantine medical and pharmacological treatises, and then supplemented by written accounts of the medical praxis of hospital personnel, physicians, and folk healers.[31] These texts are fundamental

[30] A. Tselikas, "Τα Ελληνικά γιατροσόφια: Μία Περιφρονημένη Κατηγορία Χειρογράφων," in T. Diamantopoulos (ed.), *Ιατρικά Βυζαντινά Χειρόγραφα* (Athens, 1995), pp. 57–69; D. Bennett, "Medical Practice and Manuscripts in Byzantium," *Society for the Social History of Medicine*, 13 (2000): pp. 279–91; A. Touwaide, "Byzantine Hospitals Manuals (Iatrosophia) as a Source for the Study of Therapeutics," in B. Bowers (ed.), *The Medieval Hospital and Medical Practice* (Aldershot, 2007), pp. 147–73, with extensive bibliography; C. Papadopoulos, "Post-Byzantine Medical Manuscripts: New Insights into the Greek Medical Tradition, Its Intellectual and Practical Interconnections, and Our Understanding of Greek Culture," *Journal of Modern Greek Studies*, 27 (2009): pp. 107–30.

[31] Touwaide, "Byzantine Hospitals," p. 148.

to understanding Greek medical practice from the Byzantine Empire through the early twentieth century.[32] The first *iatrosophia* were written in the early Byzantine centuries by the medical writers Oribasius (fourth century), Aëtius of Amida (sixth century), and Alexander of Tralles (sixth century); these authors took the original texts of earlier physicians and pharmacologists like Hippocrates, Galen, and Dioscorides, and made excerpts of their works.[33] Subsequent writers—for example, Paul of Aegina (seventh century) and Simeon Seth of Antioch (eleventh century)—copied these excerpts and then added contemporany recipes and medicines. From all these sources, lengthy lists of medical recipes and therapeutics were drawn up into texts for practical healers.[34] *Iatrosophia* were copied, recopied, and reproduced over the centuries, as they were not fixed documents: individual physicians or groups of physicians working in a hospital revised the *iatrosophia* they had access to in order to take into account new *materia medica*, new technology, new diseases, and clinical observations of actual case histories.[35]

After the fall of Byzantium, *iatrosophia* continued to be written and published. Evangelia Varella has counted over 700 medical manuscripts and books from the Ottoman period of Greece, of which approximately half are *iatrosophia*, although Agamemnon Tselikas lowers that number to 150 or so.[36]

---

[32] Scholars are now beginning to publish some of these texts. Patricia Clark has published a nineteenth-century *iatrosophion* by the Cretan practical doctor/folk healer Konstantinos Theodorakis: *A Cretan Healer's Handbook in the Byzantine Tradition: Text, Translation and Commentary* (Aldershot, 2011); N.E. Papadogiannakês, in his *Κρητικά Ιατροσόφιον του 19ου αιώνα* (Rhethymno, 2001), offers an excellent edition (with extensive notes) of a Cretan *iatrosophion* dated to the first decade of the nineteenth century. See too the bibliography in Papadopoulos, "Post-Byzantine Medical Manuscripts," pp. 129–30; and also A. Lardos, "The Botanical *Materia Medica* of the *Iatrosophion*—A Collection of Prescriptions from a Monastery in Cyprus," *Journal of Ethnopharmacology*, 104 (2006): pp. 387–406; cf. Clark, *A Cretan Healer's Handbook*, pp. 11–22.

[33] P.A. Clark, "Landscape, Memories, and Medicine: Traditional Healing in Amari, Crete," *Journal of Modern Greek Studies*, 20 (2002): pp. 339–65, at p. 341; J. Stannard, "Aspects of Byzantine *Materia Medica*," *Dumbarton Oaks Papers*, 38 (1984): pp. 205–11.

[34] Bennett, "Medical Practices."

[35] See in detail Papadopoulos, "Post-Byzantine"; cf. Touwaide, "Byzantine Hospitals."

[36] Papadopoulos, "Post-Byzantine," p. 109; E. Varella, "La thérapeutique byzantine dans le monde grec d'epoque ottoman," *Medicina nei secoli*, 11 (1999): pp. 577–84. Of the remaining texts, about a third are ancient texts or copies of Byzantine writers like Nemesius, Bishop of Emesus; Simeon Seth; Michael Psellus; Nicolas Myrepsus; and John Aktouarios. The rest are paraphrases or translations of earlier works. In a more recent article, "Greek Medical Manuscripts of the Period of 16th–Middle 19th Centuries," in Alfredo Musajo–Somma (ed.), *Proceedings: 39th International Congress on the History of Medicine, September, 5–10, 2004, Bari–Metaponto, Italy* (Bari, 2004), pp. 140–45, D. Karaberopoulos and A.

Iatrosophia may be found all over Greece—in monasteries, libraries, and private collections.[37]

Two basic types of *iatrosophia* were in common use. One type, linked particularly to monasteries and penned by monks (Lardos, "*Materia medica*"), contains only medical recipes and therapeutics. Most recipes consist of herbal concoctions, with the others containing minerals or animal substances. The majority of recipes derive from ancient and Byzantine formal medicine, but we also have the pharmacopoeia of folk healing. Although many of these medical *iatrosophia* were connected to religious institutions, religion is kept to a minimum, usually restricted to a simple θέλημα τοῦ Θεοῦ (God willing). The second type of *iatrosophion* also contains remedies drawn from both folk medicine and classical Greek medicine, but besides the medical recipes and treatments, there are sections on a variety of other topics such as advice on agriculture and veterinarian matters, astrology, exorcisms and spells, magic, and religion.[38] The primary concern of this type of *iatrosophion* remained the healing of bodily ailments (listed *a capite ad calcem*, that is, "from the head to the heel"), but we also have nonmedical things like magical spells and amulets etched with occult symbols and letters, alongside the medical prophylaxis.[39]

Blasius adheres to the format of the magico-medical *iatrosophion*, insofar as he gives both medical and nonmedical advice to his readers on how to avoid the various evils that their dreams predict. One method he recommends involves being on one's guard for a specific period of time. For example:

Oeconomopoulou categorize their inventory of medical manuscripts (not printed books) as follows: 123 manuscripts of medical texts of ancient Greek doctors; 95 manuscripts of Byzantine doctors; 334 anonymous medical manuscripts (*iatrosophia*); and 108 translations into Greek of European medical books. See also Bennett, "Medical Practice," and A. Touwaide, "The Corpus of Greek Medical Manuscripts: A Computerized Inventory and Catalogue," in W.M. Stevens (ed.), *Bibliographic Access to Medieval and Renaissance Manuscripts* (New York, 1992), pp. 75–9.

[37] Papadopoulos, "Post-Byzantine," with literature; cf. Touwaide, "Byzantine Hospitals," pp. 155–7.

[38] Stannard, "Aspects," pp. 206–7, 210; Clark, "Landscape"; Papadopoulos, "Post-Byzantine."

[39] See A. Tselikas, "Spells and Exorcisms in Three Post-Byzantine Manuscripts," in J.C.B. Petropoulos (ed.), *Greek Magic: Ancient, Medieval and Modern* (London and New York, 2008), pp. 72–81. For the pre-Byzantine period see R. Kotansky, "Incantations and Prayers for Salvation on Inscribed Greek Amulets" and J. Scarborough, "The Pharmacology of Sacred Plants, Herbs, and Roots," both in C.A. Faraone and D. Obbink (eds), *Magika Hiera: Ancient Greek Magic and Religion* (New York and Oxford, 1991), pp. 107–37 and pp. 138–74, respectively. See also the essays in Horstmanshoff and Stol (eds), *Magic and Rationality*.

> [fol. 89v] Snakes: If you dream of a snake, know that somebody wishes to do you harm and so be on your guard for five days or up to the changing of the sign of the zodiac; if you do not take such precautions, you will suffer greatly.
>
> [fol. 90r] Owls: If you see an owl in your dream, know that some evil person wants, and is seeking, to kill you with a small herbal concoction; be on your guard for this [poison] for two days and [the danger] will pass.
>
> [fol. 91r] Oysters and Mussels: Whenever you see in your dream oysters, mussels, mollusks, or any other sort of shellfish, I advise you to ignore the dream. But if you are married, do not sleep [fol. 92r] with your wife for four days, for she will give birth to a mute child lacking the means to walk. If you are single, you will be filled with an equivalent gain of sperm and you will be strong.[40]

Blasius also recommends acts of piety, the magical properties of substances like water, and certain ritualistic methods for transferring evil to a third party. So:

> [fol. 92r] Boats: If you dream that a boat was moving on dry land, this signifies death. But this very day give alms and fast so that God Himself may be gracious to you; perhaps you will then see that someone other than you has died, thus causing that hour of bitterness to pass.
>
> [fol. 94r] Wheat: If you dream of wheat, know that [the outcome] is bitter. [To counter this dream,] at the crack of dawn take a basin of cold water and pour it over your head; then [the dream's] outcome will pass.[41]

---

[40] The first interpretation is based on analogy (the inability of the child to move is analogous to bottom-dwelling shellfish), while the second is based on the longstanding *topos* in Greek culture that shellfish acted as aphrodisiacs (A. Dalby, *Food in the Ancient World from A to Z* [London and New York, 2003], pp. 300–301) and on the association in oneirocritic literature (from ancient Assyria through Hellenistic Greek and medieval Arabic texts) of genitals and sperm with strength and power; see Oberhelman, *Oneirocritica*, pp. 177–8, 205, and "Hierarchies of Gender, Ideology, and Power." See below for Blasius replicating ancient medical and philosophical thought that a man full of sperm will dream of having sex.

[41] The reason for water's apotropaic power is its association with the rite of baptism, which symbolically washes away sin and evil; see C. Stewart, *Demons and the Devil: Moral Imagination in Modern Greek Culture* (Princeton, 1991), pp. 199–202, 209–10, 240–45. For water and its healing and protective powers (as used in binding spells), see R. Blum and E. Blum, *The Dangerous Hour: The Lore and Culture of Mystery and Crisis in Rural Greece* (London, 1970), p. 137; and the *Iatrosophion* of Papadogiannakês, p. 83, 3–21.

> [fol. 94ʳ] Barley: If you see barley in your dream, know that you have worms or lice. And if you have fruits in your house, this [condition] will affect them as well. And so do the following. Take a bar of unused soap and scrub your head [fol. 94ᵛ]; then bury the rest of the bar among the fruit so as to excise the evil that is doggedly pursuing you. This [evil] will then enter your fowl, and so take one of them and slaughter it; dip your finger into its blood and moisten the lips of your children and then your own lips. [If you do this,] then you will see yourself being successful in every respect twice over during this year.[42]

> [fol. 98ᵛ] Falling off [a cliff]: If you dream that you fell off [a cliff], know that you will be taken up to a court of judgment. When you have this [dream], as soon as you get out of bed pour a jug of water outside your door; keep the door shut for about thirty minutes and then go wherever you like. [If you do this,] the dream will spin[43] [from you and] onto others.

As opposed to writers of magico-medical *iatrosophia*, Blasius does not mention imprecations or spells (for example, a curse against neighbors or thieves or love rivals), nor does he use magical binding words and *materia magica* alongside rites, rituals, and objects of the Greek Orthodox faith.[44] All the religious prayers

---

[42] This is a very interesting passage. The interpretation is based on the association of head lice with barley, which can be plagued by meal worms and grain lice; indeed, the dermatological condition known as barley itch afflicts people who handle barley infected with food mites (R.L. Rietschel et al. [eds], *Fisher's Contact Dermatitis* [Lewiston, NY, 2008], p. 428). Blasius recommends hygienic measures to get rid of the lice, but he also writes that because of the contagion of evil in the household, any fruit (which can be afflicted by plant lice) will be affected. There may be a further association in that fruits (e.g., atis: *Anona squamosa L.*) were, and still are, used to cure head lice. Blasius' advice to bury the soap is reflective of the longstanding Greek tradition of burying magical tablets in the ground, wells, graves, etc.; over 1,000 curse tablets, for example, survive from the ancient Greek world (see C.A. Faraone, "The Agonistic Context of Early Greek Binding Spells," in Faraone and Obbink (eds), *Magika Hiera*, pp. 3–32). The transference of the evil into the fowl has biblical overtones, a particular example being Jesus transferring demons from the man of Gedarsene into swine; for transference in a medical context, see W. Hand, "The Magical Transference of Disease," *Folklore*, 13 (1965): pp. 83–109 and "Measuring and Plugging: The Magical Containment and Transfer of Disease," *Bulletin of the History of Medicine*, 48 (1974): pp. 221–33; Blum and Blum, *The Dangerous Hour*, p. 251.

[43] The verb γυρίζειν (to turn, to rotate, to spin back) depicts disease as an entity fully capable of movement and entering/exiting a person; cf. Blum and Blum, *The Dangerous Hour*, pp. 35, 164.

[44] Papadogiannakês' *Iatrosophion*, for example, has many binding spells and prayers/imprecations (although it is hard to determine when either εὐχή or προσευχή means a "spell" or a "prayer": see Stewart, *Demons and the Devil*, pp. 222 and 243 with notes) as

in Blasius' text are positive, framed solely as pleas to Mary Theotokos to intervene and deflect physical harm:

> [fol. 91^{v}] Crabs: If you see crabs in your dream, they show that someone will bite you with words of reproach. And you, when you rise from your bed, look upon the face of Lady Mother of God and pray to her: "Lady Mother of God, I beseech you because of this dream: protect me from evil men and do not allow me to be harassed by anyone today. And again I beseech you: deliver me from the biting words of a cruel man and I will glorify you forever and ever. Amen." Do this every morning for three days and you will escape judgment. Offer up to our Lady Mother of God any other prayers you wish, for in this way she will protect you from the devil himself.

> [fol. 93^{r}] [Pray:] "Redeem me from the wrath-bearing dream that I saw in my sleep, so that I may not be handed over to any disease of soul or body." You will be delivered from the tongues of evil men if you repeat these words nine times for the nine orders of the angels.[45]

The vast majority of Blasius' recommendations for the safekeeping of one's body from illness or for preserving health revolve around dietetics and prophylaxis. As stated above, Blasius does not mention binding spells, phylacteries, inscribed amulets, or *materia magica* (plant or mineral), which

well as instructions for writing magical characters and phylacteries. For the former, examples include: p. 60, 8–16, p. 81, 11–14, p. 82, 4–14, p. 90, 9–14, p. 91, 13–15, p. 116, 23–5, p. 152, 5–p. 154, 12; for the latter: p. 56, 3–5, p. 59, 2–17, p. 73, 11–12, p. 89, 13–p. 90, 8, p. 128, 25–p. 129, 11, p. 179, 1–p. 180, 11, p. 199, 1–5. The verb ὁρκίζειν (to adjure) prefacing many of these spells was commonly used in Greek magical texts to bind demons or gods; see Faraone, "The Agonistic Context," p. 6 with p. 25, note 28. A parallel is the healing text in the fourteenth-century Codex Bibliothèque Nationale 2011, fol. 11^{r-v}: "I adjure you, the first demon of those [afflicting this person], the one called Kandan, [the demon] of the cycle of the zodiac, and Krios, the one who shakes to and fro the forehead and heads of men; in the name of Michaêl, drawn near, Ouren; immediately withdraw from So-and-So, the slave of God. I adjure you, the second demonic power, the one called Barsaphaêl, the one who causes migraines to hurt men in your [evil] hour; hear me, O Gabriêl, and confine [the demon]! And immediately, [Barsaphaêl,] withdraw from So-and-So, the slave of God. I adjure you, Artosaêl, the evil demon who injures the eyes of men. Hear me, O Ourouêl, and confine Artosaêl; and you, [Artosaêl,] withdraw from So-and-So, the slave of God." The manuscript then gives binding spells for healing other parts of the body.

45 The nine orders [τάγματα] are angels, archangels, principalities, powers, virtues, dominations, thrones, cherubim, and seraphim. Stewart (*Demons and the Devil*, pp. 198–9) reports observing a baptism where a priest prayed to God to send a guardian angel who would deliver the baby from the devil, evil, and demons.

were all too common in magico-medical *iatrosophia* and in magical papyri directed to healing.[46] Blasius' advice on healing incorporates only naturalistic (holistic, we may even say) means, mainly proper diet and drink supplemented by acts of religious piety. Thus, for the dream symbol "donkey," Blasius offers this advice:

> [fol. 88v] Donkey: If you dream of a donkey, know that this means evil; but pray to God to safeguard you from it. Also do not eat anything with salt or fruit in it, and abstain from wine, lest these things plunge you into asthenia. The reason is that whenever the blood has become languid, a donkey is portrayed in a dream, as dream interpreters say. But if the blood is restored to a peaceful state, it shakes off the [fol. 89r] asthenia.

---

[46] Blasius does make references to astrology, which is a mark of magico-medical *iatrosophia*. The author of Papadogiannakês' *Iatrosophion* recommends cutting certain roots and plants during various phases of the moon (e.g., p. 128, 5–20). The author discusses the efficacy in recipes of plants associated with specific planets; for example, "On Sunday: the sun: the sun-plant is knotgrass. Wear its root as a means to counteract the pain of a headache. On Tuesday: Ares. Pestle leaves of cinquefoil. If you put it on stings from bees, wasps, and scorpions, there will be healing. It also cures the spleen and feet. It treats dental problems, and if one chews the root, it cleanses the mind and expels kidney stones On Wednesday: Hermes. Viper's bugloss. This plant is useful for the skeleton as well as for every sort of stomach ailment, dysentery, and women's menstruation. On Saturday: Cronus. The hedge-hyssop. Take the juice and combine with storax. This will heal pain in the knees. You can fry the plant and put it on the nerves. It also cures those who are mad and treats children's dental problems" (p. 172, 12–p. 173, 18). He also describes what plants are specific to the signs of the zodiac and how they work in treating disease; for example, "The plant of Virgo is maidenhair. Pestle its leaves with a bear bone and smear it on for rheumatic pains. It is also useful for stenosis, if it is boiled with water and sugar and drunk by the patient. It is also most efficacious if the branches are frayed off onto the skin of a wolf, for this [talisman] will overcome your enemies" (p. 174, 11–15). See also the *iatrosophion* of Clark (*A Cretan Healer's Handbook*, pp. 136–41) for similar instructions. Blasius advises an interpreter to avoid giving advice on certain days during starlight, but if the interpreter goes ahead and interprets anyway, then he can deflect the resulting evil by slapping the consultant (fol. 103r). Ancient Babylonian texts detail auspicious and inauspicious days and months for purposes of divination; see R. Labat, "Hemerologien," *Reallexicon der Assyriologie*, 4 (1972–1975): pp. 317–23; cf. bloodletting and astronomy in the Babylonian Talmud as detailed in M. Geller, "Bloodletting in Babylonia," in Horstmanshoff and Stol (eds), *Magic and Rationality*, pp. 305–24, at pp. 320–21, with more on Babylonian texts. See too the extensive sections on astrology and healing found in the fifth-century AD medical text written by a Syrian Christian in E.A.W. Budge, *The Syriac Book of Medicines: Syrian Anatomy, Pathology and Therapeutics in the Early Middle Ages: With Sections on Astrological and Native Medicine and Recipes by an Anonymous Physician; Syriac Text, Edited from a Rare Manuscript, with an Introduction to the History of Hellenistic and Oriental Medicine, an Index, and an English Translation* (2 vols, St. Helier and Amsterdam, 1976).

This passage is interesting in several respects. First, Blasius' assertion that bodily illnesses can be portrayed in a dream's images reflects Greek medical theory, such as we find in the Hippocratic *Regimen* 4 and Galen. As written elsewhere in this volume, images in dreams are often analogous to the conditions of the body and should be interpreted on the basis of the imitation (ἀπομίμησις) of the microcosm of the body and the macrocosm of the universe.[47] Blasius does not delve into dream theory: he does not tell us how dream images are formed, how images are perceived (whether the soul or the mind does), or the relation between the body's disposition (here, the languid blood) and the perceiving faculty; Blasius only says that "dream interpreters" say that an image is formed (ὀνειρεύεται) of a donkey in the case of asthenic blood. Like the Hippocratic doctors who interpreted medical dreams, Blasius forms his interpretation analogically: the sluggish movements of a donkey are analogous to the movement of blood when it "languishes." He further recommends avoidance of certain foods and drink to avoid the body's condition from worsening; prayer, he adds, works well too. At each step, then, Blasius has followed the general method of interpreting dreams in the Hippocratic *Regimen*. Van der Eijk summarizes the method thusly:

1. the signs (τεκμήρια), i.e., the dream images themselves;
2. the significance of the dream, i.e., whether it is good or bad, whether it indicates particular bodily affections or disorders, etc.;
3. explanations of the relationship between sign and significance;
4. prophylactic (dietetic) measures to prevent disease; and
5. instructions as to the gods one should pray to in order to prevent disease.[48]

Thus, Blasius first states the dream image (donkey); then its significance (evil, for it predicts possibility of disease); an explanation of the sign's significance (a donkey indicates sluggishness of the blood); dietetic steps to remedy the bodily condition (avoid salty foods, fruits, and wine); and an exhortation to pray to God.

A similar schema appears in other entries in Blasius' dream-key manual. For example, if someone dreams of carrying a woman, this indicates disease, but the effect of that illness on the body can be minimized by proper prophylactic steps:

> [fol. 93^{v}] Women: If you dream of carrying a woman on your shoulders, know that a disease will befall you. And to what extent you were fatigued by the [weight

[47] See in this volume the chapters by Downie, Hulskamp, and Pearcy; see also van der Eijk, "Divination, Prognosis and Prophylaxis," pp. 199–203.

[48] Van der Eijk, "Divination, Prognosis and Prophylaxis," p. 198.

of the] woman's body is how severe [that disease] will be. Stay away from women and from meats and beverages, and do not eat anything unless it has been boiled. Do this to keep your blood untroubled.

Blasius interprets this dream through analogy: the oppressive weariness caused by carrying a burden is analogous to the debilitating condition of a body racked by an illness, whose severity is proportionate to the weight.[49] The dreamer will not escape falling sick (at least the text implies as such), but he can ease his suffering if he avoids activities that sap his body's strength (sex) and watches his diet. Blasius' analogic reasoning parallels what we read in the short treatise on dreams attributed to the Greek physician Galen. Galen (*On Diagnosis from Dreams*, p. 104, 37–9 Guidorizzi)[50] writes that a person whose humors are heavy will dream that he is carrying burdens.

Galen seems to be referenced again when Blasius associates a buildup of sperm with the dream image of having sex:

[fol. 93v] Sex: [fol. 94r] If you dream of having sex with a woman, know that your sperm has increased in amount, and this is why [the dream] occurred.

Galen had written: "So also the impression of drinking without being filled befalls those who thirst exceedingly, just as also that of eating without fulfillment happens to the famished and that of making love to those who are full of semen" (*On Diagnosis from Dreams*, p. 104, 31–2 Guidorizzi). A direct borrowing from Galen cannot be proved, however, since Blasius' analogic reasoning seems simple enough and the production of sperm as a cause for sex dreams was a *topos* among ancient writers.[51]

---

49 Analogy, especially between the macrocosm (celestial bodies, terrestrial objects, activities of the daytime, etc.) and microcosm (the patient's body), was commonly used by physicians when analyzing dreams; see van der Eijk, "Divination, Prognosis and Prophylaxis," pp. 196–203; cf. V. Langhoff, "Frühe Fälle der 'Verwendung' von Analogien in der altgriechischen Medizin," *Brichte zue Wissenschaftgeschichte* 12 (1989): pp. 7–18; see also Hulskamp in this volume.

50 References to Galen's treatise on dreams (probably spurious but based on Galenic ideas; see Hulskmap's chapter in this volume) come from G. Guidorizzi, "L'opusculo di Galeno 'De Dignotione ex Insomniis,'" *Bollettino del Comitato per la Preparazione dell' Edizione Nazionale dei Classici Greci e Latini*, 21 (1973): pp. 81–105.

51 For example, Lucretius 4.1024–36; see the commentary in C. Bailey, *Titi Lucreti Cari De rerum natura libri sex: Edited with Prolegomena, Critical Apparatus, Translation, and Commentary* (3 vols, Oxford, 1949), vol. 2, pp. 1295–301. See also S. Rousselle, *Porneia: De la maîtrise du corps à la privation sensorielle IIe–IVe siècle de l'ère chrétienne* (Paris, 1983), pp. 62 –3.

Blasius offers other recommendations of prophylaxis, but these seem more Hippocatic than Galenic:

> [fol. 92^{v}] Snow: If you see snow in your dream, know that you will become feverish. Therefore avoid eating salty foods and abstain from beverages. Take a purgative to clean yourself out and do not be afraid, whether you are dreading a fever or even λεμική.[52]

> [fol. 99^{r}] Testicles: If you dream of testicles, know that you will [fol. 99^{v}] become enervated in many ways. Do not fall into arms of a woman, but eat pastas and boiled onions with meat; drink wine early in the morning, followed by two more cups at each meal; abstain from raki and don't have cheese either.

Once again, Blasius has recommended dietary regimens for remedying a physical ailment. In the first passage, the use of a purgative for fever was commonplace in Greek medicine, going back to Hippocrates, although the advice to avoid liquids does run counter to conventional wisdom. In the second, the diagnosis of asthenia is correctly balanced by the directions for wine (prescribed by Hippocrates for most illnesses), meat and pastas (what we would call today "carbo-loading"), and avoidance of liquor (here, probably a prohibition on its overuse).[53]

At one point, Blasius goes beyond his dietary recommendations and advises the use of healing professionals:

> [fol. 95^{r}] White Vegetables: If you see white vegetables in your dream, know that bilious secretions are affecting you in the head and so draw out the bile by the skill of healers.

The association of bile and white starchy vegetables is not surprising,[54] but to what *iatroi* (healers) is Blasius referring? It is not clear, but most likely it refers to

[52] The word λεμνική means either an infectious disease generally or an epidemic or the plague specifically. The interpretation of this dream and the subsequent one is based on antinomy: the cold of the snow versus the heat of the fever, and testicles (an age-old [e.g., Egypt: British Museum Papyrus 10683] symbol of strength and power) versus enervation.

[53] If we hypothesize a little, the stricture against liquor would seem to pre-date Brunonian theory, which was popular in Greece during the eighteenth century and according to which asthenic diseases (asthenia) were to be treated by stimulants, especially the alcohol of hard liquor. This, and Blasius' references to humoral theory, could support a date for the dreambook of c. 1700, but we should not read too much into this one passage.

[54] The white vegetables would not include the potato, since the cultivation of this crop was introduced at a later date by Ioannis Antonios Kapodistrias, the first head of Greece after its independence from the Ottomans. Rather, the vegetables would be items like garlic,

people who possessed the necessary knowledge to remove bile. These "healers" need not have been physicians in the modern sense; they could just as easily have been root-cutters, wise women dispensing homegrown remedies, Greek Orthodox priests, or local practical doctors. Indeed, by his use of the plural form of *iatros*, Blasius may very well have been envisioning a multiplicity of healers, and so we may wish to translate *iatroi* as "medical practitioners" to denote healers of every ilk.

Let me conclude by adducing one final medical treatment that is quite interesting. Blasius records a conversation he had with his "teacher" over the proper way to cure catarrh:

> [fol. 91^r] All the Other Kinds [of Fowl]: If you see in your dream birds with heads but without wings, know that you will suffer some disease in your head. I asked my teacher once [about the proper treatment?] and he told me: "Well, if you wish to turn aside inflammation of the mucous membranes, go into your bedroom and cover your head with a towel; then place under your feet an incense-burner that has been set aflame; then place in it enough frankincense to fumigate yourself until you become drenched with sweat in your chair. Keep yourself well muffled up for one or two hours. [The ailment] will pass, God willing."

Frankincense (the dried resin sap of the *Boswellia carterii*), an important part of incense burning in Greek Orthodox rituals, has been used for thousands of years in aromatherapy to counteract catarrh, bronchitis, and asthma. Certain Western European and Greek medical texts, which are contemporary with our dreambook, preserve illustrations of the fumigation of ill people.[55] But two phrases in Blasius' text merit further comment. First, this "teacher" does not seem to be an instructor in oneirology (dream interpretation), but rather a medical practitioner. The word διδάσκολος, of course, can describe anyone involved in formal and informal education, from preceptor to university professor, but the treatment advocated by this διδάσκολς indicates that he was a medical practitioner. We cannot say whether he was a practical doctor or a trained physician or simply a professor with access to healing manuals (*iatrosophia*). We cannot be sure in what context Blasius received his advice. The text is unclear as to whether Blasius asked about both the dream and the treatment of the illness that the dream predicted, or whether he asked about how to treat catarrh on

---

mushrooms, onions, and turnips. As for the bile in the head, Hippocrates (*Critical Days* 3) notes that in acute diseases this is where bile settles.

[55] See the text in Papadopoulos, "Post-Byzantine Medical Manuscripts," pp. 118–20, where a patient inhales a combination of frankincense and water through the form of vapor; see also note 57 below.

another occasion and he then combined the dream and its interpretation with a proper course of medical treatment. The grammar of the Greek text actually lends support to the latter theory: the first section of this paragraph seems awkwardly joined to the second half. Perhaps, then, Blasius did not rely only on his own written sources but also on his own educational background.[56] Also of interest is the final phrase, "[the ailment] will pass, God willing" (θέλημα τοῦ Θεοῦ περνᾷ). This phrase commonly occurs in *iatrosophia* after a recipe is given, and so the "teacher" could have been acquainted with the iatrosophic tradition.[57]

Assuming that Blasius was not a trained healing practitioner himself (a possibility, to be sure), from what *iatrosophion* or practical healing manual did he draw his medical treatments? *Iatrosophia*, as stated above, are mostly composed of medical recipes taken from classical, Byzantine, and post-Byzantine formal medicine and folk medicine—none of which appears in Blasius' text. Blasius only records dietary prophylaxis and changes in lifestyle. But writers of *iatrosophia* did often give advice to patients on proper diet and regimen, such as we read in the dreambook. For example, the 1849 *Iatrosophion* of the Makhairas monastery on Cyprus offers the following instructions for those suffering from a sore throat or a swelling in the throat:

> The water that the patient should drink and the diet [δίαιτα] that he must follow. Take 50 drams of raisins, 50 drams of dried figs, and 30 drams of the sweet–root. Pestle these thoroughly and then place in two okas of water. Boil this mixture well. Let the patient drink of this water. He should also abstain from salty foods, wine, raki, vinegar oil, raw greens, walnuts, onions, garlic, cheese, hallumi cheese, and dry mizithra cheese. Fresh mizithra cheese, unsalted and mixed with honey,

56 We cannot exclude the possibility that Blasius fabricated this mentoring occasion. He could just as easily have pulled the medical treatment from a healing manual and then inserted it into a fictional dialogue so as to lend his words a sense of authority and authenticity.

57 E.g., Papadogiannakês' *Iatrosophion*, p. 132, 3–10: "[Take] cypress tree cones, oak-gall, roses, watermelon rind, and the root of milk thistle. Dry these and then make a powder. Place the powder inside a hollow belly-shaped pot containing coals. Put one dram of mercury in the middle of the powder. Have the patient [stand over the pot and] open his mouth, taking in all of the vapor; cover him well [with a towel] so that none of the vapor escapes. Do this for three days. On the first two days the patient should not eat any salty foods, as I have stated above. [Be warned that] his teeth will rattle because of the mercury, but he should not fear any harm, for if God wills it, he will be healed." For the phrase "God willing," see also note 46 above. Note that this cure, which deals with the treatment of the effects of syphilis (which the author calls "the French disease"), is very similar to the one advocated in Blasius' text for catarrh.

> does no harm. Likewise, let the patient eat butter, raisins, figs, and pomegranates, and he will be healthy.[58]

Another *iatrosophion*, written by the practical doctor Nikolaos Konstantinos Theodorakis in 1930 but based on many generations of medical knowledge that had been passed down through his family, offers similar dietary regimens in conjunction with pharmacopoeia. For example:

> **For fistula.** Take fistula herb and the root of the lily and the milky juice of phlomos,[59] pound them and work on his wound and dry the root of the lily and make a very fine powder and give to him two sips with tepid water to drink every morning, having fasted, and have him stand until he vomits, and a fasting diet only: black raisins and bread to eat.
>
> **For the frying pan disease.** The black frying pan disease—this is also a bad disease and comes out into every part of the body, at the beginning it puts out in the centre one large blister and around it many small little blisters, then the large blister sinks down and the little ones around it stay. Well, you moisten a piece of cotton with strong raki and you put it on top of the cotton and you brown it. You do it like this three times and he gets well, and he should keep a fast from salty foods, sour foods, raki, wine, and sweets. He should have only the compress and meat to eat.
>
> Whoever suffers from pleuritis, immediately take blood and use the cupping glasses, and he should not drink wine or raki or (eat) sour foods, only (drink) water from husked pearl barley, and water from cooked *polypodon* fern[60] and have him also take a clyster.[61]

58 Page 30 of the printed 1924 copy (manuscript dated to 1849); my thanks to Andreas Lardos for sharing with me a copy of this *Iatrosophikon*. This is the most extensive iatrosophic text from Cyprus.

59 The plant *Euphorbia platyphyllos L.*

60 The plant *Polypodon vulgare L.*

61 The passages are taken from pp. 53, 81, and 123, respectively, of Clark's translation of this Cretan *iatrosophion* (see note 32 above). Papadogiannakês' *Iatrosophion* also offers dietary recommendations along with the recipes. For example, "Three drams mercury, 6 drams oak-gall, 6 drams raki, 1 dram ginger, 1.5 carats of dark-blue stone, 20 drams melon seed, liquid of a rotten apple: knead all these. Place [the mixture] in the sun to dry. Turn it into powder. Fumigate the patient while he is fasting. The patient should be covered well, so that he can inhale through the mouth and nose. And if his mouth hurts, make a sharbat with honey to rinse his mouth. And if he is thirsty, let him drink warm water. He should be on his guard not to eat any acidic or salty food" (p. 130, 9–16).

These dietary measures are similar to what we read in Blasius' dreambook, but unlike the Makhairis text and other *iatrosophia*, we do not find in Blasius' text any medical recipe based on plants, minerals, and animals. The prophylactic measures we encounter are prayers (supplications and exorcisms), diet, and regimen. In this respect, Blasius has followed in the footsteps of the author of the Hippocratic *Regimen* 4, who wrote for dieticians and fitness trainers so that they could make diagnostic or prognostic determinations of a person's health and then offer the appropriate regimen.[62] The Hippocratic author's most common regimens, written from the perspective of a dietician, consisted of conducting exercises or avoiding them, vapor baths, drying and cooling, alterations in a patient's food and drink, emetics, and hellebore. To help his own readers to avoid disease, to minimize its painful effects, or prevent the illness from lingering on, Blasius drew on a variety of resources: practical healing manuals, his professors, and perhaps his own training and vocation. He emphasized a holistic approach to healing; using dreams and dream imagery as his guide to a person's physical condition, he advocated dietetics, regimens conducive to restoring health, and a strong spiritual life. In a world filled with uncertainty and turmoil, Blasius' readers could take comfort in the knowledge that they had some control, thanks to dreams, over their health and the diseases that afflicted them.

[62] See van der Eijk, "Divination, Prognosis and Prophylaxis," pp.195–6, 202–3.

Chapter 13

Fields in Dreams: Anxiety, Experience, and the Limits of Social Constructionism in Modern Greek Dream Narratives

Charles Stewart

In this chapter, I consider accounts of Greek dreams that occurred in moments of anxiety caused either by the dreamer's own illness or by the serious illness of a close relative.[1] The image of a field or *pediáda* (green meadow, pastureland) recurs in these dreams. These fields can be interpreted as simultaneously personal and collective symbols,[2] and I contend that this ambiguity reflects the synthetic, irreducible quality of dream experiences, and no doubt other emotional experiences as well. There has been a temptation to treat emotions and feelings as cognitions, thereby reducing them to culture.[3] The limitations of such a view, which cleaves the mind from the body and culture from nature, have become increasingly apparent.[4] Underlying this split is another divide that must be repaired—namely the insistence on the strict separation of the individual from the collective.[5] The image of the field that I explore here reveals the continuities between the personal and the social, the emotional and the cognitive, and thus offers an example of how these putative dichotomies merge

---

[1] This is an edited version of an article first published in *American Ethnologist*, 24 (1997): pp. 877–94 and reprinted with permission of the American Anthropological Association.

[2] G. Obeyesekere, *Medusa's Hair* (Chicago, 1981).

[3] J. Leavitt, "Meaning and Feeling in the Anthropology of Emotions," *American Ethnologist*, 23 (1996): pp. 514–39; and W. Reddy, "Against Constructionism: The Historical Ethnography of Emotions," *Current Anthropology*, 38 (1997): pp. 327–51.

[4] M. Lyon, "Missing Emotion: The Limitations of Cultural Constructionism in the Study of Emotion," *Cultural Anthropology*, 10 (1995): pp. 244–63; and N. Scheper-Hughes and M. Lock, "The Mindful Body: A Prolegomenon to Future Work in Medical Anthropology," *Medical Anthropology Quarterly*, 1 (1987): pp. 6–41.

[5] A. Kleinman and J. Kleinman, "Suffering and Its Professional Transformation: Toward an Ethnography of Interpersonal Experience," in M. Jackson (ed.), *Things as They Are: New Directions in Phenomenological Anthropology* (Bloomington, 1996), pp. 169–95.

in human experience. The challenge is to develop a sufficiently broad analytical framework to cope with the complexity of experience.

In examining experience, people's accounts are generally our primary means of access. Dreams present an extreme instance of this situation because no observer can directly share in another person's dream visions and sensations. The dreamer's retrospective narrative, based on the memory of what happened during sleep, represents the only evidence for the dream. This situation has led philosophers such as Malcolm and Dennett to doubt that dreams are really experiences at all. [6] Even psychologists who study dreams in sleep laboratories with the help of sensitive electrographic devices can only record the neurophysiological correlates of dreaming. For the actual content of the dreams, these researchers must also depend on the narratives of the dreamers. In their privateness and inscrutability, dreams stand apart from social activities such as rituals, which are publicly performed and thus allow independent observations that can be set alongside personal narratives of experience.

Anthropological approaches to dreams cannot be reviewed in detail here, but they have been the subject of recent overviews.[7] Since Lincoln's study,[8] anthropologists have often concentrated on how dreams are culturally patterned and socially interpreted. While acknowledging the personal, psychological dimension of dreams, the anthropological tendency has been to treat dreams as social facts and cultural texts, thereby sensibly placing them inside the recognized framework of anthropological expertise. The only danger here is that anthropologists may become so comfortable with the idea of dreams as cultural constructions that, like the philosophers cited above, they might begin to disregard dreams as experiences. In such cases, the semiotic dimension (representation) subordinates the phenomenological (experience) and displaces it. Anyone who has suddenly awakened from a nightmare or orgasmic dream knows that such a bias is inadequate. Dream narratives may be our only means of knowing about dreams, but few of us would consider that these narratives are dreams; surely they are but representations of dreams. Even if we are not persuaded of this, the tellers of the dream narratives I consider below are so

---

[6] N. Malcolm, *Dreaming* (London, 1959), p. 122; and D. Dennett, "Are Dreams Experiences?" in C. Dunlop (ed.), *Philosophical Essays on Dreaming* (Ithaca, 1977), pp. 227–50, at p. 249.

[7] R.I. Lohmann, "Dreams and Ethnography," in D. Barrett and P. McNamara (eds), *The New Science of Dreaming* (3 vols, Westport, CT, 2007), vol. 3. pp. 35–69; and C. Stewart, "Introduction: Dreaming as an Object of Anthropological Analysis," *Dreaming* (special double issue: *Anthropological Approaches to Dreaming*), 14 (2004): pp. 75–82.

[8] J.S. Lincoln, *The Dream in Primitive Cultures* (New York: 1970 [1935]).

convinced, and an "experience-near" ethnography requires setting their accounts at the center.[9]

The Greek images of fields, which, I shall contend, may be visions of the afterworld, help to solve the condition of illness and anxiety by refiguring the grounds of experience. The fields remain synesthetically complex images that are not fully interpreted. That these fields originated in dreams suggests that they be viewed as "presentational" (visual, experiential) as opposed to "representational" (codified, referential) symbols.[10] As images, these dream visions of fields are fantastic and yet, at the same time, all too real. They are the point at which language is unequal to the task of representing the felt intensity of emotion;[11] experience exceeds the capacity to represent it.[12] But this does not mean that there is no attempt at evocation, and the open fields in dreams can be read as the point where the imagination overloads a representation with emotional charge. I argue that the very feature of excess embedded in these fields enables them to speak powerfully both for and to anxiety.

Dreams as Private Experiences and Collective Stories

In the accounts that I analyze, the tellers all frame their stories with contextual details of going to bed and waking up. Placing a story within the framework of dreaming serves as a modal marker in at least two ways: it grounds the narrative as the report of a direct, individual experience, and it simultaneously brackets this story as extraordinary knowledge (revelatory, transcendental) that demands a different appreciation from ordinary stories, whether factual or fictional.

I draw on Bruner's outline for the anthropology of experience in approaching these dreams.[13] This involves recognizing three different levels: reality (what actually happened), experience (how this presents itself to consciousness), and expressions (the narratives). Obviously, the first two levels are difficult to know, but this is no reason to consider them irrelevant. Using the contextualizing remarks furnished directly by the dreamers in the course of their narrations, as

---

9 U. WIkan, "Toward an Experience-Near Anthropology," *Cultural Anthropology*, 6 (1996): pp. 285–305.

10 S. Langer, *Mind: An Essay on Human Feeling* (Baltimore, 1972).

11 J. Favret-Saada, "About Participation," *Culture, Medicine, and Psychiatry*, 14 (1990): pp. 189–99, at p. 198.

12 B. Good, *Medicine, Rationality and Experience: An Anthropological Perspective* (Cambridge, 1994), p. 139.

13 E. Bruner, "Experience and Its Expressions," in V. Turner and E. Bruner (eds), *The Anthropology of Experience* (Urbana, 1986), pp. 3–30, at p. 6.

well as the content of the dreams themselves, I attempt to reach backward from the narratives to the cognitive, physical, and emotional elements that might have played a role in generating the dream experience. At the same time, I also consider the social modeling and the cultural availability of motifs that influence what is dreamed and how it is recounted. I maintain that these various levels of analysis are all complementary and must be combined if we are ever to approach an understanding of experience.

Individual narrators may claim that their narratives issue from private, internal experiences, but this is unconvincing to the observer, who may notice striking similarities not only between the dreams of separate individuals, but also between these dreams and well-known folktales. During field research, I noticed that the familiarity of a story did not diminish its credibility as a personal account of a private experience in the way it might for us if an acquaintance narrated a dream that closely corresponded to the Little Red Riding Hood story. The contributors to *The Anthropology of Experience*[14] have addressed this problem of the conventionality of putatively private experience. Their starting assumption is that people make sense of their lives primarily through a reliance on historically created symbols, conventions, and stories. This is to say that they draw on their cultural background in the relating of experience. According to Turner, "Meaning arises when we try to put what culture and language have crystallized from the past together with what we feel, wish, and think about our present point in life."[15] Geertz turns the problem into a paradox near the end of the volume when he asks: "How comes it that we all start out as originals and end up copies? The answer is surprisingly reassuring: it is the copying that originates."[16]

The Anthropology of Experience charts a good course, but it produces answers in terms of very large and general forces such as culture and history. What about the moment of experience itself? How is that conditioned by cultural forms and models? Perhaps this last question is unanswerable, just as it is impossible to know precisely what images are seen by dreamers in sleep. I think, however, that we can be still more specific in addressing this quandary.

---

14 Turner and Bruner (eds), *The Anthropology of Experience*.

15 V. Turner, "Dewey, Dithey and Drama: An Essay in the Anthropology of Experience," in Turner and Bruner (eds), *The Anthropology of Experience*, pp. 33–44, at p. 33.

16 C. Geertz, "Making Experiences, Authoring Selves," in Turner and Bruner (eds), *The Anthropology of Experience*, pp. 373–80, at p. 380.

Medicine and Miracle on Naxos

Two saints have recently emerged as preeminent among miracle working saints in Greece: Saint Nektarios and Saint Irini Chrysovalantou. Pilgrims flock to their monasteries, both of which are located near Athens, and leave impressive sums of money or elaborate gifts as devotions. The followers of Saint Irini Chrysovalantou even publish a newsletter filled with stories about people who, with the saint's help, have recovered from dread diseases or crippling accidents. This is the background against which the following accounts should be set.

In the context of a discussion about dreams, a middle-aged woman from the Naxos mountain village of Kóronos described for me how Saint Nektarios once healed her:

> What a good thing it is to pray to a saint for something and for the saint to perform a miracle for you, and for you to see it with your own eyes. Many years ago, when I was still young, I had a sore on my palate. It distressed me and hurt terribly. At night it was so painful I would sit upright in my sleep. It was a bad thing, causing me continuous pain. I prayed every day to the Panagia and to St. Nektarios. I said, "Please, if it is something serious, leave me now while I have small children to raise because they are helpless. Let them mature and grow stronger. Then you can do to me what you like." I fasted continuously. I fasted for ten days. If anyone asked [me to eat] I just said, "I ate earlier." Sometimes I would eat food with oil for two or three days but then I fasted again. Seven, eight, five, or six days—as long as I could stand it.
>
> **Q**: Why did you fast?
>
> **A**: In order to beseech [*na parakaléso*] so to say. Haven't you ever heard how people fast and pray? ... I prayed and prayed continuously. Prayers and tears. Then I saw in my dreams that I was in a place, so to say, a wide, open space. How should I say it? ... on a plain [*pediáda*]. As I was standing in that place I saw a mass of people far away from me, more people than I'd ever seen in one place. I asked, "What are they doing over there?" A person replied, "It's a doctor who, they say, saves people." A doctor, they told me, not a saint, who heals people. I say to myself, "Should I go?" I was aware that I was sick and I said, "Should I go too, so that he'll save me?"
>
> When I went up close I heard people shouting. They had formed a circle around him. They didn't approach him as one would a doctor at his practice, to be given some medicine. They approached him in a different fashion. One paralytic went

> up to him and said, "I beg you doctor, save me too." One by one. Then it was my turn. I went and stood near him and said, "Please doctor, save me too, as I have small children." As soon as I went and stood close to him I recognized that he was St. Nektarios. I saw the staff he had.[17]
>
> He took me by the hand and looked at me and put his hand in my mouth and pulled a nail out of my palate. A fingernail [*nýkhi*] just as you have [gesturing to my fingernails], growing. He pulled this nail out of my palate and threw it down in front of me covered in blood. If you looked at the back part of it, it was all bloody.
>
> At this point I awoke. I tried with my hand; couldn't find it. I said to myself, "Is this something real happening, or is this a dream?" I realized I had been dreaming. But thanks to God, the saint, and the Panagia, it disappeared from my palate. When he pulled the nail out, the sore disappeared. Do you understand? I myself saw this with my own eyes. Can you possibly not believe it? ... Is it possible not to believe that the saint exists and works wonders [*thavmatourgeí*]? It is enough if you have faith [*arkeí i pístis*]. I've seen many similar things in my dreams. I am completely convinced that saints exist and work wonders. I see it in practice.[18]

The events reported in this narrative occurred in a dream, yet the narrator insisted that these things truly did happen in reality. Perhaps we should not be entirely dismissive; even Aristotle, who must have been one of the greatest skeptics of all time on the prophetic truth-value of dreams,[19] conceded some degree of veracity to dreams that told of immediate changes in health. This, he reckoned, was because dreamers were especially sensitive to changes occurring in their own bodies—far more so than when awake.[20]

---

17 On icons, Saint Nektarios is depicted as holding a staff.

18 The events described correspond remarkably to dream visions registered at the temple of Asclepius in fourth-century BC Greece. For example: "Euhippus had had for six years the point of a spear in his jaw. As he was sleeping in the Temple the god extracted the spearhead and gave it to him in his hands. When day came Euhippus departed cured, and he held the spearhead in his hands"; taken from E. Edelstein and L. Edelstein, *Asclepius* (2 vols, Baltimore, 1945), vol. 1, p. 232. For the Asclepian cult, I refer the reader to the chapters by Cilliers and Retief, Downie, and Pearcy in this volume.

19 E.R. Dodds, *The Greeks and the Irrational* (Berkeley, 1973), p. 120.

20 Early medical writings such as the Hippocratic texts and Galen also contain references to the diagnostic value of "symptomatic" dreams—dreams that communicate present or impending illnesses or humoral imbalances; see S.M. Oberhelman, "Dreams in Graeco-Roman Medicine," in W. Haase and H. Temporini (eds), *Aufstieg und Niedergang der Römischen Welt* (Berlin, 1993), part II, vol. 37.1, pp. 121–56, at pp. 128 and 142. Many

Contemporary dream research substantiates Aristotle's assertion that in sleep somatic sensations can be converted into visual dream presentations of the onset of illness.[21] Perhaps this consideration accounts for the frequency with which dreaming appears in the context of descriptions of illness, but it can only serve as an explanation where the dreamer and the ill person are the same. As will be seen, there are a number of cases where it is not the dreamer's but someone else's health that is at stake.

Dreams of the Afterworld

The Naxiote woman's miraculous healing account is framed as a personal dream experience in which her body undergoes a radical and beneficial change. It is very much an experience rather than being merely a "story." Yet it is a particular kind of invisible experience. All that her husband could say is that she was ill one moment and better the next. One striking detail of the narrative was the woman's mention of a large field (*mia pediáda*), where she met the saint and was healed. I had noticed this detail in a number of other dreams involving encounters with saints at moments of illness or anxiety. Some of these were separated by considerable periods of time. For example, the following dream account comes from General Makrygiannis, one of the heroes of the early nineteenth-century Greek war of independence. This dream (as well as numerous other visions that he experienced) was not published until 1983 under the title *Orámata kai thávmata* (*Visions and Miracles*).[22] Makrygiannis originally wrote down this account around 1851 in the journals that he used for recording his constant illnesses as well as those of his wife and his continuing disappointments with the Greek political situation.[23] Perhaps latter-day embarrassment at the pathetic emotion and religious credulity of one of Greece's national heroes delayed the publication of these notebooks for more than a century:

---

of these same writings also entertain the idea that diagnostic dreams can be divinely sent. For fuller and more substantive discussion on this topic, Hulskamp's chapter in this volume must be consulted.

[21] H. Levitan, "Dreams Which Culminate in Migraine Headaches," *Psychotherapy and Psychosomatics*, 33 (1984): pp. 161–6; R.C. Smith, "Evaluating Dream Function: Emphasizing the Study of Patients with Organic Disease," *Journal of Mind and Behavior*, 7 (1986): pp. 397–410.

[22] General Makrygiannis, *Orámata kai thávmata* (Athens, 1983).

[23] S. Gourgouris, *Dream Nation: Enlightenment, Colonization and the Institution of Modern Greece* (Stanford, 1996), p. 176.

> One evening I was sleeping among the icons (I had set up my pallet there) and Her Grace told me what Christ had told her. I was awake, but drowsy like a drunkard. They conveyed me to an old church, which was divided into many vaulted chambers. In one vault there was a ring in the middle with a chain, and a youth was hanging from it, and he was agonizing to release his soul. I saw him and was afraid and saddened. On account of my sorrow I went outside and they took me up, to a plain [*pediáda*]; yet it was a very sad place. Readers, may I be cursed if I am making this up.
>
> Arriving in this field was our Master; on his right, Christ, and to the right of Christ the Mother of God and twelve saints. I well recognized Saint John the Baptist. And they were all dressed in black—the Master and all the others. They were also seated.
>
> On the left side were all those who had committed many crimes and all those who had baptized many children and then had committed some sin with their female spiritual kin [*koumbáres*]; and all those who had deflowered virgins, as well as many other criminals. These last were in the forefront.[24]

The question is why, at moments of painful illness or distress, should the description of a field be of any particular importance? In the New Testament, the Last Judgment is nowhere described as taking place in a broad plain. The Old Testament, well known in Greece in its Septuagint translation, offers at least one important *topos* involving plains:

> A voice cries: "In the wilderness prepare the way of the Lord, make straight in the desert a highway for our God. Every valley shall be lifted up and every mountain and hill be made low; the uneven ground shall become level, and the rough places a plain. And the glory of the Lord shall be revealed, and all flesh shall see it together, for the mouth of the Lord has spoken." (Isaiah 40:3–5)

This passage connects the leveling/opening/widening of space with divine revelation, and is echoed in the New Testament (e.g., Luke 3:4–6).[25] There is,

---

[24] Makrygiannis, *Orámata*, p. 141. This is technically a hypnagogic experience since it occurs at the onset of sleep (A. Mavromatis, *Hypnagogia: The Unique State of Consciousness between Wakefulness and Sleep* [London, 1991]). Psychologists disagree on whether hypnagogic experiences should be classified as dreams. Out-of-body experiences apparently occur more frequently in the hypnagogic state than in normal dreaming.

[25] I thank Kimberley Patton for alerting me to these passages.

however, one important reference to a plain in the New Testament. This passage recounts Christ's descent from the hills together with his disciples:

> He then came down with them and stopped at a piece of level ground [τόπου πεδινοῦ] where there was a large gathering of his disciples with a great crowd of people from all parts of Judaea and from Jerusalem and from the coastal region of Tyre and Sidon who had come to hear him and to be cured of their diseases. People tormented by unclean spirits were also cured, and everyone in the crowd was trying to touch him because power came out of him that cured them all. (Luke 6:17–19)

This passage bears a close relation to the miracle account of the woman with the sore on her palate. Christ's charismatic power, according to the gospels, was transferred to the disciples who accompanied him down from the hills (the first priesthood) and who in turn have passed it on through the ages via the ordination ceremony that calls specifically for an episcopal laying on of hands. Latter-day miracle-working saints, such as Saint Nektarios, are heirs to this particular New Testament moment.

I think that the images of fields in these dreams allude generally to the afterworld, in particular to the benevolent afterworld—if not paradise, then the place where souls destined for paradise are sent to wait after death. On Naxos, people describe this zone as a wide green meadow with plenty of water and plenty of light—a fair place in all respects. According to John K. Campbell, the Sarakatsani shepherds of northern Greece perceived the good afterlife "as a plain of well-watered grass covered with flowers."[26] The landscape of the Zagori where the Sarakatsani pasture their sheep is, like the interior of Naxos, an extremely rocky, steep, and arid environment. This landscape gives rise to fierce competition over pastureland and water rights, and the idea of broad, well-irrigated plains is one of which a shepherd may wishfully dream.

The ancient Greeks also conceived of the place of the good afterlife as a "meadowy field" (the Elysian Fields).[27] The association of bright, green meadows with paradise, including an earthly paradise (Eden), is also reported in visions beginning with Pope Gregory the Great in the sixth century and continuing throughout the Middle Ages. Carol Zaleski, an authority on "otherworld journeys," writes that "motifs of paradise topography are the most constant features of Western otherworld journey narration. It is no surprise then to find

---

26 J.K. Campbell, *Honour, Family and Patronage* (Oxford, 1964), p. 325.

27 J. Puhvel, "'Meadow of the Otherworld' in Indo-European Tradition," *Zeitschrift des Vereins für Sprachwissenschaft*, 83 (1969): pp. 64–9, at p. 68.

that near-death narratives recall the pastoral meadows ... of biblical and early Christian narration."[28]

In sum, the fields in the dreams considered so far represent a space of revelation and resolution while also figuring the ultimate resolution of human suffering—salvation in paradise. These dreams order and reorder commonly held cultural knowledge of the afterworld. Although they may have features in common with texts from the New Testament or the New Testament Apocrypha, this should not necessarily be interpreted as a case of direct familiarity with these scriptural passages—although this is a possibility in a community where all are Orthodox Christians, a priest lives in each village, and Sunday liturgies can be heard on the radio. The Orthodox funeral service includes the prayer "Lord, give rest to the soul of your departed servant, [name], in a bright place (*en tópo photeinó*), in a grassy place (*en tópo khloeró*), in a place of refreshment, where there is no pain, sorrow, or groaning."[29] This formula is repeated at the frequent memorial services and Soul Saturday services for the dead, and is probably as familiar to the Greek public as the liturgical phrase "He maketh me to lie down in green pastures" is to the English-speaking public.

Illness, Dreams, and Miracles

In this section I consider a sequence of dreams told to me on a return visit to the village of Apeiranthos after my original field research. The woman who narrated this dream (here called by the pseudonym of Sophia) has two children, a boy and a girl, who are now both adults. I met Sophia at the house of a family I knew well. They summoned Sophia when our conversation turned to the subject of dreams; they were already familiar with much of what she would say. It is not unusual for people—especially for women—to share dreams the morning after they have "seen" them. Equally, they may neglect to mention a dream or vision if they consider it irrelevant at the time. Later, they may reverse this opinion in light of subsequent events that prove the importance of the vision. An example of this was the case of one of the boys sitting in the courtyard with us that very afternoon. The boy had once dreamt that he saw an old, black-clad woman carrying a can of oil as if on her way to refill the oil lamps at a neighboring chapel. He did not recognize her, became frightened, and took another route to avoid her. He did not relate this dream to anyone until a month later when

[28] C. Zaleski, *Otherworld Journeys: Accounts of Near-Death Experience in Medieval and Modern Times* (New York, 1987), p. 134.

[29] H. Hatzopoylos, *Funeral Services: According to the Rite of the Greek Orthodox Church* (Boston: n.d.), p. 12.

he was struck down by a virus affecting his nervous system. If the virus had reached his brain, villagers said, he surely would have died. While still in the hospital recovering, he finally told his mother about this dream and together they concluded that the woman he saw was undoubtedly the Evangelistria (a manifestation of the Panagia to whom a neighborhood chapel is dedicated) who had blocked the spread of the disease, limiting paralysis to only his right side, whence it eventually receded altogether.

In our general discussion of dreams before she related her accounts, Sophia remarked that although more people than expected believed in dreams, when they spoke of their dreams, they were frequently ridiculed:

> My son was always sick. He had a contracted esophageal passage and nervous spasms. He was always sick: one day well and five days sick, one day well and two sick. He was always sick. His digestive system wasn't functioning properly and if he ate something tough he would come down with fever afterwards, sometimes reaching as high as 42°C, the temperature at which people die.
>
> One evening, then, I went to bed and I saw the Evangelistria, the Panagia, in my sleep. Her Dormition. No ... her Annunciation is celebrated on the 25th of March. Her church is our neighbor. It is celebrated on the day when the angel gave the lily to the Panagia, as we say. It is both a Christian and a national holiday. Well then, I sat down and I see one evening that I went inside the church and I saw the Panagia kneeling—on her knees—and she was praying to God. She had her arms crossed like this, with a black scarf and golden slippers. She was wearing gold slippers.
>
> **Q**: Why did she have gold slippers? [A background voice calls out "like a saint."]
>
> **A**: They were silver, as in an icon. It was a dream.
>
> So I say, I say, "I have two children and they are ill." I say to her, "Can't you [here she uses the plural form of address] help them for me? And there is also a neighbor sick too." And she said to me, "Look after your own children as they are young and leave the neighbor aside." I had considered poor Manolis [the neighbor whom she wished to help]. And she says to me, "They have stolen your older child, stolen him" [*s'tó'khane souphroméno*, i.e., bewitched]. I consider his stomach. Perhaps someone has cursed me, and subsequently my child has encountered the ugly hour [*tin áskhimi óra*]. And the child? Granted that she tells me they have stolen him ... Do you understand, she said that they had stolen him.

> But she says, nevertheless, "Don't worry," and she patted me on the back. "Don't worry, now that you've come to see me I shall struggle and whatever I can, I shall do and I shall save them; I'll save them for you." But just know, she told me again repeatedly, that they have stolen your older child. Thus she was speaking to me and she picked up—there was a spool lying there—well, she picks up the spool, looked, and the thread was gray. I say that if it had been black, the child would have died. If it had been white, that means the child would have gotten completely better. If it were gray, this means the child would be continuously ill. She takes up the thread on the spool and causes the hands of the child to turn there. There, do you see? They have stolen him. But she patted me on the back again and said not to worry, "Whatever I can do, I shall, and I shall rescue your children for you." And I say, "What are you doing there kneeling?" Ach, I didn't tell you that the first thing, as soon as I saw her, the very first moment when I saw her, I say to her, "Who are you? Are you St. Sophia?" "No, my child, I am your neighbor. Don't you recognize me?" The moment I entered she told me that. She also says, "What are you [pl.] doing here?" She says, "I'm praying to God at this moment." She was kneeling and had her hands here. She also said, "How are you?" "I am your neighbor," she told me repeatedly. She set down the thread that she was collecting and my child's arms went back to their place. And I take the child ...
>
> **Q**: Was your child there with you?
>
> **A**: Yes, in the dream. And I take the child and she stood up and patted me on the back and says to me, "Go ahead home, but I shall struggle and I shall save both of your children. Don't worry." And thus it happened.

The conventionality of the symbols in this dream—thread for life, white for life, black for death—might cause one to suspect that the dream itself could have been intentionally invented in waking consciousness. The theme of the fates (*moirai*) spinning and cutting the skein of life is familiar from classical Greek mythology, but modern Greek tradition also entertains a conception of fate (*moíra*) that determines the fortunes of humans.[30] Sometimes the modern fates are also depicted as measuring life as thread or cloth. This pervasive conventionality makes it even more likely to be accessible to the dreaming imagination, where it can be drawn upon and visualized in dream images.

One notable feature of this dream is that Sophia herself delivers the interpretation of the differently colored spools of thread in the course of

---

[30] J. du Boulay, *Cosmos, Life and Liturgy in a Greek Orthodox Village* (Limni [Evia, Greece], 2009), p. 344.

narrating the dream. Apparently she arrived at this interpretation subsequently—on her own or perhaps along with others to whom she told the dream—and then interjected this interpretation into the dream account. The dream and its social interpretation become melded, exemplifying how an idiosyncratic personal dream may be converted, through contact with public canons, into a recognizably standard narrative.

Dream narratives like Sophia's share certain features with funeral laments, another primarily female discursive form in Greece. As Anna Caraveli has pointed out, lamentation is not limited to ritual funerary contexts.[31] Lament motifs may appear in other genres such as songs for those departing on long journeys. In dreams at moments of illness, elements of the lament have migrated to the genre of dream narration and interpretation, giving rise to a hybrid form that conjoins distressed complaint (lamentation) with attempts at achieving divinatory revelation that might dispel uncertainty and anxiety (dream interpretation). These dream accounts are laments for the sick.

While in the earlier example of the Saint Nektarios dream, the woman dreamt about her own physical condition, Sophia dreamt about her son's illness and her anguish over his condition. Her dreams are narrative performances of motherhood and womanhood, as well as of social caring more generally, as evidenced by her attempt to intercede on behalf of her sick neighbor. Like funeral laments, these dream visions are grounded in pain (*pónos*) and distress, and these sentiments lend extra power and legitimation to their performance.[32] The idea of "excess" returns here: the suffering so exceeds the capacity of an individual to contain it that it must be distributed, primarily to the community of women who can most appreciate and feel the problems—the "sisterhood of pain," as Caraveli calls it.[33]

Those who see these dreams and mediate their contents to the public partake of a Christian grace, or "illumination" (*phótisi*), which commands respectful attention from co-villagers. One could well imagine that a drive to demonstrate the ability to gain divine illumination might impel women to see more and more dreams. Indeed, Dubisch has drawn attention to "competitive suffering" in the performance of womanhood.[34] Such spiritual competition may be discerned,

---

31 A. Caraveli, "The Lament as Social Protest," in J. Dubisch (ed.), *Gender and Power in Rural Greece* (Princeton, 1986), pp. 169–94, at p. 191.

32 Caraveli, "The Lament as Social Protest," p. 172; C. Nadia Seremetakis, *The Last Word: Women, Death and Divination in Inner Mani* (Chicago, 1991), p. 120.

33 Caraveli, "The Lament as Social Protest," p. 181.

34 J. Dubisch, *In a Different Place: Pilgrimage, Gender and Politics at a Greek Island Shrine* (Princeton, 1995), p. 214.

for example, in the political drive of female devotees to experience illumination from Saint Constantine in the cult of the Anastenaria.[35]

The manifest liveliness of dream traditions in the mountains of Naxos suggests that women utilize a common, empowering cultural resource, one that is diffusely distributed locally and perennially within their grasp. In these narratives, which are part and parcel of a "poetics of womanhood,"[36] mothers emerge as heroes, able to open a connection with the sacred via their saintly visions. As Sophia's next dream clearly shows, a woman is also able to take command in a dream in ways that exceed her position in everyday life. For example, she can diagnose her child and tell the doctor what to do, or leave the village and travel. Aside from pilgrimages and travels related to the schooling of children, illness is one of the few other reasons women have for leaving the island—and Sophia did accompany her son to England for surgery. The fields in these dreams thus take on yet another meaning: they are images of broad open spaces of which a woman, toiling away most of her life in a dark house tucked away in a steep-terraced, narrow mountain village neighborhood, might dream. They are images of openness and release from the conditions of daily life onto an open space where women perform heroics.

After Sophia asked about my research (I explained that it concerned dreams and their interpretation), she continued with the following account:

> Another time ... again, I'll tell you another dream. Well then, the child, my son, well then, the doctor told us to go and have surgery, as it was necessary to have surgery on the esophagus because it had a nervous spasm. The constriction was cured. We took him to England and had him operated on. The nervous spasm, however, is not curable. That's something natural. It's not curable, but the constriction that he had they opened up, brought it into proper alignment, and it does digest.
>
> **Q**: What's a nervous spasm?
>
> **A**: That's when the stomach makes spasms like this [smacks hands together]. Doesn't the stomach digest like that [*alései*, literally 'to mill' as in 'to mill grain']? In the meanwhile my child had grown heavy [i.e., close to death]. The doctor told us to have surgery, but it is very difficult and he was afraid it would not be successful; he didn't want it.

---

35 L.M. Danforth, *Firewalking and Religious Healing: The Anastenaria of Greece and the American Firewalking Movement* (Princeton, 1989); and C. Stewart, "Strategies of Suffering and their Interpretation(s)," *Culture, Medicine and Psychiatry*, 16 (1992): pp. 107–19.

36 Dubisch, *In a Different Place*, p. 212.

He was about 19 years old. Both he and we were tormented. May no other mother have to go through what I went through, nor another child get sick. Meanwhile we took the child to the hospital. We stayed there for three days; three days we stayed at the clinic of St. Nikolaos in Athens. And they said we should take him to England, perhaps he would be saved. Otherwise he would become like a thread, just like a thread.

Q: So thin?

A: You could see him and you wouldn't know he was a person: a skeleton. Well then, one evening I fell down [on my knees? The same verb, *ípesa*, was used earlier for "to go to bed" before the dream began] and said, "Panagia," I said, "illuminate me as to what will happen."

They told us, then, to go to England. Perhaps the child could be saved. He was running a continuous fever: fever, fever, fever ... 40 days without it going down even one degree. And the doctor says that he might even have consumption. So they perform the test for tuberculosis. Negative. Then he says perhaps he has "far and away and distant from here" cancer. They perform the test for cancer. It was negative. Then the doctor says ... I say to him, I say, "Listen to me and I'll tell you since I am his mother. Whatever ails my child comes from the stomach." They stop giving him food and give him only water to stop the circulation of the stomach in digesting. They gave him a little yogurt to eat and the fever rose again.

Then the doctor says to take him to England, perhaps. They pumped his stomach and put him on an intravenous feeding system. Great sufferings. One evening, then, I go to bed and I say in my sleep, I say, "Panagia, illuminate me. Will my child live or will he die?" And I see in the same room where the Evangelistria was [in the earlier dream?] in Manolis' courtyard ... I bend down there and find an egg. Instead of the egg being white, that one was this color [indicates a yellow object]. It had shriveled up. It had lost its color and it was cracked: cracked, cracked [makes knocking noise]. Just like when we pick up an egg and we strike it, we strike it to crumble it when we go to eat it. That's how the egg was, exactly the color of Katerina's hair [indicating a blondish-brown-haired girl sitting nearby and listening to her].

The same thing inside the church, where she has a church over here and the Panagia came down and I saw the dream and I see a field, all clean, with clean stones and the earth was blond—not the color of dirt—it was all white just like the girl's hair. That's the way it was: the egg, the field—clean as could be. And there I see

> pebbles arranged down on the ground, very beautiful and clean, these rocks. And we passed by and when we neared England in order to go to London, before we got to the city I saw from the airplane. It looked a lot like those [English] fields.
>
> By this cross that I'm making if I'm telling lies. Exactly those fields they were. It was, after all, here at our neighbor's [the Evangelistria], right next to the church. I saw the field in this manner. And I found the egg and I grab it and I say, there, I say, is an egg. Should I break it, I say, to see what is inside it? And so I break it and out comes a bird; and out comes a bird with legs like a partridge's—how do they call them there?—with long legs [she indicates just how long these were, "down to there"]. Its legs were like a spindle, just a little bit thicker, a little bit thicker than that and long. And I say, "O Panagia," I say, a bird that came out and the bird came to life immediately. It seems as if it were years inside the egg; as if the bird were years inside the egg and now I broke it, I say, and it came out and came alive. No, it wasn't dead after so many years. And then I awoke.
>
> I awoke in the morning and thought to myself. I said, "My child won't die, he'll live." And he was inside for years with the sufferings and the sicknesses and in breaking the egg he emerged. I awoke.

Her final word, *xýpnisa* (I awoke), repeated several times near the end, expresses more than just simple emergence from sleep; it suggests an arrival at a new understanding. Someone who is intelligent is *éxypnos*, literally "awake, alert" in Greek. Although her son will continue to be intermittently ill, she will no longer worry about his imminent death. The lack of understanding—and with it, anxiety—lifts.

Again, the imagery of fields in these dreams is striking.[37] In the open, peculiarly clean, seemingly bleached fields of her dreams, Sophia finds the egg that communicates the positive news regarding her son's future. At the same time, this field reminds her of England, where technology and medical knowledge were brought to bear on her son's ailment. The image of the field conjoins the mysterious and the scientific.

[37] In the highly successful film *Field of Dreams* (1989), a man sees visions of famous baseball players in a field, where they deliver inspiration and insight. Perhaps the connection between fields and revelation uncovered in Greek dreams also holds for American dreams—and those of the Japanese and other international tourists who have been flocking at a rate of 65,000 visitors per year to the Iowa cornfield where the film was shot.

Anxiety, Cognition, and Experience

The fields in all the dreams considered thus far provide the context within which beneficial action takes place or where reassuring omens are received. In themselves, the fields have no particular meaning; the narrators did not pick them out for decipherment as signs of anything. In Freud's terms, the field could be considered "the navel of the dream, the spot where it reaches down into the unknown."[38]

In modern Greece, books of dream symbols and their interpretations, called *oneirokrítes*, circulate in cheap and readily available editions. Of the various *oneirokrítes* that I have consulted, only about half contained an entry for field (*pediáda*). In general, these books focus on the issue of whether the field is green, fertile, and inhabited (good), or dry, rocky, and barren (bad). According to one dreambook:

> If you see that you are in a field filled with greenery, and cultivated, and with trees, etc., you will have successes in your life, in your endeavors, and generally in matters that concern you. If the field is dry and uncultivated, unforested, and devoid of greenery, then you will be tormented by great tedium [*plíxi megáli tha se vasanízei*].[39]

A desert may be an open space, but it extends anxiety rather than solving it. This is illustrated by the following dream, recorded from a Greek-Canadian woman in the waiting room of a general practitioner:

> I came to the doctor about my nerves [*névra*]. I'm tired and really nervous. I get headaches and pain down the back and recently I've been screaming around the house a lot and fighting for my life by myself. There's nobody to help me out. I'm in a vast desert with no way back and I have this dream several times a night. I see it more and more these days.[40]

Like Sophia's dreams and the dream of the woman with the sore on her palate, this woman's dreams occur after a long period of suffering or illness—indeed, they are still part of that suffering. In all these narratives, certain linguistic devices serve to highlight the frustrating persistence of distress. In Sophia's accounts, the repetition of words such as "fever" and "sick" emphasize the exasperating

38 S. Freud, *The Interpretation of Dreams* (New York, 1965 [1900]), p. 564.

39 S. Zambouke, *Mégas oneirokrítis* (Athens, n.d.), p. 311.

40 M. Lock, "Nerves and Nostalgia: Greek-Canadian Immigrants and Medical Care in Quebec," *Curare*, 7 (1991): pp. 87–103, at p. 92.

duration of the situation. The early parts of Sophia's dreams, as well as the early part of the first dream of Saint Nektarios, also contain descriptions using the continuous verbal aspect.[41] These aspectually imperfect descriptions emphasize the internal experience of suffering and yield to the perfective descriptions of encounters with saints, and awakening.

What is solved in these dreams is the excessive worry, the anxiety, the wrenching uncertainty generated by illness, whether one's own or that of a loved one. In the case of the sore on the palate, the dream apparently did cure a physical ailment. Fundamental to all my examples, however, is that dreams work on, represent, and sometimes heal the experience of distress. It is often difficult to know when an illness will spontaneously go into remission or be cured, or when pain will subside. This is part of the human predicament. But not all such aporias cause anxiety: those that trap attention and propel one into a desperate recursion of thought are the ones that may be termed "intractable." Intractability arises in a situation of imperfect knowledge in the face of an apparently unchanging situation.

After each of the dreams I have described—with the exception of the Greek-Canadian woman's dream, which is still in recursive, intractable process—each dreamer awakens to a different perspective on life, accomplished by placement in a wide, open space. This should be read as a leveling of the prior condition of anxiety. The word for "distress" or "worry" is *stenokhória* in Greek, literally "a tight or constricted space." The English word *anxiety* similarly reveals etymological associations with tightness and lack of space. It is a cognate of the German word *eng* (tight) and the Latin *angina* (a choking throat infection), and comes from the ancient Greek verb ἄγχω (to strangle, to squeeze tightly). The image of an open field is exactly the converse of associations with anxiety.

Hirschon's and Danforth's[42] rich ethnographic discussions amply demonstrate how "open" and "closed" are conceived in the context of Greek culture as ideal states indicative, respectively, of happiness and sadness, release or constraint. Nevertheless, I contend that the field is not itself the solution, but rather is the

41 The modern Greek verb may be formed in continuous or simple/perfect aspect. As A. Leontis ("'The Lost Center' and the Promised Land of Greek Criticism," *Journal of Modern Greek Studies*, 5 [1987]: pp. 175–90, at p. 189) explains, "The perfective looks at the situation from the outside, without necessarily distinguishing any of the internal structure of the situation, whereas the imperfective looks at the situation from the inside, and as such is crucially concerned with the internal structure of the situation."

42 R. Hirschon, "Open Body/Closed Space: The Transformation of Female Sexuality," in S. Ardener (ed.), *Defining Females: The Nature of Women in Society* (London, 1978), pp. 66–88, at p. 76; and Danforth, *Firewalking*, p. 122.

ground on which a resolution may occur. The field situates the dreamer in a new space for relating to experience; it erases the former relation of intractability.

The mechanics of this transaction should not strike us as a mystical *deus ex machina*, for we know that dreams are a particularly visual form of thinking. In the Greek language, people say that they "see" dreams, not that they "have" them. Whether or not all thought possesses a visual component is a point that is still debated among psychologists and philosophers. At the very least, it appears that visualization—and thus some degree of spatiality—are important for memory and other cognitive operations, such as the grasping of metaphor.[43] As Levinson argues, "When an intellectual problem can be spatialized, it can be conceived clearly."[44] Consider, for example, Sacks' case of the autistic twins who could instantly assess multidigit prime numbers. The twins themselves said that they could "see" the numbers and, according to Sacks, when they calculated an answer, they rolled their eyes "as if scrutinizing an interior landscape."[45] Likewise, the mnemonist who was studied by Luria[46] could remember long lists of random numbers or arbitrary words by picturing them spread along a street down which he imagined himself walking.[47] In these examples, open space does not in itself mean anything, but is a necessary precondition for thinking and memory to work—for knowledge to become manifest. In the Greek case, then, *stenokhória* (distress, lack of space) correlates with the inability to think properly and productively. The appearance of fields in dreams introduces space, and this facilitates problem solving.

Nightmares, by contrast, are bound up with constriction, and in traditional Greek lore they are caused by demonic figures called *vrakhnás* or *móra* who jump on the sleeper's chest and cause a suffocating sensation.[48] Nightmares are sometimes described as "heavy sleep" (*ýpnos varýs*). Dreams of fields are the opposite of classic nightmares; they create space and allow for movement.

---

[43] D. Holland and N. Quinn, *Cultural Models in Language and Thought* (Cambridge, 1987), p. 28.

[44] S. Levinson, "Primer for the Field Investigation of Spatial Description and Conception," *Pragmatics*, 2 (1992): pp. 5–47, at p. 5.

[45] O. Sacks, *The Man Who Mistook His Wife for a Hat* (London, 1985), p. 187.

[46] A.R. Luria, *The Mind of a Mnemonist* (Cambridge, 1987).

[47] The technique of distributing memories in space is, of course, akin to the Graeco-Roman "art of memory" studied by Frances Yates in *The Art of Memory* (Chicago, 1966).

[48] N. Politis, *Neoelliniki mythologia* (Athens, 1979 [1874]), p. 439; and C. Stewart, "Erotic Dreams and Nightmares from Antiquity to the Present," *Journal of the Royal Anthropological Institute*, 8 (2002): pp. 279–309.

Conclusion

I suggested earlier that fields in dreams could be understood as a conventional image of the afterlife. This meaning is sometimes referenced directly in dream narratives, such as the one cited from Makrygiannis. It can thus be said that miracles may contain a glimpse of death—but only a glimpse, because death is quickly elided from the picture. People deftly jump to the other side—to immortality. Freud offers a reason why this should be the case:

> It is indeed impossible to imagine our own death; and whenever we attempt to do so we can perceive that we are still present as spectators. Hence the psychoanalytic school could venture on the assertion that at bottom no one believes in his own death, or to put the same thing in another way, that in the unconscious every one of us is convinced of his own immortality.[49]

As Freud further explained,[50] fantasy and trauma stand in a direct and balancing relationship to each other: the greater an individual's unhappiness and discomfort, the more that person will try to compensate with imaginative flights, such as visits made to the benevolent afterworld in the sort of dreams I have been discussing. Instead of dwelling on their anxiety and uncertainty, individuals incorporate images of the afterlife into their dreams to help resolve the tense uncertainties surrounding illness. Borrowing from one sphere of the unknown palliates another sphere of unknowability.

The perennial appearance of fields in dreams of anxiety and suffering could, according to the anthropology of experience, be understood as the result of the cultural motifs available through oral and literate traditions that began with the Old and New Testaments. These motifs are reworked at the local, neighborhood level by women who listen to each other's narratives of *pónos*, grace, and illumination, and then perennially draw on these themes as they rise to confront, express, and encompass their own personal or family misfortunes.

Cultural anthropologists often stop here at the level of collective representations as these are socially expressed in public narratives. These representations can easily be considered as culture pattern dreams, and it is interesting that, like culture pattern dreams in so-called shamanic societies,

[49] S. Freud, "Thoughts for the Times on War and Death," in J. Strachey (ed. and trans.), *The Standard Edition of the Complete Psychological Works of Sigmund Freud* (24 vols, London, 1957 [1915]), vol. 14, p. 289.

[50] S. Freud, "Beyond the Pleasure Principle," in A. Richards (ed.) and J. Strachey (trans.), *On Metapsychology: The Theory of Psychoanalysis*, Penguin Freud Library (15 vols, Harmondsworth, 1984 [1920]), vol. 11, pp. 275–330.

they involve knowledge-gathering visits to the otherworld.[51] Furthermore, these visions are largely experienced by a particular category of person, primarily women at a certain stage in life: motherhood. In this view, the dream narratives are the experiences. Nevertheless, there is more to experience than merely the story, the gender position, the cultural tradition, the environment, or the social structure. I suggest that we should seriously consider these dream accounts as indications of personal experiences of anguish and suffering that generate, or independently reinvent, what are, from an analytical perspective, constant, collective symbols and narratives. Fields in dreams are individual and collective symbols.

At the physiological level, I have considered the idea that dreams symbolically communicate the effects of symptoms on the body, particularly the onset or lifting of illness. Nightmares involve feelings of constriction and dreams that undo trauma and anxiety contain images of open space. In light of the supposition by Freud and others that the dreaming imagination works linguistically, turning words into images, individual submersion in constricted states of *ángkhos* and *stenokhória* might lead to reversal in which the experiential production of images of openness (for example, fields) obliterates and dispels this tightness.[52]

Finally, the cognitivist view holds that the production of dream images of fields, or open spaces more generally, serves to facilitate problem solving. Such spatializing strategies are evident in the operation of mnemonists. Still more interesting for our purposes, however, is Silberer's idea[53] that sleep imagery often represents not only what a dreamer is thinking, but also depicts the dreamer's own cognitive processes in visual form.[54] In this view, fields in dreams are pictorial imitations of the cognitive spatializing of thought that are undertaken in actual thinking and problem solving. Silberer described the field in the dream as a fairy-tale space created and entered by the imagination—"a *pratum felicitatis*

---

[51] M. Eliade, *Shamanism: Archaic Techniques of Ecstasy* (New York, 1964), p. 102; and Lincoln, *The Dream in Primitive Cultures*, p. 68.

[52] On the linguistic basis of dreaming from a cognitive viewpoint, see D. Foulkes, *A Grammar of Dreams* (New York, 1978). From a Jungian perspective, but again with an emphasis on etymology and image, see J. Hillman, *The Dream and the Underworld* (New York, 1979).

[53] H. Silberer, *Hidden Symbolism of Alchemy and the Occult Arts* (New York, 1971 [1917]), p. 46.

[54] R. Arnheim, *Visual Thinking* (Berkeley, 1969), p. 112; and H. Hunt, *The Multiplicity of Dreams: Memory, Imagination and Consciousness* (New Haven, 1989), p. 149.

[meadow of felicity] in spite of the dangers and accidents which we have there to undergo."[55]

An acceptance of dreams as complex human phenomena requires an admission that there exist multiple approaches involving simultaneous avenues of interpretation: cognitive psychological, psychoanalytic, anthropological, and so on. All these different theorizations can account for the appearance of these fields. The meaning of fields in dreams is "overdetermined" theoretically, but not semantically, since the field is consistently understood as a space of freedom and resolution.

A constructionist may ignore these complementary approaches and insist that it is strictly the socialization into familiarity with cultural images and the demands of particular contexts of dream narration that constrain the repetition of standard single images (such as the depiction of open space), or standard narrative motifs (such as the visit to the otherworld). In my view, the field may equally be rooted in common physical and psychological experiences of anxiety. Pursuing this individual experiential basis does not contradict social constructionism, but instead balances it against the phenomenology of experience.

The images of fields in dreams, then, are ultimately more than just motifs that people select in order to tell stories. Tangles with the intractable may necessarily involve traversing a space of emptiness on the way to resolution. The image of the field is thus a condition of experience—one that I hold to be discoverable and repeatable at the personal level. This realization adds a personal dimension to our attempts to understand the manifest historical and cultural consistency of certain story traditions.

[55] Silberer, *Hidden Symbolism*, p. 47.

Chapter 14
Dream Healing for a New Age

Jill Dubisch

Introduction

The New Age movement has adopted or revived a number of spiritual and healing practices from other cultures, both past and present. One such practice is the use of dreams and dreaming as a source of both guidance and therapy. While the practices and ideas surrounding dreams are often drawn from non-Western cultures, there has also been a revival of interest in the ancient Greek practices of Asclepian dream healing, particularly through the work of Dr. Edward Tick, an American psychotherapist. Through his writings and through organized pilgrimages to Greece, Tick has sought to connect to ancient spiritual sites and mythology, focusing on dreams in order to effect physical, psychological, and spiritual healing among the participants in these journeys.

While healing pilgrimage is a common Greek Orthodox practice,[1] and while many pilgrimage sites draw foreigners as well as Greeks, the dream-healing journeys I will describe here differ from more conventional religious pilgrimage in several ways. For one thing, while contemporary Greek Orthodox pilgrims openly conduct rituals at established pilgrimage sites and sometimes stay overnight at churches to connect with the healing power felt to be present at the site, pilgrims on Tick's journeys must imagine and connect with a long-vanished time and with no longer observed ritual practices by visiting archaeological sites and by reading or hearing about a past in which they cannot directly participate. And while Orthodox pilgrims visit sites sacralized by both contemporary religious authority and popular faith, the pilgrims on a dream-healing quest must create their own sacred space, as their places of contact with the spiritual are desacralized archaeological sites. Here also they are limited by the regulations governing such sites. Performing rituals, especially at the more popular and heavily visited (and more strictly supervised) sites, is problematic, while spending the night at even the more remote Asclepian healing centers

---

[1] See, for example, J. Dubisch, *In a Different Place: Pilgrimage, Gender, and Politics at a Greek Island Shrine* (Princeton, 1995).

is not possible, as, like all archeological sites, such sites are closed at night. Therefore, each of these pilgrimages involves acts of creation and re-creation. Out of visits to ruins, invocations of gods and goddesses, recounting of myths, guided meditation, and other practices, participants work to create a journey that, through ritual and dreams, seeks to accomplish what every pilgrimage seeks: the spiritual, emotional, and/or physical transformation of those who journey to a sacred place.

Based on anthropological participant observation and drawing on the writing of Edward Tick and others, this chapter analyzes contemporary dream-healing pilgrimages to Greece. Each of the three pilgrimages in which I participated, as well as most of the other journeys led by Tick, concluded with a dream-healing incubation conducted in a hotel room, converted, through ritual and sacred objects, into a healing dream space. Within that space, those pilgrims who wished to experience dream healing underwent individual dreaming, watched over during the night in shifts by the rest of the group. Although a ritual designed by and participated in mostly by foreigners, these dream-healing journeys, and the rituals that accompany them, have attracted the attention of some Greeks who, seeking spiritual alternatives to Orthodoxy, look to the past for inspiration.

Spiritual Journeys and the New Age

Greece's past draws many foreign visitors. For the most part, this past is the Greece of antiquity, as imagined by the West and constructed by contemporary Greeks.[2] While the tourist focus on pre-Christian Greece is mainly secular in nature and satisfied by visits to the many archaeological sites and museums located throughout Greece, more recently this period of Greek history has drawn another sort of attention, that of those who are interested in the spiritual life of the centuries before Christianity. While this interest may be part of a general paganism that looks to pre- and non-Christian deities for its basis, it can also be more specifically focused on Greece itself, with the pantheon of Greek gods and goddesses providing its spiritual subject matter. This variety of paganism can be found both outside Greece and in a small, and controversial, movement within Greece.[3] Certain archaeological sites, such as the temples and religious complexes of Delphi and Eleusis, as well as the Acropolis and the

[2] See, for example, M. Herzfeld, *Anthropology through the Looking Glass: Critical Anthropology in the Margins of Europe* (Cambridge, 1987). Greece as the land of the New Testament has also drawn pilgrims.

[3] See M. Brunwasser, "Letter from Greece: The Gods Return to Olympus," *Archaeology*, 58(1) (2005): pp. 63–70.

Parthenon, are especially important to pagans, not simply as evidence of pre-Christian spiritual practices and inspiration for their revival, but also as sites for contact with ancient spiritual forces believed to be still present there—or at least capable of being invoked when one is within the sacred premises. A few pre-Christian sites visited by those interested in pagan spiritualities remain in use by local Orthodox populations (for example, the cave of Skotino in Crete), while other places that are not national archaeological sites have acquired a spiritual reputation and are in covert or at least unpublicized use. Any or all of these may become destinations for the sort of pilgrimage discussed here, as well as for other pagan or New Age practices.

People drawn to Greece for such pilgrimages seek not only alternative spiritualities (for example, a goddess-focused pilgrimage), but also, more specifically, the experience of Asclepian dream healing as reconstructed by Dr. Ed Tick, a Jungian psychotherapist, who since the 1990s has been leading groups of pilgrims to Greece. While these groups are composed mainly of Americans, Tick's work has also drawn the attention of Greeks attracted to the idea of an alternative spirituality—alternative, that is, to the Orthodox Church, the official and predominant religion of Greece. One of the attractions of Greek-focused paganism for these Greeks is that, unlike such "New Age" practices as yoga and Reiki (both also found in Greece today), it is, as one Greek woman said to me, quintessentially Greek.

An important difference, however, between Greeks and non-Greeks drawn to these journeys is that while the latter are likely to engage in a variety of New Age or "alternative" practices (Reiki, shamanism, goddess spirituality) in addition to their participation in the dream-healing pilgrimage, the former are usually interested in the revitalization (or one might say "spiritualization") of ancient Greek practices and ideas. As one Greek woman who participated in our journeys said to me, "We Greeks know the ancient myths but we don't know what to do with them." For such individuals—and for both Greeks and non-Greeks on these journeys—the museums and archaeological sites, which purport to connect the observer with the ancient Greek past, serve instead to disconnect insofar as the spiritual purpose that informed so many of these sites is no longer invoked or felt. The search for reconnection, for a re-enchantment of the ancient world and by extension of the present world, is thus an important part of the journey. For the woman quoted above, to make this connection is, as she put it, to "experience the Hellenic spirit."

I use the term "New Age" to refer to these dream-healing pilgrimages (and to other contemporary spiritual pilgrimages in which I have engaged), a term that requires some explanation in order to make clear the significance of the pilgrimages' focus on ancient spiritual beliefs and practices (at least as such beliefs and practices are re-imagined in the present). And while many who engage in such activities (including the pilgrims I will be describing here) would probably reject the label "New Age," scholars who take the beliefs and practices of "alternative" spirituality seriously see the term as an appropriate designation for a diffuse and yet significant spiritual movement, a movement that is characterized by several features.[4]

The first feature is, as the name implies, the sense of the coming of and/or need for a "new age," one that offers a new relationship with the world and the cosmos, and that seeks to overcome the dualism and materialism that characterize contemporary life.[5] Second, the search for such a new age often draws on ideas about past cultures (I say "ideas about" because, as noted above, these are particular contemporary reconstructions of the past), as well on beliefs and practices of cultures loosely termed "primitive" or "tribal." This reflects the idea of "ancient wisdom," an important theme in much New Age spirituality, whether that wisdom is seen as embodied in past cultures or preserved today in traditional practices of certain contemporary societies. In addition, this drawing on other cultures is eclectic in nature (a feature that has led to some of the criticisms of New Age). This eclecticism is justified by the idea that truth is not the exclusive property of any particular religion or culture and that all or most spiritual traditions have some wisdom to offer. Thus, in the dream-healing pilgrimages to be described here, Tick, who himself has had training as a shaman, utilizes such practices as smudging with sage in the rituals in which the pilgrims engage. Other participants contribute their own ritual additions to the ceremonies, some of them drawn from Native American spirituality, others from other spiritual traditions.

I should point out, however, that this does not mean that all participants in these journeys are pagans. In these, as well as in other New Age activities in which I have engaged, there have been individuals who, although considering themselves Christians, sought within their faith spiritual paths that provided alternatives to those offered by conventional practice and who did not exclude elements from other traditions in their search.[6]

This raises another point about New Age: the importance of individual experience. One finds one's way to the spiritual by experience—not through

---

[4] See, for example, W.J. Hanegraaff, *New Age Religion and Western Culture: Esotericism in the Mirror of Western Thought* (Albany, 1998); and J.A. Herrick, *The Making of the New Spirituality: The Eclipse of the Western Religious Tradition* (Downers Grove, IL, 2004).

[5] In this sense, the New Age movement might be considered a revitalization movement, as A.F.C. Wallace would call it; see his *Religion: An Anthropological View* (New York, 1966).

[6] Such individuals have been described as "spiritual but not religious"; see R.C. Fuller, *Spiritual But Not Religious: Understanding Unchurched America* (Oxford, 2001).

dogma or the teachings of others (though these can serve as guidance or inspiration), but through what Heelas terms "the wisdom of the experiential."[7] At the same time, as I will show here, other individuals can serve to interpret or validate this experience, which is an important part of the process that occurs in these dream-healing journeys.

Edward Tick's Vision

Ed Tick came to lead dream-healing pilgrimages to Greece through his work with Vietnam veterans.[8] Dissatisfied with the approaches of conventional psychotherapy and with what he felt was their ineffectiveness in dealing with veterans' post-traumatic stress disorder (PTSD), Tick, a Jungian psychotherapist, searched other traditions for archetypes that might be helpful in his therapeutic work. He felt that he had found these in the mythologies of classical and pre-classical Greece, especially in the warrior archetype, and in the various Greek gods and goddesses of mythology. He also discovered a healing tradition in the rituals of Asclepian healing as practiced in a variety of sites in the classical Greek world—a healing tradition he considered more holistic and profound than that practiced by contemporary Western medicine.

Tick's own healing journey began with a visit to Epidaurus, where he attended a performance of *The Trojan Women*. The performance provided a profound spiritual catharsis and gave him insight into the nature of healing, particularly into the mythic immersion he came to see as crucial to the healing process for the veterans he counseled, and indeed for all who wish to be healed. Such re-enactment, then, is part of the dream-healing journeys to Greece, journeys involving veterans and others seeking healing, both physical and spiritual. He has described these journeys, and the mythology underlying them, in his book *The Practice of Dream Healing: Bringing Ancient Greek Mysteries into Modern Medicine*. In his journeys, Tick and those traveling with him seek the "mythic immersion" mentioned above. Such immersion, however, is not an attempt to simply re-create past practices. As Tick puts it in his book, "We do not forget that we are a modern people with a modern consciousness. But we accept and believe that the ancients had access to transpersonal dimensions that we have

---

[7] P. Heelas, *The New Age Movement: The Celebration of the Self and the Secularization of Modernity* (Cambridge, MA, 1996), p. 9.

[8] He has also led veterans' pilgrimages to Vietnam and more recently has come to work with veterans of the Afghan and Iraq wars as well, though there were none of these more recent veterans in the journeys I describe here.

lost, and that by following their teachings, we may regain and achieve such access as well."[9]

The itineraries of these journeys of immersion vary according to the interests of the participants and to the theme Tick has chosen. One journey's theme, for example, was "Gods and Goddesses." The pilgrimages always begin in Athens with a visit to the Acropolis, including the Parthenon and the Theater of Dionysus, as well as the Asclepieion located on the south slope of the Acropolis. The three journeys in which I participated also all included Eleusis. Other sites visited varied from one journey to another—Delphi, Troy, Ephesus, Poros, Corinth, Samos, Mytilene, Epidaurus, Kos—according to the theme of the journey, its length, and the interests of the participants. Though these journeys were not necessarily focused on dream healing per se, during the course of those in which I participated, there were requests for a dream-healing incubation, as most of the participants were familiar with Tick's work on dream healing and had been drawn to the journey for that very reason. Although individual meditation and guided visions could sometimes be carried discreetly at the archaeological sites that the group visited, actual incubation and dreaming could not, since sites are closed at night; moreover, in some cases, visitors' activities are closely monitored to prevent the very sort of activities in which the group wished to engage. Therefore, incubations were set up in hotels near the archaeological sites, with pre-incubation rituals conducted in or just outside, and the dreamers placed in rooms rented for this purpose.

The Journeys and the Dreams

The several days spent in Athens at the beginning of the journey allow the participants to recover from jet lag and to introduce themselves, discuss their individual backgrounds, and declare their goals for the journey. A communal dinner at a Greek restaurant the first evening serves both to introduce everyone to Greek life and to allow for individual conversation. (Introductions and some discussion have already taken place by email before the journey begins.) The groups that I joined (in 2005, 2006, and 2010) were composed of 12–18 participants from a variety of backgrounds. Some were in therapeutic professions, such as chiropractic, massage, or counseling. Some were retired, others involved

[9] Ed Tick, *The Practice of Dream Healing: Bringing Ancient Greek Mysteries into Modern Medicine* (Wheaton, IL, 2001), p. 40. I do not analyze the accuracy of his interpretations here, as other chapters in this volume address Asclepian healing in antiquity; see the chapters by Cilliers and Retief, Downie, and Pearcy. Rather, my concern is with the way in which the interpretations of the past are utilized in present-day practice.

in a variety of spiritual practices. One participant, for example, had led women's spiritual pilgrimages to Morocco, while another taught tai chi. Although affluent enough to afford the journey, most could be described as middle class rather than wealthy, and some of those less well to do had made financial sacrifices in order to make the trip. There were Vietnam veterans on the journeys (including a woman who had been a nurse in Vietnam), but also individuals connected in other ways to war and whose wounds also required healing. One woman, for example, whose husband had been a marine in the Vietnam War, was on the first journey I took, while another woman who worked with veterans participated in a subsequent trip. Participants were mostly middle-aged, but in each of the three trips that I joined, there was also at least one young woman in her twenties or early thirties (in two cases, a mother–daughter pair). Participants came on the trip for a variety of reasons. Veterans came in search of healing for PTSD. Those who worked with veterans were also drawn to the journey by Tick's own work with veterans. Others were motivated by interest in Asclepian healing and Greek mythology. A doctor who has always identified with Asclepius (and who even resembled busts of Asclepius) has made this pilgrimage several times. A woman whose husband had been a pioneer in the holistic health movement came to scatter his ashes in Greece. Some sought healing for physical ailments, others for psychological or spiritual needs or concerns. And still others were at crossroads in their lives—changing careers, facing personal crisis, or simply wishing to alter the direction of their lives—and were seeking guidance and direction in the course of the journey. One woman had dreamed that she had an empty suitcase and that she should come on this journey to fill it. Another was told by a psychic that she should go to Greece.[10] Many who make the journey have read Tick's book and, no matter the theme and itinerary of the particular pilgrimage, want to experience a dream-healing incubation as part of their pilgrimage.

As I said, the first and second days are spent visiting several of the major sacred sites in Athens: the Acropolis (the Parthenon, the Theater of Dionysus, and the Asclepieion), the Agora, and, in the last two journeys in which I participated, the Kerameikos.[11] The group gathers for collective ritual at some sites and/or individuals are left to move or meditate individually as well.

---

[10] While each group of pilgrims, and each pilgrimage, has unique features, this sort of mix of participants seems to be fairly typical. It is also not unusual for participants to have dreams pertaining to their pilgrimage before the journey begins. See Tick, *Practice of Dream Healing*; and J. Giannini, "Pilgrimage to the Ancient Healing Sites of Greece: A Journey with Edward Tick," *San Francisco Jung Library Journal*, 23(1) (2004), pp. 75–91.

[11] The Kerameikos was the site of the cemetery for state tombs and battle heroes, as well as plots for wealthy citizens and buildings used in conjunction with the great festivals of Athens (the Panathenaia and the Eleusinian Mysteries).

A point to note here: meditative visions, guided visualizations, and dreams all merge in these journeys as sources of spiritual insight, inspiration, and healing. Thus, it is not only the dreams of sleep that provide the material for individual experience and collective discussion, but "waking dreams" as well. Sacred sites can be the setting for the latter, depending upon the site. The Parthenon, for example, always extremely crowded with tourists and, in recent years, noisy with construction, as well as vigilantly patrolled by guards, is not a place particularly conducive to meditation. But on the lower slopes of the Acropolis, the Asclepieion offers a more peaceful setting, one in which individuals can sit and meditate and connect with the god of healing, with little interruption from tourists passing by. While only licensed guides can conduct tours, it is possible in more quiet or secluded sites to carry out quiet collective or personal rituals as well, with guidance from Ed Tick and sometimes from other participants. The reading at Kerameikos of Pericles' funeral oration, for example, attracts little attention.[12] On one journey, the group gathered in a circle here to give ritual support to a veteran who had a psychological and spiritual crisis in this place in which so many warrior spirits are felt to dwell.

The recounting of myths and explanations of the healing practices and beliefs of antiquity, as well as Tick's recitations of his own experiences and visions before or during our visits to sites, set the stage for individual experiences and for collective rituals. On my first journey, which included sites in Anatolia, Turkey, as well as Greece, at the Asclepian temple near Pergamum several people lay on the grass and some fell asleep in a simulation of the dream healing that once took place in the still-visible *abaton* located here. At Eleusis, also on my first journey, we did a guided meditation led by Tick's wife, Kate Dahlstadt, in a shallow cave at the site, a meditation in which we were to imagine ourselves, like Persephone, descending into the underworld, and to reflect on the mother–daughter relationships through the myths of Demeter and Persephone.

Although sites serve as places of ritual and spiritual inspiration and, for some, as places to connect with ancient spiritual powers, there are limitations on what can be done there. Some sites are too crowded for such activities to be comfortable, and of course all sites are closed off at night, so that nocturnal Asclepian dream-healing incubations are not possible at the sites themselves. Additionally, there is official oversight of these places that limits activities.[13] However, it is not only activity that might damage the ruins themselves which

---

[12] Pericles delivered a speech for the dead from the first year of the Peloponnesian War fought between Athens and Sparta (431–404 BC). See the account in Thucydides 2.35–46.

[13] At the Parthenon, guards are ready with shrill whistles that they blow at any sight of a tourist infraction, such as stepping into the Parthenon itself or even picking up a pebble.

is a focus of official concern. One year, a group of young Greeks joining us at Eleusis reported that before our arrival at the site, the guard had become very upset that they had taken their shoes off and were walking around barefoot. He made them put their shoes on again, presumably out of fear of some "pagan" ritual, since being barefoot hardly poses a threat to the physical integrity of the site. (One of the Greeks told us that some dead black cats had been found a few months earlier at the site.)

On my first journey, some young Greek actresses who had been inspired by Tick's work put on a performance for us on Philopappou Hill. They had the group form a circle and, chanting in ancient Greek, enacted a ritual they had created themselves, using wheat, flour, and bread to symbolize the substance of life. They then performed Clytemnestra's dream scene from Sophocles' *Electra*, chosen, they told us afterward, because it involved both dreams and ritual, the two themes of our journey. (Indeed, for them, the performance was itself a ritual, just as theater was part of the healing ritual at ancient Asclepian sites.) We concluded the ritual by partaking in turn of the bread the women themselves had baked.

Rituals and visions occur not just at archaeological sites; they can be conducted on ships, in hotels, and even on the beach. Individuals can have healing and spiritual experiences in these settings, and significant dreams at any point along the journey. These experiences and dreams may be discussed in the group gatherings that usually take place every day, gatherings in which people speak of their feelings, experiences, and any problems or issues that confront them.[14] Depending on the composition of the particular group and their knowledge of the individual speaker, others may offer observations or analysis as dreams and other experiences are recounted. On one trip, for example, a woman who was facing a critical transition point in her life had a dream one night filled with classical scenes that Tick and several others in the group interpreted in light of her own situation and in terms of classical and mythological archetypes.

Dream Incubation

The dream incubations in which I participated occurred at the end of the journeys in two cases, and in the middle of the other, as the latter journey was divided into two parts, with several individuals leaving the group after the first

[14] What is revealed in these gatherings is confidential, so that what I report here is either already published in some form or something that I have been given permission to repeat. Other accounts I have rendered anonymous or have combined into general statements.

part.[15] The first incubation in which I participated took place on the island of Samos, the second on Kos, and the third on Poros. Each was carried out in a hotel room, with Ed Tick arranging for rooms or suites according to the number of individuals who wished to participate. Those who did not wish to undergo a dream incubation took turns as watchers during the night.

While the rituals connected with the dreaming varied somewhat, there were certain common goals: to create a sacred space in what would otherwise be a mundane setting; to induce a spiritually receptive state in both dreamers and watchers; to invoke the dream-healing power of Asclepius; and to induce a state that would create the dream that would provide healing for the incubant.

Ed Tick encouraged the incubants to fast during the day before the incubations as part of their spiritual preparation. In the first incubation in which I participated, on the island of Samos, the group met on the hotel terrace in the late afternoon, forming a circle and offering prayers. This was the opportunity for anyone who did not want to participate in the night's events to opt out, but no one did. The four incubants each chose a supporter from among the others in the group, someone to whom they could turn for particular help during the night.

Around 9:30 that evening, we met again on the terrace and then walked singing in a line up a stairway to the back of the hotel. We formed a circle around the incubants, who each stated what he or she wished from the night's dreaming. Everyone was smudged with sage and Tick invoked Asclepius with the *Homeric Hymn to Asclepius*:

> Doctor of our ailing, Asklepios, I begin your praise.
> Son of Apollo, awakened through Mother Koronis
> Of the Dorian Plains, daughter of King Flegion
> Great to humanity, soother of cruel suffering.
> And thus you are welcomed, Master.
> By this song I beseech you.[16]

The incubants were instructed to close their eyes and then were led by the others into the hotel, up the stairs, and to the room where the incubation was to take place.

Inside the room, an altar had been prepared on which various objects had been laid: personal spiritual and healing items such as crystals or jewelry, statues

---

15 For an account of this journey, see J. Dubisch, "Encountering Gods and Goddesses: Two Pilgrimages to Greece," *CrossCurrents*, September 2009: pp. 283–99.

16 For this *Hymn*, see G. Evelyn-White, *Homeric Hymns* (Cambridge, MA and London, 1914), where it is listed as *Hymn* 16.

of gods or goddesses purchased on the journey, and natural objects such as stones or feathers collected along the way. A candle was lit on the altar. The incubants lay on the beds and were wrapped in sheets to ready them for their night's journey. As part of preparing the incubants, several members of the group did energy-healing work on them. Then those who were to take the later shifts left to get some sleep, and the first shift of non-incubants remained to watch over the incubants. Although the incubants were restless at first, eventually they settled into sleep and the room grew still. The flickering candle was the only light, the hotel was quiet, and only the occasional sigh or faint snore interrupted the stillness of the room. It was easy for the watchers to fall into a meditative state, and in this and other incubations, watchers have even had visions themselves, or at least a sense of the presence of spiritual forces. The watchers changed shifts in the night, and with the dawn the sleepers awoke or were awakened. Everyone broke their fast together and, when all were ready, the incubants gathered to recount their dreams, while the watchers recounted their own nocturnal experiences as well. On this first journey, for example, and on another trip in which she participated, one woman delivered messages from Asclepius to each of the incubants, messages she received as she sat watching during the night. Ed Tick, too, has seen Asclepius entering the incubation chamber and has had other visions as well (see below).

The dreams that individuals experience are not necessarily dramatic or in and of themselves transformational, but they can be. Perhaps the most dramatic incubation experience during one of my journeys with Tick's groups involved a Vietnam veteran who had severe PTSD. This was on my second trip, in 2006, in the incubation on the island of Kos. During the night, this individual had a series of dreams in which he relived all the traumas of his wartime experience. He awoke refreshed and, as he recounts it, cured of his PTSD. (This veteran, John Fisher, has gone on to work with Tick and to lead veterans' healing pilgrimages to Vietnam.)

During this same incubation, Tick had a powerful vision of a giant serpent swallowing and then regurgitating one of the dreamers, himself a healer who had long identified with Asclepius, whose symbol is a serpent. Interestingly, the person incubating mentioned to me in the morning that John (the veteran) had a restless night, and that he even threw up during the night. In fact, no such thing had happened to John, and it was not until we gathered later that morning to recount our dreams and experiences that we learned what Ed had seen and understood that the vomiting the dreamer had heard was not another incubant but his own regurgitation by the serpent.[17]

[17] This theme also emerged in other dreams during the journeys in which I participated. For accounts of snakes and dreams during earlier journeys, see Tick, *Practice of Dream Healing*, pp. 219–21, 224–9.

The pilgrims themselves are not the only ones involved in the incubation. During the incubation on Samos, a Greek woman who had joined us for the first part of the journey but who was unable to stay for the entire trip said she was supporting the group with candles and prayers at home in Athens during the night of the incubation. And on the third trip I took, Tick's wife, who was unable to come, carried out her own rituals at home during the time when the incubation took place in Greece in order to support the pilgrims in their spiritual quest.

It is important to emphasize that the dream incubation, like the ancient ritual on which it is modeled, is the culmination of a series of rituals and experiences, including the ritual of group therapy, or "sharing," which occurs throughout the journey, and the rituals and meditative experiences at the various sites visited during the pilgrimage. In some cases, these experiences might be considered "mini incubations." This was clearly stated by Tick when the group visited the Cave of the Muses near Delphi on my first trip. Descending into the darkness of the cave and after singing, prayer, and guided meditation, we doused the lights and each entered into his or her own dream world individually, mimicking the descent into the *abaton*. When we emerged from our dream state, we weaved our way single file out of the cave, singing as we made our way from the dream world into the light. We then enjoyed a ritual communal picnic lunch at the cave's mouth.

The incubation, then, reflects a process that consists of ritual preparation, mythic immersion, instruction and guidance, and the development of group support and solidarity. The rituals along the way prepare pilgrims for the final dream incubation, which is itself a journey, a descent into another world. The emergence from the incubation then signals the beginning of the return to the pilgrims' normal, everyday life that marks the journey's end.[18]

The Dreams

The individual dreams that are recounted on the journey, whether along the way or during the incubation, take a variety of forms. They are usually interpreted in light of their significance to the concerns and goals that had induced participants to make this pilgrimage journey. Sometimes they directly incorporate symbolism related to the mythological context of the journey and to the sights and experiences encountered along the way. For example, in his book *The Practice*

[18] On the stages of pilgrimage, see V. Turner, *Dramas, Fields, and Metaphors: Symbolic Action in Human Society* (Ithaca, 1974); and A. Van Gennep, *Rites of Passage* (Chicago, 1960).

of Dream Healing, Tick (pp. 181–2) recounts one person's dreams of dogs, an animal associated with Asclepius. (It is not uncommon to encounter dogs at the sites that the pilgrims visit. One joined us for the ritual on Philapappou Hill, for example, and followed us afterward down into the Plaka.) Other symbols may be interpreted in the light of other spiritual traditions or Jungian archetypes, or may represent personal situations more directly. These dreams come to form a sort of narrative as the journey progresses, with an individual moving through the various stages of the healing process, represented by the dreams he or she has along the way. This process begins with the search for healing or for a new self that comes from the seeker's sense of having reached the limits of the therapy offered by conventional forms, whether they be psychotherapeutic approaches to PTSD or conventional Western medicine or established religion. Through dreams and visions, the seeker encounters symbols of spiritual powers (such as animals representing gods and goddesses), often descends into an underworld in which he or she grapples with powerful forces, and then emerges with a new alignment of the self.[19] Objects or events from the journey may play a role in this process, providing both insight into the individual's issues and pathways for healing. For example, on one of Tick's journeys, a woman dreamt that her face was covered by a golden mask, similar to the gold death mask of Agamemnon. Not wishing to fuse with the rigid metal, she fled. Recounting the dream, she speculated that it was indicative of her desire to flee artifice and lead a more authentic life.[20] For others, dreams of snakes are symbolic of rebirth into a new life, of shedding the skin of the old. In all of the dreaming and other experiences during this healing journey, the individual seeker is supported by group members, who provide not only interpretation of specific dreams but also validation for the significance of dreams themselves and for the healing power of dreaming and ritual.

Dreaming does not end once the journey is over, however. The pilgrims may report further dreams related to the journey after they return home, while the effects of the pilgrimage and its dreams may be experienced in various ways. Some returnees make significant life changes. Some are cured of physical ailments; others undergo healing from the psychic wounds that serious illness such as cancer or other life-threatening conditions often bring. One woman on the first journey I undertook had stomach cancer that had been diagnosed as terminal. The message she received on the journey, she told us, was, "Live your life, not your death." She died some months after her return, surrounded by friends (her last days and death were shared with her fellow pilgrims via email). A man with potentially fatal hemochromatosis (an excess of iron in the blood)

---

19 Tick, *Practice of Dream Healing*, p. 184.

20 Ibid., p. 174.

who was on one of Tick's earlier trips returned home, if not cured of his disease, at least having achieved a balance that allowed him to live a healthy life.[21]

Conclusion

Dissatisfaction with what they see as a fragmented and materialistic contemporary world has led many to seek inspiration in the ways of life of other times and places. Whether driven by the search for alternatives to Western biomedicine, by the desire for more satisfying spiritual experience than that provided by organized religion, or by personal existential crises, the pilgrims on the journeys I have described here are, like all pilgrims, seeking some sort of transformation in their lives. Drawing on the dream-healing traditions of Greek antiquity, as interpreted by a contemporary psychotherapist and experienced in guided journeys through the Greek landscape, these pilgrims seek connections with spiritual sources of guidance and healing through a process of "mythical immersion." Dreams become a key part of this mythical personal journey and enable the construction of a narrative of the self and its relation to the visible and invisible world that, in Tick's words, allows us to see that "disease and destiny are two serpents twining around the central wand that is our soul."[22]

I would like to conclude on a personal note. Although my own dreaming during these journeys was somewhat disappointing (as usual, I seldom remembered my dreams on awakening), I had one interesting dream in Athens in 2005, just before I joined the first dream-healing pilgrimage in which I participated. Although I have been to Greece many times, beginning with my early fieldwork in a small Greek village and continuing with my later research on pilgrimage at the Church of the Annunciation on the island of Tinos,[23] when I returned in 2005, it had been a number of years since my last visit. Arriving a few days before the pilgrimage was due to begin, I found myself experiencing a certain amount of culture shock from being back in Greece and from the changes that had occurred since my last visit, as well as some anxiety about the journey ahead, a journey that would begin a new research project for me. The night before the group was to arrive, I had the following dream:

> I am going down the steps into one of the small Byzantine churches in the Plaka. Inside I find, not the dimly lit interior, old icons, and iconostasis I expected, but

---

21 Ibid., pp. 185–6.

22 Ibid., p. 267.

23 See Dubisch, *In a Different Place*.

> rather a big well-lighted shop with many gold and silver items laid out on tables and trays. (I have the sense that many of these were religious items but this was not clear.)

At the time I interpreted this dream as a metaphor for what Greece had become, moving away from the more traditional Greece I had first known and into the modern, consumer world that I was now experiencing on this return trip. But upon rereading my account, I now wonder if the dream perhaps held another significance. Like the descent into the *abaton* of the Asclepieion, my descent into the little church revealed the treasures that can be found when one journeys into the hidden world of dreams.

Index

References to illustrations are in **bold**